Contents

The New Politics of the NHS

From creation to reinvention

Fifth Edition

Rudolf Klein

Radcliffe
Oxford • S

Radcliffe Publishing Ltd
18 Marcham Road
Abingdon
Oxon OX14 1AA
United Kingdom

www.radcliffe-oxford.com
Electronic catalogue and worldwide online ordering facility.

Reprinted 2007, 2008

First Edition 1983
Second Edition 1989
Third Edition 1995 (published by Pearson Education)
Fourth Edition 2001 (published by Pearson Education)

British Library Cataloguing in Publication Data

A catalogue record for this book is available from the British Library.

ISBN-10: 1 84619 066 5
ISBN-13: 978 184619 066 7

Typeset by Anne Joshua & Associates, Oxford
Printed and bound by TJ International Ltd, Padstow, Cornwall

Preface

With the new millennium a new era started for the National Health Service. After decades of Treasury parsimony, and complaints about underfunding, extra billions started to flow into the NHS at an unprecedented rate. At the same time the Labour Government launched its ambitious programme for 'reinventing' the NHS. The monolithic, paternalistic 1948 model was to be transformed into a pluralistic, consumer-led model. A command and control system was to be replaced by the dynamics of the market as money followed the patient. However, radical change was contained in a cocoon of institutional continuity. The NHS remains a tax-funded service that provides comprehensive, universal health care free at the point of delivery. The values that had inspired the founding fathers, and shaped the NHS in the first place, still drive the reinvented service.

To make sense of this combination of change and continuity, radicalism and conservatism, means making sense of the NHS's political history: the aim of this book. It is the history of the NHS which explains why the foundations of the NHS are set in the concrete of popular support and political consensus: why the NHS has become a much cherished national monument. It is the history of the NHS which also explains, however, why successive governments have over the decades struggled to cope with the flaws in the 1948 model, itself the product of political controversy and compromise. For only ideological piety can sustain the notion that the NHS's survival for so many decades simply reflects the perfection of the original design. To interpret the policies adopted by the Blair Government requires therefore an understanding of its inheritance: of both the strengths and weaknesses of the 1948 model as they emerged subsequently. From this perspective the reforms of the post-2000 era can be seen as one more step, albeit a particularly radical one, in the evolution of policy over the decades as successive governments sought to adapt the structure of the NHS to changing medical technology, changing demography and a changing society – developments which were not, and could not have been, anticipated by the founding fathers.

This book concentrates on the policy-making process in the NHS and the accompanying political debates over the past 60 years. It examines the influence of ideology and the role of interest groups in shaping policy. But it does so in the wider context of the NHS's changing environment. Many of the problems confronting the NHS are specific to it. So are many of the constraints facing policy makers. But the NHS is also a mirror of society. As society changes, so will perceptions of the NHS and the assumptions of policy makers. The 1948 model accurately mirrored a society strong on collectivism, reconciled to scarcity and with a firm faith in the technocratic rationality of planning. The tide of collectivism receded; scarcity yielded to rampant consumerism and faith in planning evaporated. In turn, policy makers began to operate with a new set of ideas and assumptions about how to manage the public economy: intellectual fashions matter. The wider transformation of society and the changes in the dominant public philosophy are therefore an essential element in any analysis of the evolution of health care policy.

In preparing this new edition I have not tried to re-write the past with the benefit of hindsight or to take account of the literature that has been published since I first wrote the text. I would not, in any case, wish to make any major modifications to my interpretation of events, and there seems little point in engaging in scholarly niggles. So the first seven chapters taking the story up to 2000 remain as they were written in 1982 and subsequent editions. Two new chapters deal with events since the turn of the millennium. Their length reflects the fact that this was a period of unprecedented activity and policy drama as the Blair administration abandoned its attempt to fit the last remaining monument to Old Labour into New Labour's Third Way strategy and struck out on a new course, in effect resurrecting Mrs Thatcher's internal market even while repudiating the label.

Edition-by-edition, the perspective shaping the analysis has shifted somewhat as new questions have come to the surface. However, the book remains structured around themes and preoccupations that have organised the text from the beginning and continue to do so. It is shaped, above all, by the assumption that the NHS (and the wider health care policy arena) can be seen as a laboratory for a whole range of social, institutional and organisational experiments with implications for other areas of policy and perhaps other countries as well. To quote the preface to the first edition:

> The NHS illustrates with special sharpness, for example, one of the main policy dilemmas faced by all modern societies: how best to integrate experts into the policy machinery – how to reconcile policy-making seen as the product of political processes and policy-making seen as a search for an abstract rationality based on expertise. Again, the NHS's experience underlines the tensions between policies designed to achieve national standards in the pursuit of equity and other policy aims, such as the encouragement of local participation: it can be seen as a case study of conflicting values in the design of social policy. Lastly, the NHS provides an opportunity to study the classic question of political analysis: who gets what? In short, a health care system can be seen as a political world in its own right, where the balance of power will determine the distribution of resources.

Other themes run through the text. One is the tension between central government and delivery agencies, between the State and the professions, between the requirements of public accountability and professional autonomy. How is political overload to be avoided in a tax-funded service which inevitably pulls decision making to the centre? Should rationing be explicit or implicit? What should be the currency of performance evaluation? Finally, edition-by-edition, it has become increasingly clear that if the NHS is a laboratory in which the micro-politics of a specific policy arena can be studied, it is also an example of how macro-politics can reshape an arena.

In exploring these themes, the book is written to appeal both to those with a special interest in health care policy and those interested more broadly in the policy-making process. Accordingly, it is assumed that the reader does not necessarily come equipped with any knowledge of the NHS.

A final disclaimer. This book is not a history of the NHS but, as its title implies, a history only of the politics of the NHS. Accordingly it is highly selective. It concentrates on those policy issues which seem best to illuminate the analytic questions and to provide the most insight into political processes. Others have provided more comprehensive accounts. And it is selective in another respect as well. The organisation of health services in Scotland and Northern Ireland, and to a lesser extent Wales, differs in important respects from that in England, and divergence has become more marked since devolution. To make the task of analysis manageable, a Little Englander approach has therefore been adopted.

Rudolf Klein
London
April 2006

Acknowledgements

Over the years and editions, I have incurred many debts. My analysis throughout is informed by interviews and conversations with policy makers in central government, in the NHS and in professional and trade-union organisations. All interviews were conducted on a 'lobby' basis; that is, on the understanding that the information given was for use but not attributable. The conversations were all the more useful for being informal but, for that very reason, the insights yielded are once again not attributable. Which is why no sources are given in the text for quotations drawn from such interviews and conversations and why, furthermore, I cannot name all those who have helped me. Those currently or recently involved in policy-making – whether as civil servants or politicians – probably would not thank me if I identified them.

The following list of those who have helped me, and to whom I would like to express my gratitude, is therefore very incomplete. It includes only those no longer active in the policy arena. My thanks (in many cases, alas, posthumously) go to: Lord Aberdare, Michael Alison, Barbara Castle, Richard Crossman, Sir George Godber, Sir Roy Griffiths, Sir Graham Hart, Douglas Houghton, Dr Gordon Macpherson, Sir Alan Marre, Sir Richard Meyjes, Sir Patrick Nairne, Audrey Prime, Kenneth Robinson, Dame Enid Russell-Smith, Simon Stevens and Dr Derek Stevenson.

I am also grateful to the Keeper of the Public Record Office for permission to quote Cabinet and other papers. I have tried throughout to quote from original sources wherever possible since policy-making is dialogue and it is important to catch the tone of voice, the intellectual style and assumptions used by those involved. In this respect, the analysis of policy-making is rather like the analysis of literature: to paraphrase documents is to risk losing precisely what gives them their distinctive character.

I owe another debt of gratitude to academic colleagues in this country and abroad, as well as to commentators like Nick Timmins. Some of these are acknowledged in the footnotes. But more important than the printed word has been the challenging question in a discussion over lunch or at a seminar which has forced me to re-examine my own assumptions. This is a form of creative subversion at which North Americans excel and I owe much in this respect to friends like Ted Marmor, Carolyn Tuohy and Dan Fox, with whom I have enjoyed a transatlantic dialogue over the decades. At home, I owe much to Patricia Day: the final chapters draw heavily on a succession of research projects carried out in collaboration with her and on the common stock of ideas developed in the process. Lastly, I must apologetically acknowledge the help and stimulus of those whose ideas I have unconsciously appropriated: originality is, as the saying goes, a function of forgetfulness.

In the first edition I acknowledged the help of Sylvia Hodges and her efficiency in organising me and in typing the manuscript. That was 1982. Since then the computer has gradually emancipated me from dependence on secretarial help.

But at various times Janet Bryant, Thelma Brown and Kim Stirling have rescued me from my technical incompetence, a role more recently taken over by Freya Moffat, my 12-year-old grand-daughter. So my thanks go to them. Finally, this book was only made possible by a succession of helpful librarians at the Centre for Studies in Social Policy, the University of Bath and the King's Fund.

Chapter 1

The politics of creation

> If many simultaneous and variously directed forces act on a given body, the direction of its motion cannot coincide with any of those forces, but will always be a mean – what in mechanics is represented by the diagonal of a parallelogram of forces. If in the descriptions given by historians . . . we find their wars and battles carried out in accordance with previously formed plans, the only conclusion to be drawn is that those descriptions are false.
>
> Leo Tolstoy, *War and Peace*

Britain's National Health Service (NHS) came into existence on 5 July 1948. It was the first health system in any Western society to offer free medical care to the entire population. It was, furthermore, the first comprehensive system to be based not on the insurance principle, with entitlement following contributions, but on the national provision of services available to everyone. It thus offered free and universal entitlement to State-provided medical care. At the time of its creation it was a unique example of the collectivist provision of health care in a market society. It was destined to remain so for almost two decades after its birth when Sweden, a country usually considered as a pioneer in the provision of welfare, caught up. Indeed, it could be held up as 'the greatest Socialist achievement of the Labour Government', to quote Michael Foot, the biographer of Aneurin Bevan who, as Minister of Health in that Government, was the architect of the NHS.[1]

The transformation of an inadequate, partial and muddled patchwork of health care provision into a neat administrative structure was dramatic, even though the legislative transformation was built on the evolutionary developments of the previous decades. At a legislative stroke, 1,000 hospitals owned and run by a large variety of voluntary bodies and 540 hospitals operated by local authorities were nationalised. At the same time, the benefits of free general practitioner care, hitherto limited to the 21 million people covered by the insurance scheme originally set up by Lloyd George in 1911, were extended to the entire population. From then on, everyone was entitled, as of right, to free care – whether provided by a general practitioner or by a hospital doctor – financed by the State. At the summit of the administrative structure there was the Minister of Health. Under the terms of the 1946 Act setting up the NHS, the Minister was charged with the duty 'to promote the establishment in England and Wales of a comprehensive health service designed to secure improvement in the physical and mental health of the people of England and Wales and the prevention, diagnosis and treatment of illness, and for that purpose to provide or secure the effective provision of services'. The services so provided, the Act further laid down, 'shall be free of charge'.

How did this transformation come about? It is not the aim of this chapter to provide a history of the creation of the NHS: other sources are available, giving a detailed blow by blow account of what happened in the years leading up to 1948.[2] The intention, rather, is to analyse the political dynamics of the creation: to identify the main groups of actors in the arena of health care politics and to delineate the world of ideas in which the plans for a national health service evolved. In doing so, it is necessary to explore the complex interplay between the ineluctable pressure on politicians and administrators to do something about the practical problems forced on to their agenda by the clamouring inadequacies of health care in Britain, as it had evolved over the previous century up to 1939, and their resolution of the policy puzzles involved in accommodating competing values and insistent pressure groups. It was the historical legacy which made it inevitable that *a* national health service would emerge by the end of the Second World War. It was the ideological and practical resolution of the policy puzzles which determined the precise shape taken by the NHS as it actually emerged in 1948.

The emerging consensus

First, let us examine the nature of the consensus that had emerged by 1939: the movement of ideas which made it seem inevitable that some kind of national health service would eventually evolve – dictated, as it were, by the logic of circumstances, rather than by the ideology of politicians or the demands of pressure groups. Basically, this consensus embodied agreement on two linked assumptions. These were that the provision for health care in Britain, as it had grown up over the decades, was both inadequate and irrational.

Health care, it was agreed, was inadequate in terms both of coverage and of quality. Lloyd George's 1911 legislation had provided insurance coverage only for general practitioner services. In turn this coverage was limited to manual workers, excluding even their families. Hospital care was provided by municipal and voluntary institutions on the basis of charging those who could afford to pay and giving free care to those who could not. Even though the bewildering mixture of State insurance, private insurance and the availability of free care in the last resort meant that everyone had access to some form of medical treatment, the quality varied widely. The general practitioner, operating usually on the small shop-keeper principle of running his own practice single-handed and relying mainly on the income from the capitation fees of his insured patients, was isolated from the mainstream of medicine. 'It is disturbing to find large numbers of general practitioners being taught at great trouble and expense to use modern diagnostic equipment, to know the available resources of medicine and to exercise judgement as between patient and specialist', the 1937 Political and Economic Planning (PEP) survey of health care in Britain commented,[3] 'only to be launched out into a system which too often will not permit them to do their job properly'. In the case of the hospital sector, the quality of specialist care varied greatly; indeed there was no officially agreed definition of who should be considered a specialist – the title of consultant being attached to specific posts, mostly in the prestigious teaching hospitals, rather than being a generally accepted description of doctors with special skills recognised according to explicit criteria. In many of the smaller voluntary hospitals, especially, it was general practitioners who carried out both medical and surgical procedures, with no check on their qualifications or competence for the job.

The system, it was further agreed, was irrational. Specialists gravitated to those parts of the country where the population was prosperous enough to pay for private care, since hospital consultancies were honorary and they were thus dependent on income from private practice. By definition, the most prosperous parts of the country were not necessarily those which generated most need for medical care. Voluntary and municipal hospitals competed with, and against, each other. The distribution of beds across the country was determined by historical hazard, not the logic of the distribution of illness: Birmingham, for example, had 5.7 beds per 1,000 population, while Liverpool had 8.6. Hospitals shuffled off responsibility for patients to each other: the voluntary hospitals regularly dumping chronic cases onto the municipal sector. Municipal hospitals could, and indeed did, refuse admission to patients coming from outside their local authority area. A further article of faith in the emerging consensus was, therefore, the need to co-ordinate the various systems – voluntary and municipal – that had emerged, and to introduce some rationality into the distribution of resources.

The consensus had another ingredient. There was widespread acceptance of the fact that the voluntary hospital system was no longer viable financially. By the mid 1930s traditional forms of fund-raising from the public – the appeal to altruistic charitable instincts – were not yielding anything like enough to support their activities: only 31 per cent of the income of London teaching hospitals and 20 per cent of the income of the provincial teaching hospitals came from this source. More important was income from charges to patients, financed – on a 50:50 basis – either out of their own income or out of contributory insurance schemes. The bankruptcy of the voluntary sector was staved off by the Second World War, when these hospitals drew large-scale benefits from the Government's scheme of paying for stand-by beds for war casualties. But it was clear that, in the long term, their dependence on public finance was both irremediable and likely to increase.[4] Equally, it had long since become clear that the original purpose of the most prestigious of the voluntary hospitals – to provide free care for the poor – could not be fully carried out, since financial pressures were forcing them to rely on attracting precisely those patients who could afford to pay. The price of survival was, to an extent, the repudiation of the inspiration which had led to their creation in the first place.

Not surprisingly, therefore, the years between the two world wars – between 1918 and 1939 – were marked by the publication of a series of reports from a variety of sources, all sharing the same general perspective. In 1920 the Minister of Health's Consultative Council on Medical and Allied Services (the Dawson report) enunciated the principle that 'the best means of maintaining health and curing disease should be made available to all citizens' – a principle to be later echoed by Aneurin Bevan when he introduced the 1946 legislation – and elaborating this principle in a detailed scheme of organising health care; a hierarchy of institutions starting from the Primary Health Centre and culminating in the Teaching Hospital.[5] In 1926 the Royal Commission on National Health Insurance came to the conclusion, although it baulked at spelling it out in its immediate recommendations, that 'the ultimate solution will lie, we think, in the direction of divorcing the medical service entirely from the insurance system and recognising it along with all other public health activities as a service to be supported from the general public funds'.[6] In 1930 the British Medical Association (BMA) came out in favour of extending the insurance principle to the dependents of the working population and supported a co-ordinated reorganisation of the hospital system, while in 1933 the Socialist Medical Association added its radical treble to the conservative bass drum of the BMA and published its plan for a comprehensive, free and salaried medical service, to be managed by local government but with a regional planning tier.[7]

There are a number of strands within this consensus which need disentangling. In the first place, the consensus speaks with the accents of what might be called rationalist paternalists, both medical and administrative. This is the voice not so much of those outraged by social injustice as of those intolerant of muddle, inefficiency and incompetence: a tradition going back to the days of Edwin Chadwick, via the Webbs. It is further, the voice of practical men of affairs, trying to find solutions to immediate problems. In the second place, the consensus reflects a view of health care which was rooted in British experience, though not unique to it: an intellectual bias which helps to explain why the institutional solution devised in the post-war era was unique to Britain.

The second point requires elaboration. When, confronted by the muddle of health care, men started thinking about possible solutions, they had before them two models – either of which could have been developed into a fully-fledged national system. The first model was that of Lloyd George's insurance scheme for general practice: an import from Bismarck's Germany. In theory, there was no reason why such a model could not have been elaborated into a comprehensive national insurance scheme: the road followed by nearly all other Western societies in the post-war period, and advocated by the BMA not only in the 1930s but also subsequently (*see* Chapter 3). The other model, however, was that of the public health services, developed and based on local authority provision in Britain in the nineteenth century: a model based on seeing health as a public good rather than as an individual right. While the first model emphasised the right of individuals to medical care – a right to be based, admittedly, on purchasing the appropriate insurance entitlements – the second model emphasised the obligation of public authorities to make provision for the health of the community at large. While the first model was consistent with individualistic medical values – given that the whole professional ethos was to see medical care in terms of a transaction between the individual patient and the individual doctor – the second model was consistent with a collectivist approach to the provision of health care. Indeed throughout it is important to keep in mind the distinction between medical care in the strict sense (that is, care and intervention provided by doctors with the aim of curing illness) and health care in the larger sense (that is, all those forms of care and intervention which influence the health of members of the community).

Thus the whole logic of the Dawson report was based on the proposition that 'preventive and curative medicine cannot be separated on any sound principle. They must likewise be both brought within the sphere of the general practitioner, whose duties should embrace the work of both communal as well as individual medicine'. Nor was this just a matter of intellectual tradition. Local government was already in the business of providing health care, ranging from curative medicine in its hospitals to chronic care for the elderly and mentally ill in its institutions, from the provision of maternity clinics to looking after the health of schoolchildren. Organisational bias thus reinforced intellectual bias in the sense that the services provided by local government would have to be incorporated into any national scheme that might emerge. To have adopted an insurance-based scheme would therefore have meant actively repudiating the service-based legacy of the past.

Given this convergence of views on the necessity of devising some form of national health service, as distinct from some form of national health insurance, it is tempting to interpret the eventual emergence of the 1948 NHS in a deterministic fashion: to see it as the child not of Labour ideology, not as a Socialist triumph, but as the inevitable outcome of attempts to deal with a specific situation in the light of an intellectual consensus, both about what was desirable and about what was possible. Equally, given this convergence, it would seem redundant to search for explanations in Britain's wartime experience, whether administrative or emotional. The acceptance of the need for a national health service long predates, as we have seen, the wartime administrative experience of running the emergency medical service: an experience which, at best, can have generated confidence that it was actually possible to run a complex web of hospitals and services. Similarly, this acceptance long predates the wartime commitment to a collectivist solution of welfare problems: a commitment epitomised in the 1942 Beveridge report which assumed, without elaborating in detail, the creation of a 'comprehensive national health service'.

Accepting a general notion is, of course, one thing. Devising and implementing a specific plan is, however, a very different matter. The consensus may have provided a foundation. It did not provide a blueprint: when it came to detail, the various proposals put forward during the inter-war period had all come up with somewhat different schemes. To examine the evolution of plans from the out-break of war in 1939 to the enactment of the 1946 legislation for setting up the National Health Service is to identify a whole series of clashes not only between interest groups but also between competing values. If everyone was agreed about the end of policy in a general sort of way, there was little by way of consensus about means – and much awareness of the fact that the means chosen might, in turn, affect the end. It was a conflict of a peculiar sort: conflict contained, and limited, by an overarching consensus – a constraint which forced compromise and caution on all the protagonists. Indeed, as we shall find, the theme of conflict within consensus is one which runs through the entire history of the NHS.

The curtain goes up

An appropriate starting point for tracing the evolution of policy is a memorandum written only a few days after the outbreak of the Second World War, on 21 September 1939 by the Ministry of Health's Chief Medical Officer, Sir Arthur MacNalty. This formed part of a series of papers[8] prepared for discussion by a small group of civil servants who, already in 1938, had started considering the future development of health services. At the first meeting, the Permanent Secretary – Sir John Maude – had outlined two possible lines of approach: 'either the gradual extension of National Health Insurance to further classes of the community and by new statutory benefits, or the gradual development of local authority services.' But in his memorandum, MacNalty addressed himself to a third option: 'the suggestion that the hospitals of England and Wales should be administered as a National Hospital Service by the Ministry.'

Since it was precisely this suggestion which prevailed – in so far as the 1948 NHS was, essentially, a national hospital service – it is worth examining MacNalty's arguments in some detail. First, he pointed out that a National Hospital System 'is already practically established for purposes of a national emergency'. Second, he argued that 'it will be difficult and in many cases be impossible for voluntary hospitals to carry on owing to the high costs of modern hospital treatment and the falling off of voluntary subscriptions after the war'. But then, turning to the case against such a solution, MacNalty outlined the possible objections. First, 'the nationalisation of the hospitals would dry up the flow of voluntary subscriptions which largely contribute to relieving the rate-payer and the taxpayer of the cost of hospital provision'. Second, 'the majority of the medical profession would be bitterly opposed to it. This would cause much dissension, controversy and ill-feeling at a time when it is vitally important that national unity should be preserved'. Third, the proposal implied 'a radical change in the policy of the Ministry. Hitherto, we have always worked on the assumption that the Ministry of Health was an advisory, supervisory and subsidising department, but had no direct executive functions'. Lastly, 'from the point of view of local authorities executive control of all hospitals by the State might excite opposition and present difficulties'.

In conclusion, however, MacNalty came out on the side of nationalisation, if only tentatively. He wrote:

> It is a revolutionary change, but it is one that must inevitably come, because the voluntary system with all its excellent attributes is unsuited to the modern needs of the whole population. . . . As I have mentioned, the proposal may meet with much opposition from the medical profession. But I am certain they would, for the most part, welcome national control in preference to being controlled by local authorities. We have a very good method of approach to them in showing that even before the war the voluntary system was breaking down, that it has failed in wartime to cope with modern conditions and has necessitated general hospital control by the State. I suggest then the time is ripe that we should approach the medical profession in this way, not as seeking to impose a national system upon them, but taking them into council, saying, for example, these are our difficulties. Will you help us find a way out of them? On these lines it might be possible to get a National Hospital Service established by negotiation with the general agreement and support of the medical profession.

There was, of course, yet a further option, discussed in a memorandum written the subsequent day by Sir Arthur Rucker – a senior civil servant, later to be the Ministry's Deputy Secretary. As between the Permanent Secretary's option of municipalisation and the Chief Medical Officer's option of nationalisation, there was the possibility of establishing a mixed-economy system. This could be done by establishing 'joint hospital boards', which would be responsible for planning both municipal and voluntary hospital services. Financial support to the voluntary hospitals would be contingent on them co-operating. The advantage of such an approach, Rucker argued, was that it offered the 'most practical solution' since it would build on existing developments. Further, it would avoid the administrative problems of nationalisation: 'We simply have not the medical or administrative staff that could cope with so enormous a task and it is difficult to see how such a staff could be recruited from outside the Ministry at the present moment.'

So here, in 1939 already, we have set out most of the main assumptions, issues and factors that shaped the discussions over the next six years, in so far as they affected hospital as distinct from general practitioner services, at any rate. The exchange of notes is revealing in a number of respects. It shows civil servants taking the initiative in generating policy options unprompted, as far as can be judged from the records, by the politicians. It also indicates their operating assumptions: the emphasis is on seeking 'practical' solutions which will be acceptable, on bringing about change through agreement. It reveals the bias of the Ministry of Health: a department with a tradition of regulatory rather than executive functions, reluctant to take on direct administrative responsibilities for a complex service. It shows the natural inclination of civil servants to build on existing developments and organisations, rather than to invent new institutions. However, it also shows a civil service engaged in a wide-ranging search operation, as it examines a wide range of possible policies: if the style is evolutionary, radical solutions are not excluded.

But these notes not only define the rules of the game, as interpreted by the Ministry of Health hierarchy. They also define the arena of health care politics: those considered to be legitimate actors, with a claim to participate in the negotiations. The cast-list is as significant for those left out as it is for those included. Among the excluded are the Approved Societies which administered the existing national insurance system: an exclusion all the more notable given the dominant role of these societies in the formation of the system in the period between 1911 and 1913.[9] So, too, are the majority of those actually working in health services: from nurses to floor sweepers. But included are the voluntary hospitals, local authorities and, above all, the medical profession. The key to successful change is seen to be, as is clear from MacNalty's memorandum, the support and co-operation of the medical profession. Even allowing for the fact that as Chief Medical Officer, and thus the middleman between the Ministry and the profession, MacNalty was bound to put particular stress on the role of doctors, this is a recurring theme. It is further reflected in the records of the Ministry over the next few years: records which document a seemingly endless series of meetings between Ministry officials and representatives of the medical profession, as well as with the voluntary hospital and other interests.

One set of characters remains to be introduced: the politicians – the political masters of the Ministry of Health. This late introduction of those who might be expected to be the central actors may seem perverse in a book devoted to the politics of health. In fact, however, it is entirely appropriate. For most of the time in the period covered, politicians play the role of Fortinbras: when he comes on stage in the last scene, the trumpets may sound – but all the protagonists of the action are dead. Only occasionally, and exceptionally, do the politicians play a central role in the drama. The point is well illustrated by the evolution of policy between 1939 and 1946: a story which breaks into two sharply distinguished sections – the politics of compromise under the Coalition Government, during which politicians are fringe figures, and the politics of innovation under the Labour Government, when politicians take the centre of the stage.

Coalition compromises

The best starting point for considering the evolution of policy under the wartime Coalition Government is to examine the end-product of the years of negotiation: the 1944 White Paper setting out the plans for a National Health Service,[10] written by Sir John Hawton, subsequently the Ministry of Health's Permanent Secretary. This was based upon two principles, which were to remain the foundation of the National Health Service as it finally emerged in 1946. First, that the new service should be comprehensive: that 'every man and woman and child can rely on getting all the advice and treatment and care which they need. . . . and that what they get shall be the best medical and other facilities available'. Second, that the service should be free: that 'their getting these shall not depend on whether they can pay for them, or on any other factor irrelevant to the real need – the real need being to bring the country's full resources to bear upon reducing ill-health and promoting good health in all its citizens'.

Although the proclaimed ends of the 1944 White Paper were the same as those of the 1946 Act, yet the institutional means were different. As the White Paper argued, there were two alternative strategies for achieving change: 'One, with all the attraction of simplicity, would be to disregard the past and the present entirely and to invent ad hoc a completely new reorganisation for all health requirements. The other is to use and absorb the experience of the past and the present, building it into the wider service.' It was the second approach which shaped the White Paper, not surprisingly perhaps given the fact that the Minister of Health, Henry Willink, was a Conservative and given also the intellectual bias of the civil servants.

More important still the White Paper was an attempt to reconcile the views of the principal coalition partners: the Conservative and Labour parties. When the Prime Minister, Winston Churchill, had last-minute qualms about publishing the White Paper, he got a sharp reminder about the political realities from Lord Woolton, the Minister for Reconstruction.[11] The latter pointed out:

> This is a compromise scheme, but it is a compromise which is very much more favourable to the Conservatives than to Labour Ministers and when it is published, I should expect more criticism from the Left than from Conservative circles. . . . If discussion of the whole scheme is to be reopened . . . I fear that the Labour Ministers may withdraw their support of the scheme and stand out for something more drastic which would be far more repugnant to Conservative feeling.

The White Paper was also an attempt to minimise opposition from the various interest groups in the arena of health care politics. Indeed any solution would be politically acceptable to the extent that it avoided a clash with those interests, particularly since each of these tended in turn to have their links with the political parties: a link which was, for example, strong in the case of the Conservative Party and the voluntary hospital movement. To a large extent the records of the negotiations that took place in the years before the publication of the White Paper, as reflected in the files of the Ministry of Health, show the civil servants and the representatives of the three major interest groups (in particular, the medical profession) engaged in searching out the limits of the acceptable: trying to identify the sticking points in each other's position and to devise ways of reconciling the different points of view.

Lastly, though, the White Paper was an attempt to solve certain basic dilemmas of policy. It was a compromise document because it sought to reconcile various aims of policy, all desirable in themselves, which pointed in different directions. It thus incorporated judgements both about the relative weights to be given to considerations of feasibility (maximising political agreement within the Government, minimising opposition from interest groups) and different policy values.[12] So perhaps the most illuminating way of analysing the White Paper proposals is to look at them in the context of the specific dilemmas – the kind of choices between competing tactical considerations and policy aims – faced by those involved in producing the document: dilemmas which provide themes running through the entire history of the NHS, and which still provide an agenda for political debate 60 years later.

First was the dilemma of how to reconcile government acceptance of the principle of national responsibility for the health care system and the desire to avoid a centralised service actually operated by the Ministry of Health. Not only did the Ministry, as already noted, lack both the experience and the inclination to engage in such an exercise, but, implicit in the debate, was also the further question of the appropriate balance between central and local government, between bureaucratic control from the centre and freedom at the periphery to respond to local demands. Here the White Paper's solution was to assign responsibility for planning the service to the Minister, but executive responsibility to local government which could maintain its function of running hospitals and providing personal health services.

This solution, however, only created a second dilemma. Devolution of responsibility to the periphery assumes the existence of administrative units which are appropriate, in terms of their boundaries and size, to deliver a particular kind of service. In the case of health services, it was generally agreed, the existing structure of local government was inappropriate. In particular, the administrative division between town and country created problems, since the major hospital resources tended to be concentrated in the former. So here the solution was to propose the creation of 30–35 joint authorities, as foreshadowed in Rucker's 1939 memorandum, combining counties and country boroughs, though the option of other permutations of combined local authorities was left open. It would be the responsibility of the new joint authorities to assess the needs of their areas and to plan 'how those needs should best be met'. The plans would, in turn, have to be submitted to and approved by the Ministry of Health (a scheme of things which foreshadows the 1974 reorganisation of the NHS, as we shall see). The new joint authorities would be directly responsible for running hospital and consultant services; responsibility for local clinics and other personal health services would remain with the existing local authorities. The overall objective would be to 'unify and co-ordinate the service' by means of a 'rational and effective plan'.

Third, however, was the dilemma of how it would be possible to devise a 'rational and effective plan' if the voluntary hospitals were left outside the system. Was there a middle way between a national and a pluralistic system? Here the solution was to make government financial help to the voluntary sector dependent on their joining in the planning exercise, a proposal which can also be traced back to Rucker's 1939 memorandum. The joint authorities would be in a contractual relationship with the voluntary sector 'for the performance of agreed services set out in the plan' – a scheme which appears to be a direct descendant of Rucker's ideas put forward in 1939. The local plans would cover the totality of resources within any given area, irrespective of their actual ownership. The Minister's control over the system would, in addition, be strengthened by the creation of a hospital inspectorate.

Fourth was the dilemma of how to reconcile public accountability and professional participation in decision-making. The basic principle enshrined in the White Paper was that 'effective decisions on policy must lie entirely with elected representatives answerable to the people for the decisions that they take' – the local government councillors. But the medical profession demanded representation for its views in the formulation of policy, and there was general agreement that the voice of expertise should be heard. The White Paper sought to resolve this dilemma by establishing a Central Health Services Council to advise on national policy and equivalent local bodies to advise on local policy: in short, it established a hierarchy of professional expertise parallel to the institutional hierarchy of public accountability through elected representatives.

Fifth was the dilemma of how to integrate hospital and general practitioner services.[13] If the aim of policy was to secure more efficiency and rationality, it was impossible to exclude general practitioners from the planning process. In particular, as the White Paper stressed, there had to be an effective means of 'ensuring a proper distribution of doctors'. The logic of such an approach pointed in the direction of making general practitioners employees of local authorities. The logic of political feasibility, of minimising opposition, pointed in the opposite direction, however, since the medical profession – through the BMA – was fiercely opposed to such a solution. So here the White Paper proposed to abolish the local Insurance Committees, which had administered general practice since 1913 and were composed of medical representatives as well as lay members. The responsibilities of the Committees would be transferred to a Central Medical Board, which would be responsible for planning the distribution of doctors: thus it would have the power to refuse consent to a general practitioner to practise in areas considered to have a sufficiency of doctors.

Sixth, there still remained the dilemma of how to reconcile the inherited system of general practice based on individualistic, small-shopkeeper principles, with the aim of promoting 'developments in the modern technique of medical practice'. The system of capitation payments encouraged competition between general practitioners: the more patients they had, the bigger their income. Further, the less they spent on equipping their surgeries, the greater was their take-home pay. Yet there was widespread agreement that the quality of general practice could only be improved by groups of general practitioners practising in well-equipped premises, a view in whose support the White Paper could even invoke the 1942 Interim Report of the BMA's Medical Planning Commission. So how was the demand for a new pattern of service to be reconciled with an inherited system of payment which seemed to be in contradiction with the aims of policy? Here the White Paper again proposed a compromise: a compromise which reflected the extreme hostility of the BMA to any proposal which appeared to turn general practitioners into public servants. General practitioners would be encouraged to group themselves in Health Centres to be provided by the new joint local authorities, though they would be employed by the Central Medical

Board: the method of payment was left for future decisions, though the White Paper argued that 'there is a strong case for basing future practice in a Health Centre on a salaried remuneration or some similar alternative which does not involve mutual competition'. But other general practitioners would continue in independent practice. The principles of free choice of doctors by patients and complete medical autonomy were to remain sacrosanct.

Like all compromise proposals designed to reconcile multiple and conflicting objectives, the White Paper left most of the actors involved feeling dissatisfied. For all of them, the final compromise left them to tot up a complex balance sheet of gains and losses: the White Paper indeed was a triumph mainly for those, in particular the civil servants, whose prime objective lay precisely in achieving some kind of compromise formula which, even if it did not satisfy any of the actors fully, at least minimised the chances of continued conflict. The medical profession had reconciled itself to accepting a comprehensive health service, abandoning its earlier insistence on limiting coverage to 95 per cent of the population and thus institutionalising the scope for private practice. Again, the medical profession had lost its battle to make the Central Health Services Council representative of the medical profession – an elected rather than a nominated body – which would have an actively directing role in the operations of the health service. But it had successfully fought off the threat of direct local authority control over general practice, and it managed to compel the Coalition Government to produce a fudged formula on the vexed question of payments.

The local government lobby had averted the danger of nationalisation, but was left dissatisfied by the prospect of the new joint authorities actually taking over control of their hospitals: Herbert Morrison, the Home Secretary and the voice of local government in the administration, warned the War Cabinet's Reconstruction Committee that the 'proposed arrangements would undoubtedly be criticised by local authorities'. The voluntary hospitals, too, were unhappy: although they would nominally maintain their independence, they believed that they would suffer a 'mortal blow through the cessation of income from patients', as the Minister of Health told the Reconstruction Committee.[14]

The White Paper also embodied compromises by the political partners in the Coalition Government. Labour Ministers continued to grumble to the last during the sessions of the Reconstruction Committee involved in the final drafting of the White Paper about conceding the right to private practice for general practitioners in the public service. 'There would be a danger that some doctors would devote their energies to maintaining their private practice at the expense of their public patients', Clement Attlee, the leader of the Labour Party, pointed out. The Minister of Labour, Ernest Bevin, argued that the 'White Paper did not sufficiently emphasise the need for a vigorous development of Health Centres, served by a salaried medical staff'. Again, Labour Ministers had been forced to accept a postponement of any decision about the controversial issue of the buying and selling of practices, and whether or not this right should be expropriated.

Similarly, Conservative Ministers had been pushed into accepting policies which, once their Labour partners had left the Coalition Government, they were quick to change. In June 1945, the Cabinet accepted a revised policy programme devised by Henry Willink with the aim of modifying 'certain features in the original plan which had been unpopular with local authorities, voluntary hospitals and the medical profession'.[15] First, there was a major concession to the medical profession. The proposal for a Central Medical Board was dropped, for this had always been regarded with extreme suspicion by the medical profession, who saw it as an attempt by the central bureaucracy to gain control. The local Insurance Committees, though retitled, were reinstated. Finally, the power to prevent general practitioners from moving into well-provided areas was dropped; instead, distribution was to be improved by offering 'positive inducement by more attractive terms in less attractive areas'. Health Centres were to be experimental only; doctors working in them were to be paid on the same basis as independent general practitioners – that is, by capitation fees. Local authorities were also placated: the new joint authorities were to be limited to the planning function, with control over hospitals left with the existing units of local government.

Finally, the most prestigious of the voluntary hospitals were given a concession they had long sought: in order to give 'the principal medical teaching centres . . . a suitable place in the machinery for co-ordinating the specialised services', it was proposed to set up 'expert regional bodies' to advise on the planning of services. This was, of course, not only a gesture towards the teaching hospitals. It was also a response to the arguments of what might be called the 'medical technocracy': those whose concern had long been to achieve a more rational structure of services in terms of the quality of medical care – a concern which can be found in many of the documents published between the wars and which was reinforced during the war by a series of inquiries, sponsored by the Nuffield Provincial Hospitals Trust, into the state and distribution of health resources.[16] If the logic of the joint authorities was the need to make some sort of sense of the existing local government structure, the logic of the regional bodies was the need to plan the more specialised medical services – particularly consultant services – on a larger scale than the administrative units produced by the amalgamation of existing local authorities. The functional geography of local government, it was clear, did not necessarily coincide with the functional geography of the health service: a dilemma which, once again, provides a further theme for the history of the NHS over the next decades.

Within two months of getting the Conservative Cabinet's agreement to his revised proposals, Willink had been replaced by Aneurin Bevan as Minister of Health: a Labour Government, with a triumphant majority, had swept into office. The fragile consensus which had constrained Labour Ministers in the Coalition Government appeared to be shattered. The way was open for the politics of ideology to take over from the politics of compromise.

Private negotiation into public controversy

In retrospect, the most remarkable aspect of the controversies that attended the enactment of the National Health Services Bill in 1946 and the setting up of the National Health Service in 1948 is the disparity between the anger generated and the actual changes introduced by Aneurin Bevan. In a sense, the virulent hostility of Bevan's critics – both on the Conservative benches in Parliament and among the medical profession – flattered his achievement and exaggerated the extent to which he broke with the sedimentary consensus that had been built up over the preceding years. From today's perspective, the 1946 legislation was as remarkable for the degree of continuity it represented as for its departures from the agreed compromises of the Coalition Government. In turn, the departures from the agreed compromises reflected as much a defeat for some of Bevan's own colleagues in the Labour Cabinet as an assertion of Socialist ideology at the expense of Conservative ideology.

It is tempting to argue, indeed, that it was in the political interests of everyone concerned to overstate the extent of disagreement. For Bevan, opposition was a testimonial to his own radicalism; and for the Conservatives, and the medical profession, it was an opportunity to wash their hands in public over some of the compromises they had accepted during the years of private negotiation. It was Bevan's style of self-presentation – the aggressive insistence that it was the Labour Government's duty to present its proposals to Parliament, rather than hammering them out in private conclave with the representatives of the interest groups – which not only brought the latter's latent suspicions and resentments to the surface, but also gave them the pretext for adopting a stance of public hostility. Compromises which might just about be acceptable as part of an agreed package no longer were so once the package itself had been unwrapped by the Minister without consultation. Indeed this interpretation is strengthened by the otherwise very curious contrast between the relatively easy passage given to Bevan's most radical proposal, that for the hospital service, and the long-drawn-out battle over general practice, where Bevan in fact hardly departed from the previously agreed compromise. It is therefore helpful to consider these two facets of the 1946 legislation separately.

Bevan's plan represented one dramatic break with the immediate past – to the extent that it represented a return to MacNalty's 1939 proposal. His entire scheme was based on 'the complete takeover – into one national service – of both voluntary and municipal hospitals', as his October 1945 memorandum to the Cabinet put it.[17] In turn this would mean, Bevan's memorandum continued, 'the concentration in the Ministry of Health of responsibility for a single hospital service, coupled with the delegation of day-to-day administration to new regional and local bodies appointed by the Minister (after consultation with the appropriate local organisations) and responsible to him'. Equally, it would imply 'the centralising of the whole finance of the country's hospital system, taking it right out of local rating and local government'.

In other words, the dilemma of combining national responsibility with responsiveness to local need was to be resolved in a way totally different to that envisaged in the 1944 White Paper: there was to be no split of responsibilities between central and local government, but an attempt to solve the problem of achieving an appropriate balance between the centre and periphery by a process of delegation. It was a solution which was immediately challenged within the Labour Cabinet. The arguments involved deserve close attention, since once again they have continued throughout the history of the NHS and the issue of the appropriate balance between centre and periphery continues to be a major political issue.

The main opposition to Bevan came from Herbert Morrison, Lord President of the Council and, as in the days of the Coalition Government, the voice of local government. In his counter-memorandum to Bevan's,[18] Morrison argued that the Minister of Health is:

> on the horns of a dilemma. If the Regional Boards and District Committees are to be subject to the Minister's directions on all

questions of policy, they will be mere creatures of the Ministry of Health, with little vitality of their own. . . . Yet it is difficult under a State system to envisage the alternative situation in which, in order to give them vitality, they are left free to spend Exchequer money without the Minister's approval and to pursue policies which at any rate in detail may not be the Minister's, but for which he would presumably be answerable.

Further, Morrison argued that the Bevan scheme would weaken local government:

It is possible to argue that almost every local government function, taken by itself, could be administered more efficiently in the technical sense under a national system, but if we wish local government to thrive as a school of political and democratic education as well as a method of administration – we must consider the general effect on local government of each particular proposal. It would be disastrous if we allowed local government to languish by whittling away its most constructive and interesting functions.

In conclusion, Morrison conceded the drawbacks of joint authorities – 'I dislike them thoroughly' – but urged that while nationalisation might be superior to a local authority system 'judged purely as a piece of administrative machinery', this consideration was outweighed by the political consequences of incurring the antagonism of local government.

So here there is a clear ideological split, not in party terms but in terms of perceived values. On the one hand, there are Morrison's political values: the emphasis on local government as a school of political education, with considerations of efficiency and administrative rationality coming a poor second. On the other hand, there is Bevan's stress on a different set of values: the values of paternalistic rationalism. For one of the principal justifications advanced by Bevan in his October memorandum to the Cabinet was precisely that nationalisation would be a more efficient and rational system. His scheme, he argued, would enshrine the principle of 'public control following public money'. And it was the only way of achieving 'as nearly as possible a uniform standard of service for all'. As he pointed out, 'Under any local government system – even if it is modified by joint boards or otherwise – there will tend to be a better service in the richer areas, a worse service in the poorer.' So considerations of equity reinforced considerations of rationality, and Labour's commitment to equality went hand in hand with arguments based on efficiency.

Nor was Bevan prepared to concede that his scheme would produce bureaucratic over-centralisation. 'A centralised service must, indeed, be planned so as to avoid rigidity', he wrote in his counterblast to Morrison's memorandum,[19] 'that is why I have proposed that the hospital service shall be administered locally by Regional Boards and District Committees. . . . It is precisely by the selection of the right men and women to serve on these bodies that I hope to be able to give them substantial executive powers, subject to a broad financial control, and so prevent rigidity.' But, he conceded that, 'admittedly, this is a field in which there is room for development in the techniques of governments, but the problems that will arise should not be incapable of solution'. The search for new techniques has proved to be one of the themes running through the history of the NHS, as the problems prove themselves remarkably resistant to the various solutions that have been tried since Bevan wrote his memorandum.

Bevan's view prevailed in the Cabinet. But there was a price to be paid; predictably enough, given that any policy choice involved trade-offs between competing considerations. One of the arguments against divorcing control over hospitals from local government was that this would ensure the continued co-ordination, under the same authority, of hospital and personal health services. In his October memorandum Bevan had tentatively, if logically, raised the possibility of transferring responsibility for the personal health services, as well as the hospitals, from local to central government:

> the future allocation of the other local government health services – child welfare, district nursing, the provision of health centres for general medical and dental care, and so on – can be considered in detail once a decision in principle has been reached on the hospital services. It looks at first sight as though the ultimate responsibility for these should rest with the Minister, to ensure a unified health service, but there should be provision for delegation to existing persons and agencies for doing the day-to-day job.

However, this suggestion quickly disappeared from view in the subsequent discussions of the legislation: a concession, no doubt, to the Morrisonian advocacy of the local government role. Much of the criticism in the following months, from both the Conservative Opposition and from the medical profession, concentrated precisely on Bevan's failure to achieve a 'unified health service'. Nor was this criticism confined to Bevan's political opponents: one of Labour's backbenchers, Frederick (later Sir Frederick) Messer, argued in the Second Reading debate[20] that Bevan's measure was 'not a health service Bill; it is a medical service Bill'. The divorce between medical services in the strict sense and health services in the wider sense was to become one of the major themes in the continuing debate about the NHS over the coming decades.

Bevan's legislation embodied other concessions as well. There was no concession to the voluntary hospitals as such: unlike local authorities these did not have any spokesmen in the Labour Cabinet, nor did they carry any weight with the Party. But his plans did incorporate some features designed specially to appeal to the most prestigious medical specialists, represented by the Royal Colleges, as part of an overall political strategy of splitting the medical profession. This strategy consisted of buying off the potential opposition of the Royal Colleges, and enlisting their support against the BMA – the voice, essentially, of the general practitioners.

Not only were teaching hospitals given special status: with governing bodies of their own directly under the Minister of Health, instead of being integrated into the administrative structure of the hospital service. Not only were the regional authorities given executive status, instead of being merely advisory bodies as envisaged in the 1945 proposals of the Conservative Government. But, in addition, the right to private practice in hospital pay beds was enshrined in the legislation, to the dismay of many Labour backbenchers. A new system of merit or distinction awards was also introduced – the brainchild of Lord Moran of the Royal College of Physicians and one of the key actors in Bevan's manoeuvres to enlist the support of the hospital specialists. This was to give consultants deemed to be meritorious by their peers special financial rewards, over and above their basic salaries. Lastly, once the principle of limiting the bodies responsible for the health service to elected local government representatives had been abandoned, the way was open for doctors to serve on the new authorities: something the profession had long fought for, but which the 1944 White Paper had explicitly rejected. 'The full principle of direct public responsibility must, of course, be maintained, but we can – and must – afford to bring the voice of the expert right into direct participation in the planning and running of the service', Bevan wrote in his October memorandum to the Cabinet, introducing his scheme for a National Health Service. As between accountability to elected members and professional participation, the balance had decisively been tilted towards the latter, though in the Second Reading debate Bevan did warn against 'the opposite danger of syndicalism'.

Interestingly, Bevan was not prepared to extend the participation principle conceded to the medical profession to other health service workers. When the Trades Union Congress raised this possibility, Bevan was quick to quash it.[21] No one, he pointed out in a letter to Sir Walter Citrine, the TUC's General Secretary, would be on the Regional Boards and Hospital Management Committees in a representative capacity:

> I attach great importance to the principle that these bodies shall consist of members appointed for their individual suitability and experience, and not as representatives or delegates of particular, and possibly conflicting, interests. This means that members of Regional Boards and Management Committees could not be appointed to 'represent' the health workers, and I could not agree to an alternative suggestion that has been put forward – that a proportion of members of these authorities should be appointed after consultation with the health workers. The difficulty here would be to draw any line which would keep membership of the Boards and Committees down to reasonable numbers. If the nurses were to be consulted, why not also the hospital domestics? the radiotherapists? the physiotherapists? and so on.

So while doctors were to participate in the running of the new NHS, representing 'expertise' rather than the medical profession, the same principle was not to be applied to other health service workers: a disparity which was to fuel argument in the 1970s when this issue once again surfaced.

Given these concessions, it is not surprising that the initial opposition to Bevan's proposals for the hospital service soon melted away. Nor, of course, is it surprising that the concessions so made were to become the raw material of future political controversy, in so far as they represented the victory of tactical considerations over administrative and political logic, coherence and consistency. However, it was issues involving general practitioners which aroused the fiercest passions and opposition between 1945 and 1948: so much so, that the ability of the Minister to launch the NHS on the appointed day in July 1948 remained in doubt until almost the last month. Yet, paradoxically, in the case of general practice, Bevan was for the most part content to accept the negotiated compromise that had emerged when he inherited his post.

The single most important feature of Bevan's proposals for general practice was

the acceptance of the 1945 Conservative plan for maintaining Insurance Committees in the new incarnation of local Executive Committees (with a stronger
representation for the medical profession than under the previous machinery).
All doctors would be in contract with this Executive Committee, thus removing
any threat of general practitioners becoming either part of a national corps of
doctors employed by a Central Medical Board, as envisaged in the 1944 White
Paper, or of becoming local authority employees. In this respect, then, Bevan's
plan marked a major retreat since 1944, in the face of the medical profession's
objections. The medical profession's suspicions were roused by three other aspects
of Bevan's proposals. First, it was laid down that Health Centres would be
provided by local authorities: this not only fulfilled a long-standing Labour
commitment to this kind of practice, but also was designed to serve as a bridge
between medical services and the health services provided by local authorities.
The change was one more of emphasis than of substance: the 1944 White Paper
had stated that Health Centres should be given a 'full trial', while even the
Conservative plan had suggested that there should be a 'controlled trial'. But even
this was enough to arouse the latent paranoia of the BMA, which scented the
danger of local authority control.

This paranoia was further reinforced by another proposal: this was that general
practitioners should be remunerated on the basis of a mixture of part-time salaries
and capitation fees. This was not as threatening as the 1944 White Paper, which
had proposed full-time salaries for all doctors employed in Health Centres. But it
marked a change from the Conservative plan, which had dropped any salaried
element. Here the BMA were quick to seize on the thin end-of-the-wedge
argument: once even partial salaries were introduced, the way would be open
to turn all general practitioners into salaried State bureaucrats. In logic, the BMA
was wrong: part-time salaries were in fact introduced in the 1960s (see Chapter 3)
without turning general practitioners into salaried officials. In their reading of
Bevan's long-term intentions, however, the BMA were right. At a meeting of the
Cabinet's Social Services Committee, Bevan said that he looked forward towards
the establishment of a full-time salaried medical service in due course, but felt
that it would be impracticable to make such a major change in established
practices at once.[22] The BMA's ire was further fuelled by the reinstatement of
the 1944 White Paper proposal – dropped by the Conservative Government – to
set up a central Medical Practices Committee which would have the power to
prevent doctors from setting up in practice in areas which already had their fair
share of medical manpower. Lastly, and this was the only point on which Bevan
was more radical than the 1944 White Paper, the Labour Government proposed
to prohibit the sale and purchase of practices, and to compensate existing general
practitioners accordingly.

It was these proposals which threw a lighted match into the BMA's smoulder-
ing discontent. In the long-drawn-out battle that followed, the BMA raised a
number of further issues – invariably dressed up in the rhetoric of the threat to
the sacred principles of the freedom of patients to choose their own doctors and of
the right of doctors to practise their craft free from interference (neither of which
were, in fact, threatened by the Labour Government's proposals). The details of
the controversy are of little concern here. But two points require noting. First, in
April 1948 – when it seemed that the opposition of the BMA would prevent the
NHS from getting off the ground on the appointed day – Bevan made what was

apparently a dramatic concession. Amending legislation would be introduced to make it clear that it was no part of his intention to create a whole-time, salaried service: general practitioners would continue to be paid on a capitation fee basis – and part-time salaries would be limited to new entrants to the profession for their first three years. Whether or not this represented a defeat for Bevan is arguable: this depends on just how committed he was to the 'establishment of a full-time medical service', and what he envisaged the timetable of progress towards this policy aim to be – something which cannot be established conclusively on the basis of the available evidence. But the concession was certainly a victory for the doctors, in that it recognised the principle that the medical profession could veto any proposals to change the methods of remuneration: a phenomenon which appears to be international.[23]

Second, the years between 1945 and 1948 help to illuminate the complex nature of intra-medical politics. Indeed the politics of the medical profession, as distinct from the politics of health care, would require a study in their own right to do them anything like justice. The BMA's constitution included, in the words of the Webbs, 'all the devices of advanced democracy'. That is, neither the BMA bureaucracy – led by its Secretary, Charles (later Lord) Hill – nor the elected leadership could commit the Association: all deals had to be referred back to the BMA's representative body. Thus it is not surprising that 25 years later Hill could write, reflecting on that confrontation with Bevan:

> It is undeniable that emotional outbursts in public at critical times, inevitable in a large body at times of crisis, did sometimes embarrass the profession's spokesmen by the headlines they stimulated and the somersaults of policy they encouraged. . . . Furthermore, the Representative Body did declare itself – in advance of any Government plans – in favour of many features of a health service which it subsequently rejected. It did tend sometimes to ignore such gains as its representatives had secured and immediately to switch its attention to the points on which it had not won, however important or unimportant they were. Balance sheets of gains and loss are not always judged dispassionately in large assemblies, where oratory and emotion prevail. Tactics are better devised in private by the few than publicly by the many.[24]

This emphasises the danger of 'reifying' the medical profession: to see it as a phalanx of disciplined troops defending clearly defined interests and objectives. The interests of the medical profession were by no means homogeneous: we have already noted the division between the BMA, representing mainly general practitioners, and the Royal Colleges. The objectives, also, differed: as between those who were concerned to promote a technically efficient, high-quality medical service based on consultants and those whose main aim was to conserve a particular way of life based on the GP surgery – between the technicians and the individualists in the profession. Moreover, on any questions of tactics, the profession tended to be split: in the final plebiscite organised by the BMA, to decide the profession's response to Bevan's promise of amending legislation in 1948, 54 per cent were against further discussion with the Minister, while 46 per cent were in favour (with the consultants split evenly, and the general practitioners opposing further negotiations by nearly two to one). Given the constitutional machinery of the profession's organisation, it was always easier to mobilise support for outright opposition rather than to secure agreement on specific proposals – with the consequence that the difficulty in getting agreement on what was or was not acceptable would in turn eventually tend to undermine the commitment to outright opposition. It is, once again, a pattern which provides a leitmotif for the history of the NHS: one which helps to explain, for example, the outcome of the protracted negotiations about consultants' contracts in the 1970s (*see* Chapter 4).

Whose victory was it?

So, in July 1948, the National Health Service was launched. It was designed, as Aneurin Bevan told the House of Commons when introducing the Bill, 'to universalise the best': to divorce the ability to get the 'best health advice and treatment' from the ability to pay and 'to provide the people of Great Britain, no matter where they may be, with the same level of service'. It is thus easy to see why the creation of the National Health Service has been seen as a triumph of Socialist ideology, inspired as it appeared to be by egalitarian ideas: a model of institutionalising the principle of allocating resources according to need. From this perspective, if we try to explain the political processes which resulted in the creation of the NHS, there is no need to look further than the election which brought the 1945 Labour Government into power and Bevan into office.

Yet, as the previous account should have made clear, the question of whose victory the creation of the NHS represented allows of no clear-cut answer. For Eckstein,[25] the creation of the NHS represented a victory not so much for Socialist ideology – in the strict sense of being concerned with remedying distributional inequities – as a victory for a 'radically managerial' ideology. Admittedly, the creation of the NHS was part of a long, evolutionary process, in which both the paternalistic rationalists within the civil service and the medical technocrats – the professional élite which sought to maximise the opportunities to deploy the tools of medical science – played a leading role. From their point of view, the health services as they existed in 1939 presented a policy puzzle: how to make sense of a ramshackle, partly bankrupt, incoherent and incomplete system. As we have seen, much of the process of policy-making represented a series of attempts to test out the 'fit' of various solutions: to reconcile different aims of policy and to minimise opposition. To a large extent, then, the creation of the NHS can be seen as an example of social learning.[26]

Social learning is not, however, a neutral process which takes place in a vacuum of preconceptions and assumptions. What people learn depends on their perceptions of the situation with which they are trying to deal, and the assumptions they bring to bear on problems. The years between 1939 and 1948 show that different actors in the policy machine had very different perceptions and assumptions, and that these differences played a large part in shaping their actions. Thus civil servants tended to put much emphasis on the engineering of consensus, and in particular on avoiding a clash with the medical profession. In this, they were at one with the Conservative politicians. In contrast, Bevan and the Labour Government were prepared to move out of the private arena of health care politics – the engineering of consensus through negotiations in Whitehall – into the public arena of political conflict. The extent of the break with the past, represented by Bevan's arrival at the Ministry of Health, must not be exaggerated: Bevan did not abandon the politics of compromise. If his plans represented a striking innovation in one respect, he largely built on the compromises that had been hammered out over the previous years and paid a heavy price in terms of concessions made to buy off opposition, both from consultants and local government. But there was nothing inevitable about the final shape of the NHS as it emerged in 1948: the same aims of policy could have been achieved through different organisational and institutional means.

Equally, to concentrate on the terms of the debate is to risk missing out on what was, surely, at least as important: those issues which were not debated precisely because all the actors were agreed in their assumptions. If much of the debate was about technical issues – that is, about the appropriate administrative machinery – this was because certain crucial aims of policy were taken for granted. If there was little evidence of Socialist ideology in the debate, if there appeared to be little emphasis on distributional issues, this was at least in part because this was common ground. Nothing is more remarkable than the shared assumption that the health service should be both free and comprehensive – and that it should be based on the principle of the collective provision of services and the pooling of financial risks through the public financing of the service. Even in the years of the Coalition Government, when the Conservatives might have been expected to take a different view, one of the few issues of controversy in the arguments of the Cabinet Reconstruction Committee was the limited question of whether or not there should be hotel charges in hospitals[27] – a question prompted not by ideological considerations but by the practical problem of how best to ensure an independent source of income for voluntary hospitals.

Most important of all, perhaps, the discussions reflected a shared assumption about the past achievements and future potentials of medical science. Implicit in the consensus about the general aims of policy was a shared, optimistic faith in progress through the application of diagnostic and curative techniques. In turn, this mirrored the belief that medical science had not only triumphed over disease and illness in the past but would continue to do so in future. On this view, the only problem was how best to create an institutional framework which would bring the benefits of medical science more efficiently and equitably to the people of Britain. There might be disagreement about specific policy instruments, but there could be little argument about the desired goal or about the eventual rewards.

Again, it is all too easy to present the evolution of policy as though all the sets of actors involved were discrete and homogeneous. This is to miss the flow of ideas across the different categories: to assume that the ideas of, for example, the Socialist Medical Association did not influence the attitudes of the civil servants or the medical technocrats. This is surely to ignore the extent to which all the actors were drawing from a common pool of ideas: the extent to which certain assumptions were important precisely because they had ceased to be controversial and had become part of the conventional wisdom.

If the consensus about the ends of policy has to be stressed, so too has the conflict about means. For it was the question of the means to be used which brought the policy-makers into conflict with the interests that would be affected by the organisational and institutional devices chosen to translate the general aims of policy into practice. The battle was about the instruments of policy: a battle in which the main protagonists were the medical profession. Once more, the question of who 'won' this particular battle allows no simple answer, if only because the medical profession itself was a collection of different (and sometimes conflicting) interests. In the case of general practice, the doctors were in effect conceded a right of veto: a right which they used to maintain the status quo. In the case of the hospital services, the NHS was designed to accommodate certain specific interests within the medical profession. But in both cases the power of the medical profession consisted less in being able to impose its will in a positive sense than in being able to block changes. Most important perhaps for the future, the medical profession obtained a monopoly of legitimacy among the health service providers: a unique position, reflected in the participation of doctors in the running of the NHS.

The conflict about means did not, however, simply reflect a clash of interests. It also represented a clash of values. In its final form, as it emerged in 1948, the NHS represented the victory of the values of rationality, efficiency and equity: it was designed to be the instrument of national policies for delivering health care in a rational, efficient and fair way across the country. But as the debates between 1939 and 1948 showed very clearly, there are other values. The case for local government control was based not just on the defence of a particular interest – the existing local authorities – but on a view of the world anchored in the values of localism: a view which stressed responsiveness rather than efficiency, differentiation rather than uniformity, self-government rather than national equity.

Built into the structure of the NHS, therefore, were certain fundamental contradictions. Some of these contradictions reflected political concessions: the deliberate acceptance of imperfections in the grand design in order to minimise opposition. Other contradictions, however, reflected the incompatibility of certain objectives. The history of the NHS since 1948 can largely be seen as the working out of these contradictions: a continuing and never-ending attempt to reconcile what may well turn out to be irreconcilable aims of policy.

References

1. Michael Foot, *Aneurin Bevan*, vol. 2, Davis-Poynter: London, 1973.
2. In many ways the best account remains Harry Eckstein, *The English Health Service*, Harvard UP: Cambridge, Mass. 1958. At the time of writing, the government documents were not accessible and the book is perhaps biased by the sources that were available: Eckstein's exclusive emphasis on the central role of the medical profession reflects the fact that the main sources available were the published accounts of negotiations in the medical press. Another account based on published sources is AJ Willocks, *The Creation of the National Health Service*, Routledge & Kegan Paul: London 1967. The first book to be based on the documents now available in the Public Records Office is John E Pater, *The Making of the National Health Service*, King Edward's Hospital Fund for London: London 1981. Pater himself was a civil servant at the Ministry during the period in question, and his book therefore is a most authoritative (if extraordinarily discreet and self-effacing) account.
3. Political and Economic Planning, *Report on the British Health Services*, PEP: London 1937.
4. Brian Abel-Smith, *The Hospitals in England and Wales, 1800–1948*, Harvard UP: Cambridge, Mass. 1964.
5. Ministry of Health, *Interim Report on the Future Provision of Medical and Allied Services*, HMSO: London 1920, Cmnd. 693.

6. Royal Commission on National Health Insurance, *Report*, HMSO: London 1926, Cmnd. 2596.

7. British Medical Association, *A General Medical Service for the Nation*, BMA: London 1930; Socialist Medical Association, *A Socialized Medical Service*, SMA: London 1933.

8. Public Records Office, MH 80/24, Minutes of 'The first of a series of office conferences on the development of the Health Services', dated 7 Feb. 1938; Minutes by the Chief Medical Officer, dated 21 Sept. 1939.

9. Bentley B Gilbert, *The Evolution of National Insurance in Great Britain*, Batsford: London 1966.

10. Ministry of Health, *A National Health Service*, HMSO: London 1944, Cmnd. 6502.

11. Public Records Office, CAB 124/244, Memorandum dated 10 Feb. 1944.

12. Sir Geoffrey Vickers, *The Art of Judgment*, Chapman & Hall: London 1965.

13. For a detailed study of this issue, see Frank Honigsbaum, *The Division in British Medicine*, Kogan Page: London 1979.

14. Public Records Office, CAB 87/5, Minutes of the War Cabinet Reconstruction Committee, 10 Jan. 1944 and 11 Jan. 1944. The quotations in the following paragraph also come from the records of these two meetings.

15. Public Records Office, MH 77/30 A, Draft Cabinet Paper by Minister of Health, June 1945.

16. Sir George Godber, *The Health Service: Past, Present and Future*, Athlone Press: London 1975.

17. Public Records Office, CAB 129/3, Memorandum by the Minister of Health: The Future of the Hospital Services, 5 Oct. 1945.

18. Public Records Office, CAB 129/3, Memorandum by the Lord President of the Council: The Future of the Hospital Services, 12 Oct. 1945.

19. Public Records Office, CAB 129/3, Memorandum by the Minister of Health: The Hospital Services, 16 Oct. 1945.

20. Hansard House of Commons 5th Series, vol. 422, 30 April 1946. All subsequent quotations from the Second Reading debate refer to this source.

21. Public Records Office, MH 77/73, Letter dated 18 July 1946.

22. Public Records Office, CAB 134/697, Minutes of the Cabinet Social Services Committee, 29 Nov. 1945.

23. TR Marmor and D Thomas, 'Doctors, Politics and Pay Disputes', *British Journal of Political Science*, no. 2, 1972, pp. 421–2.

24. Lord Hill, 'Aneurin Bevan Among the Doctors', *British Medical Journal*, 24 Nov. 1973, pp. 468–9.

25. Eckstein op. cit. (see ref. 2), pp. 2–3.

26. Hugh Heclo, *Modern Social Politics in Britain and Sweden*, Yale UP: New Haven, Conn. 1974.

27. Public Records Office, CAB 87/5, Minutes of the War Cabinet Reconstruction Committee, 10 Jan. 1944.

Chapter 2

The politics of consolidation

In 1958 the House of Commons held a celebratory debate to mark the tenth anniversary of the creation of the National Health Service.[1] It turned out to be an exercise in mutual self-congratulation as Labour and Conservative speakers competed with each other in taking credit for the achievements of the NHS. Aneurin Bevan proclaimed that the service 'is regarded all over the world as the most civilised achievement of modern Government'. Derek Walker-Smith, the Conservative Minister of Health, produced a statistical litany of success. Since 1949, he pointed out, 'Effective beds are up by 6½ per cent; inpatients admitted are up by 29½ per cent; the ratio of treatment to beds is up by 22 per cent, and the waiting lists are down by 11½ per cent'. Diphtheria had been conquered; tuberculosis was about to be conquered. 'We have to aim', he concluded lyrically, 'at the prevention and, where possible, the elimination of illness, resulting in a positive improvement in health, reflected in the factory, the foundry and the farm, and not merely in the convalescent home.'

Not all was self-congratulation. Some of the issues which were to emerge more strongly over the following decades provided an element of dissonance, if in a minor key. Bevan spoke of the poor state of the mental health service: 'Some of our mental hospitals are in a disgraceful condition', he pointed out. Similarly, he touched on the politically sensitive issue of pay beds in hospitals, where consultants could treat their private patients. The system was being abused by some consultants, he claimed, to allow their private patients to jump the waiting list. In turn, Walker-Smith qualified his optimistic vision of progress by conceding that success was creating its own difficulties for the NHS. 'If one is less likely to die of diphtheria as a child, or from pneumonia as an adult, one has a greater chance of succumbing later to coronary disease or cancer', he argued. 'By increasing the expectation of life, we put greater emphasis on the malignant and degenerative diseases which are characteristic of the later years.' An ageing population, and a new pattern of disease, were generating new problems for the NHS.

This anniversary debate provides a convenient, if necessarily arbitrary, watershed in the political history of the NHS. Ahead lay the politics of rational planning: a series of endeavours to adapt the machinery of the NHS in the light of the experience gained and problems revealed during the first decade. This is the theme of the next chapter. Behind lay the politics of consolidation: the transformation of what started out as a controversial experiment in social engineering into a national institution anchored in consensus. This provides the theme for the present chapter. By 1958 the transformation was indeed complete. 'The National Health Service, with the exception of recurring spasms about charges, is out of party politics', wrote Iain Macleod – a former Conservative Minister of Health – in 1958.[2] Some controversies might occasionally disturb the calm of the political pond: charges was one such issue, pay beds was another. But as an institution, the

NHS ranked next to the monarchy as an unchallenged landmark in the political landscape of Britain. Public opinion polls consistently showed a high degree of enthusiasm for the NHS, with 90 per cent or more of the respondents declaring themselves to be satisfied with the service. More surprisingly, perhaps, two-thirds of the medical profession declared that – given a chance to go back ten years and to decide whether or not the NHS should be started – they would support the creation of the service.[3]

The contrast between this consensus and the political furore that attended the launching of the NHS is striking. But it is more apparent than real. The rhetoric of battle in the years between 1946 and 1948 served largely to conceal, as we saw in the previous chapter, the very considerable degree of continuity and compromise involved in the creation of the NHS. Until Bevan's arrival on the scene, the norm and style had been closed arena politics: private negotiations between the various interests within the health care arena. Moreover Bevan himself, once he had won his victory of principle, quickly reverted to this style: negotiations about the detailed implementation of the general principles laid down in the 1946 Act were conducted in the customary discreet manner between Ministry of Health civil servants and the representatives of the medical profession.[4] The depoliticisation of the NHS after 1948 can thus be seen simply as the re-emergence of organisational routines anchored in the British tradition of government; in particular, the emphasis on resolving disagreement by the incorporation of interest groups in the processes of decision-making.[5]

It is, of course, misleading to talk about the depoliticisation of the NHS in a general sense. In the period in question, and indeed later, it was depoliticised only in a very specific sense: that of party politics. The NHS remained a political system in its own right: a political system with its own actors, rules and dynamics. Moreover, even given the absence of party controversy about the fundamentals of the NHS, it was inevitable that the health care system would be influenced by the political environment in which it was operating: the ideological and intellectual assumptions which shaped attitudes not only towards, but also within, the NHS.

This chapter, then, examines the internal politics of the NHS in the decade or so that followed its launching. In doing so, we shall develop some of the themes that emerged in the discussions that led up to the formation of the NHS: to see how the problems and policy dilemmas then identified were, or were not, resolved. But before exploring specific areas we must, however, look at the evolving character- istics of the health care policy arena. Throughout the 1950s, the policy process bore the imprint of three shocks. First, there was the harsh discovery of the gap between the commitments of the NHS and the resources available. Second, there was the gruelling experience of actually getting the NHS off the ground: of putting administrative flesh on the legislative skeleton of 1946. Lastly, the NHS, con- ceived in an era where the dominant ideology favoured collectivist planning, grew up in an intellectual climate that leant towards minimal government. All three factors helped to shape the assumptive worlds of the policy-makers – their perceptions of what was possible and desirable, what administrative tools could be used – and thus, in turn, influenced the development of the NHS.

Infinite demands, finite means

In December 1948, only four months after the NHS had been launched, Bevan addressed what was to be the first of a series of self-exculpatory memoranda to his Cabinet colleagues explaining why the service would cost much more than anyone had expected.[6] The original estimate of £176 million for 1948–49 would, he warned his colleagues, turn out to be £225 million:

> The rush for spectacles, as for dental treatment, has exceeded all expectations. . . . Part of what has happened has been a natural first flush of the new scheme, with the feeling that everything is free now and it does not matter what is charged up to the Exchequer. But there is also, without doubt, a sheer increase due to people getting things they need but could not afford before, and this the scheme intended.

More important still, he stressed, the cost of salaries and wages had proved much higher than anticipated. He concluded:

> The justification of the cost will depend upon how far we get full value for our money; and that in turn will depend on how successfully my Department administers the service, eradicates abuse – whether by professional people or by the public – and is able to control the inevitable tendency to expand in price, which is inherent in so comprehensive and ambitious a scheme as this.

In the event, the Ministry of Health did not appear to be able to 'control the inevitable tendency to expand in price'. A supplementary estimate of £59 million for 1948–49 was followed by one of £98 million for 1949–50. NHS expenditure appeared to be out of control. In 1949 the Government passed legislation giving it power to impose a shilling prescription charge, with the aim both of raising £10 million in revenue and of reducing the 'cascades of medicine pouring down British throats', in Bevan's own phrase.[7] In 1950 Bevan, who despite his public support for prescription charges had fought a private Cabinet battle against their actual introduction, agreed to a compromise whereby a ceiling was imposed on NHS expenditure. Later the same year a special Cabinet Committee, under the chairmanship of the Prime Minister, was set up to 'keep under review the course of expenditure on this Service'.[8] Finally in 1951 the Chancellor of the Exchequer, Hugh Gaitskell, announced charges for dental work and optical service with the aim of containing spending within the £400 million limit set: an announcement which led to the resignation of Bevan from the Cabinet.

In retrospect, the political furore may seem disproportionate to the cause: a battle fought over paper figures and symbols, rather than real issues. The 1956 report of the Guillebaud Committee, set up in 1952 to inquire into the cost of the NHS, showed that much of the anxiety aroused both by the seeming extravagance of the NHS and by the policy responses had been exaggerated.[9] Much of the apparent increase in spending, it pointed out, was due to general price inflation: 'the rising cost of the Service in real terms during the years 1948 to 1954 was less than people imagined.' Indeed expenditure on the NHS actually fell as a proportion of the national income in the climacteric political year of 1950–51.

As far as charges were concerned, the Guillebaud Committee tended to be agnostic. Charges for dental treatment, the report concluded, had acted as a deterrent and were, in the long run, undesirable; however, given the current shortage of dentists, the Committee thought it would be a mistake to abolish them. Charges for spectacles also acted as a barrier to use, and the Committee recommended that a 'fairly high priority' should be given to a 'substantial reduction' in the level of charges when more resources became available for the NHS. Lastly, the Committee favoured, on balance, the retention of pre-scription charges (introduced by the Conservative Government in 1952): '. . . we have no reason to think', the report concluded, 'that the charge hinders the proper use of the Service by at least the great majority of its potential users.' Overall, with some reservations that will be discussed later, the Committee threw out the indictment of extravagance and inefficiency against the NHS: '. . . allowing for the manifold shortcomings and imperfections inherent in the work-ing of any human institution, we have reached the general conclusion that the Service's record of performance . . . has been one of very real achievement.'

Despite this retrospective vindication, the days of financial innocence for the NHS were over. The original sin of health care utopias – the contrast between infinite opportunities for spending money and all too finite availability of resources – had been revealed. With the benefit of hindsight, this may be an all too obvious point. Yet nothing is more striking in the voluminous files of the discussions that led up to the creation of the NHS, drawn upon in the previous chapter, than the lack of consideration given to the financial implications of setting up the NHS: even the Treasury dog did not bark. The assumption was that the cost of the NHS could be calculated simply by extrapolating pre-war health care expenditure: hence, of course, the gross under-estimate for the first year of the NHS's operation. No thought appears to have been given to the possibility that a national health service would have a financial dynamic of its own; on the contrary, the assumption was rather that expenditure on health care would tend to be self-liquidating by producing a healthier population. Equally little thought seems to have been given to the income side: the long-term implications of the methods chosen to finance the NHS. It therefore came as all the more of a shock to realise that the logic of the NHS's commitment to providing a free service and to 'universalising the best', in Bevan's phrase, ran counter to the logic of its dependence on the Treasury and tax revenue for funds.

The case for accepting the NHS as an institution which inevitably and rightly generated extra expenditure demands was put by Bevan in a memorandum he wrote for the Cabinet in March 1950.[10] In this he argued that:

> Allowing for all sensible administrative measures to prevent waste, the plain fact is that the cost of the health service not only will, but ought to, increase. Most of the hospitals fall far short of any proper standard; accommodation needs to be increased, particularly for tuberculosis and mental health – indeed some of the mental hospitals are very near to a public scandal and we are lucky that they have not so far attracted more limelight and publicity. Throughout the service there are piling up arrears of essential capital work. Also it is in this field, particularly, that constant new development will always be needed to keep pace with research progress (as, recently, in penicillin, streptomycin, cortisone etc.) and to expand essential specialist services, such as

hearing aids or ophthalmic services. The position cannot be evaded that a nationally owned and administered hospital service will always involve a very considerable and expanding Exchequer outlay. If that position cannot, for financial reasons, be faced, then the only alternatives (to my mind thoroughly undesirable) are either to give up – in whole or in part – the idea of national responsibility for the hospitals or else to import into the scheme some regular source of revenue such as the recovery of charges from those who use it. I am afraid that it is clear that we cannot have it both ways.

Moreover, there was yet a further reason for expecting the pressure for more NHS expenditure to continue: the demands generated by the professional providers of the service. The whole point of the NHS was, after all, supposedly to eliminate all financial considerations which might inhibit treatment according to need. From the patient's point of view, this meant that there should be no financial barriers at the point of access. From the doctor's point of view, this implied that he should be free to carry out his professional imperative of doing his utmost for the individual patient without regard to the cost. Not surprisingly, therefore, Bevan complained to the Cabinet that: 'the doctors had secured too great a degree of control over hospital management committees, and were pursuing a perfectionist policy without regard to the financial limits which had necessarily to be imposed on this Service as on other public services.'[11] Professional perfectionism, clearly, was not compatible with the public financing of the NHS: a source of stress and tension throughout the history of the NHS – as doctors discovered that a hospital service, which many of them had entered on the presumption that it would free them from all financial inhibitions in the exercise of their craft, had in practice turned them into the State's agents for rationing scarce resources.

The difficulties of containing the rise in costs were compounded by another factor. In the case of the hospital service, the Ministry of Health was in a position to determine total budgets: although, as we have seen, it was not entirely successful in this respect in the first years of the NHS. But hospital service spending accounted for just over half of total NHS expenditure: £229 million out of £367 million in 1950–51. The rest of the expenditure was accounted for by the cost of the general practitioner, pharmaceutical, ophthalmic and dental services: drugs alone cost £38.5 million in 1950–51, or over 10 per cent of the total NHS bill. Here the expenditure commitment was – as in the case of the ophthalmic and dental services – effectively open-ended. If general practitioners prescribed more, if demand for spectacles or dental treatment increased, then inevitably spending would go up. In this respect, then, governments were on a financial escalator which they could not stop. Charges might be introduced to limit demand; general practitioners might be exhorted to prescribe cheaper, non-proprietary drugs. In the last resort, however, general practitioners were independent contractors. If they decided to prescribe more, or to refer more patients to hospitals for expensive treatment, there was little that anyone could do. The irony of the NHS as set up in 1948, and perpetuated since, was precisely that it could exercise least control over the gatekeepers to the system as a whole: the general practitioners, through whom all referrals to hospitals were channelled.

Not only had the financial dynamics of creating the NHS been ignored, so had the political dynamics of the system chosen to finance it. By rejecting an insurance-based health service – whose revenue would come from ear-marked contributions – the founders of the NHS ensured that it would have to compete with other government departments for general tax revenue: with education, housing and all the other claims for resources. If Socialism was the language of priorities, in Bevan's words, it did not follow that the NHS would be at the head of the queue: indeed rival spending ministers collectively might have an incentive to squeeze the share of the NHS in the total public expenditure budget (though they might also have a collective interest in maximising the total spent). Even if the public were well disposed towards the NHS, it did not follow that they would cheerfully accept higher taxes to pay for it, since there could be no direct relationship between higher spending on the NHS and higher taxation – given that all the revenue went into the general Treasury fund.

The reasons for rejecting an insurance-based system of finance were expounded by Bevan in the tenth anniversary debate. First, there were considerations of equity. The nature of the treatment given should not have to depend on the contributions made: 'We cannot perform a second-class operation on a patient if he is not quite paid up.' Second, the aim was to make the financial basis of the NHS redistributive. By drawing on general taxation, the system would ensure that those who had the most would pay the most: 'What more pleasure can a millionaire have than to know that his taxes will help the sick?' 'The redistributive aspect of the scheme was one which attracted me almost as much as the therapeutical', Bevan concluded in his retrospective reflections (although even the assumption that general taxation must necessarily and inevitably be progressive is questionable: in practice, the distributive impact depends on variable political decisions about the level and structure of taxes).

The outcome of the decision to reject an insurance-based finance was that the NHS at this period, and subsequently, was financed overwhelmingly out of general tax revenue. In 1950–51, 88.3 per cent of its income came from this source – a proportion which has fluctuated over the years but never fallen below 77 per cent.[12] Health insurance contributions were not dropped – what Treasury would ever agree to abandon a money-raising device once it had been introduced? – but became a sort of vestigial financial appendix: once the insurance principle had been scrapped, they were merely another means of raising what was in effect tax revenue. In 1950–51 they accounted for 9.4 per cent of the NHS's total income, a proportion which rose to 17.2 per cent in the early 1960s but subsequently declined to something approaching the original figure.

Another way of raising revenue for the NHS was, as we have already noted, to impose charges on users. The attraction of this was, and remains, that it allows the NHS to generate income in a way which is not competitive with other departments: in theory, it provides a magic formula for raising the spending-power of the NHS while not increasing public expenditure – pleasing both the advocates of higher health spending and the Treasury. In the event, however, charges have never contributed more than marginally to the NHS's income, even though the Conservative Government which came into office in 1951 did not share Labour's ideological commitment to the principle of a free health service and soon introduced prescription charges. In 1950–51, revenue from this source was less than one per cent of the NHS's total budget and reached only 5.3 per cent at its peak in the 1950s.

The reasons were simple and, although the controversy about charges continued to simmer away throughout the history of the NHS, were fully explored in an exchange of notes between Bevan and the Treasury in 1950.[13] If charges were more than nominal, there would have to be ways of exempting the least well-off. Any system of exemptions would mean, Bevan argued, 'administrative complexities and costs', as well as bringing back the means test into the health service. Equally, exemptions would reduce the total yield. Even a hotel charge of ten shillings a week for hospital patients, Bevan pointed out in response to Cabinet pressure, would yield a total revenue of only £10 million. It is precisely this balance between high administrative costs and relatively low yields which helps to explain why hotel charges – which were to be considered by subsequent Conservative Governments almost as a matter of routine – have never been introduced: an example of ideology yielding to administrative expediency. Indeed the reconciliation of ideological considerations and financial necessity was to depend on administrative ingenuity and innovation: the Labour Government of the 1960s managed to reconcile itself to prescription charges by introducing an automatic system of exemptions for certain broad categories – such as the young and the old – so avoiding both the costs and the political stigma of the means test. But, as always, there was a trade-off: administrative simplicity meant a lower income, since 60 per cent of prescriptions fell into the exempt category. There was no magic formula, as it turned out, for solving the NHS's financial dilemma.

The nature of this dilemma was clear by the beginning of the 1950s. On the one hand, there were the collective, environmental pressures to restrain expenditure: an alliance of Cabinet Ministers and taxpayers, as it were. On the other hand, there were the ever-present, institutionalised pressures for higher spending. As the Guillebaud Committee pointed out: 'It is still sometimes assumed that the Health Service can and should be self-limiting, in the sense that its own contribution to national health will limit the demands upon it to a volume that can be fully met. This, at least for the present, is an illusion.' There was no way of setting a financial target, the report further commented, which would ensure that an 'adequate service' would be provided: 'There is no stability in the concept itself: what might have been held to be adequate twenty years ago would no longer be so regarded today, while today's standards will in turn become out of date in the future. The advance of medical knowledge continually places new demands on the Service, and the standards expected by the public also continue to rise.'

Politicians, in short, had invented a financial treadmill for themselves when they created the NHS: whatever their political investment in raising funds, they would be chasing a metaphysical, ever-elusive concept of adequacy. They could never do enough. The NHS was a machine for generating new demands: a point recognised in Walker-Smith's tenth anniversary speech quoted at the beginning of this chapter. It is therefore scarcely surprising that in the 1950s the NHS evolved from being an instrument for meeting needs (as conceived by the founding fathers) to becoming an institutional device for rationing scarce resources.

There is another aspect of the debates about NHS finance which requires stressing. This is the language used. Bevan, as we have seen, fully accepted the existence of 'abuse' in the use of services. Moreover, he had talked about the 'cascades of medicine' pouring down British throats. It was imperative, everyone agreed, to stop waste and extravagance. In short, by the beginning of the 1950s, the NHS was stereotyped as a spendthrift organisation: a service which, moreover, had exploited its lack of financial control to grab more scarce public resources than those government departments which had actually managed to keep within their budgetary allocations. From the point of view of the Treasury, vice had been rewarded in the 1940s, and the 1950s were marked by a determination not to allow history to repeat itself. In the assumptive world of the Whitehall policy-makers, the NHS remained for most of the decade an undeserving case.

Not surprisingly, therefore, the NHS had to live on short-commons for most of the 1950s although this was a decade of booming economic growth by British standards at least. In 1958, its income (in cost terms, at 1970 prices) was only three per cent higher than it had been in 1950, while expenditure on education had soared.[14] Moreover, as the Guillebaud Committee pointed out, it had been starved of money for capital investment: its capital investment programme was running at a much lower level than that, even, of the pre-war hospital system. In turn, this slow rate of growth – and the perception of the NHS as a penitent financial sinner – affected the policy-makers both at the Ministry of Health and at the periphery: the subject of the next section.

Whatever is best administered is best

In the 1940s, the Ministry of Health was a department which was breaking exciting new ground. In the 1950s, it was the department which had to be stopped from doing things: in particular, as we have seen, from spending money. So it is not surprising that, if the years leading up to 1948 represent a case study in the politics of innovation, the decade that follows represents a case study in the politics of exhaustion. The emphasis switched from political to administrative decisions: from maximising the opportunities for change to minimising the dangers of turbulence. In a very real sense, the 1950s thus represent a breathing space between the crisis of creation in the 1940s and the renewed interest in change that characterised the 1960s. They are a period in which the stress was on achieving organisational stability: financially the new NHS had shown a cloven hoof, and now the emphasis was on seeking respectability.

In forging this new style, three sets of actors were involved: the politicians, the civil servants and the NHS administrators. Perhaps a fourth set of actors should also be considered: the medical profession. Their role is analysed in a subsequent section. Here we concentrate on the first three sets of actors. All had rather different interests and ideologies. However, in the 1950s – though not always subsequently – they shared, if for different reasons, the same quietist orientation. Taking first the political actors, the most important factor was also the most obvious one: in October 1951, a Conservative Government was voted into office. It had been elected on the slogan of 'Set the people free'. The thrust of Tory policy was to disengage from intervention in the workings of the economy. The remnants of wartime controls were scrapped; the process of nationalisation was reversed. The rhetoric of free market economics replaced that of national planning. Although the existence of the NHS was not threatened, it was operating in a different ideological and intellectual climate from that of the 1940s: from being the favourite child prodigy of the Government, it had become the somewhat embarrassing legacy of a previous liaison between Labour politicians and over-enthusiastic planners.

Whether as a direct consequence or not, the status of the Minstry of Health diminished. The process had already begun under the Labour Government. Following Bevan's translation to the Ministry of Labour in January 1951, the department's local government functions were grafted onto the new Ministry of Local Government and Planning. Its staff was, at a stroke, cut from 5,300 to 2,724: from being one of the most impressive mansions in Whitehall, it had become a semi-detached villa. At the same time, the Ministry lost representation in the Cabinet: a status it did not regain until its fusion with the Ministry of National Insurance under Richard Crossman in the late 1960s. But the process of decline in status accelerated under the Conservative Government when the Ministry became something of a revolving door for politicians. For the ambitious career politicians, it was only a resting place on the way to higher things. For others, it became a consolation prize on the way to back-bench oblivion. Between 1951 and 1958, there were no less than six different occupants of the ministerial post.[15]

Of these Iain Macleod, Minister of Health from 1952 to 1955, was the outstanding figure. Not only did he stay longer than anyone else in the 1950s, more than three years, he was also the only political heavyweight: a future Conservative Prime Minister who was never to be. It is therefore all the more significant that he saw his role at the Ministry as one of consolidation, not innovation. Within a fortnight of arriving at the department, he told his officials that he wanted the health service to enjoy a period of tranquillity, with no drastic reorganisation.[16] Too much legislation had been passed, and too many instructions had been issued, he argued in a speech in 1952: 'It is about time we stopped issuing paper and made the instructions work. I want to try and recreate local interest and above everything to get a complete partnership between voluntary effort and the State.' The encouragement of voluntary work became one of Macleod's main themes, just as it became the theme of another Conservative Minister – Patrick Jenkin – at the end of the 1970s: again a period of financial stringency for the health service, when invoking voluntary effort could be seen as a way of overcoming the inadequacies of public finance (and also a period when an ideology of minimal government was dominant).

Macleod's recessive style at the Ministry of Health accurately mirrored the prevailing mood of the Government as a whole. In turn, if for somewhat different reasons, his approach chimed well with the administrative biases of the department in the 1950s. Its senior officials – led by Sir John Hawton, Permanent Secretary from 1951 to 1960 – were veterans of the battles of the 1940s and the subsequent investment of effort in getting the NHS off the ground. 'After 1948', one of them remarked, 'a great many people felt that they had had as much change as they could take.' It was perhaps not surprising that the shell-shocked survivors of encounters with the medical profession in the 1940s – who decades later could still remember the angry representatives of the doctors pounding the table with their fists at meetings and shouting in unison – did not want to risk repeating the experience. Moreover, the strain had been carried by a very small number of officials. In 1951, the Ministry still only had 21 men and women above the principal rank, backed by 48 principals and assistant principals. Nor did this handful of civil servants engaged in policy work have much in the way of support. It was not until 1955 that the Ministry appointed its first statistician; the

Guillebaud Committee recommended, with some asperity, the creation of a statistical and research department. Qualitatively, too, the Ministry of Health was perhaps lacking, though here the evidence is at best tentative. Among successful candidates for the administrative civil service, it came low in the pecking order.[17] In the view of one BMA participant in negotiations with the Ministry, the department 'became the dumping ground for third-rate civil servants': an example, possibly, of how the Whitehall perceptions of a department as being something of a backwater, whose main achievements lie in the past, may become self-reinforcing.

Above all, though, there had been the sheer administrative slog of getting the NHS off the ground. The NHS, as conceived in the 1946 legislation, was hardly more than an outline sketch. It is only in trying to grasp the sheer enormity of the administrative task involved in the late 1940s that it is possible to understand the department's style and stance in the subsequent decade. For the Ministry of Health, the creation of the NHS involved the setting up of a new administrative structure and devising a new set of rules and regulations for making it work. The members of the new authorities had to be selected. A new machinery of negotiation for dealing with the 55 professional associations or trade unions that represented the NHS's workers had to be set up: the Whitley Council system which brought together the spokesmen of the employees and the employers. Regulations embodying conditions and terms of work had to be negotiated not only with the medical profession but with a 'bewildering variety of professional societies, covering workers as diverse as chemists and chiropodists, matrons and midwives, physicists and pharmacists, radiographers and remedial gymnasts'.[18] A vast range of administrative questions, concerned with the detailed delivery of the NHS's services, had to be hammered out in consultation with the representatives of the medical profession. Just taking the year 1948–49, these included such issues as the fees to be paid to general practitioners for vaccinations and immunisation, the layout of the Health Service prescription book, the supply of pessaries and Dutch caps, mileage allowances for rural practitioners and problems regarding certificates to enable patients to obtain surgical corsets.[19] All this was in addition to the ever-interesting, all-absorbing topic of levels of pay, about which more in a following section.

To set out this agenda for action, if only selectively, is not only to underline the burden involved. It is also to indicate the technical nature of many of the issues involved. In turn, the special nature of decision-making at the Ministry of Health was reflected in the departmental structure. Parallel to the civil service hierarchy culminating in the Permanent Secretary there was a professional hierarchy culminating in the Chief Medical Officer (CMO): the voice of expertise within the department. Like his lay counterpart, the Chief Medical Officer had direct access to the Minister (although one Permanent Secretary described the relationship between himself and the CMO as follows: 'We walk through the corridor arm-in-arm, but when we come to a door, I go through first').

From the point of view of the medical administrators, the problem of running the NHS was essentially that of concerting the activities of the consultants and general practitioners, all of whom were intensely individualistic and all of whom saw themselves as accountable only to their professional peers. From this perspective, the role of a central government department could only be to prompt and to encourage the evolution of medical practice: 'You help professional opinion to form itself spontaneously', as one experienced medical administrator put it. The point is well caught in the following quotation from Sir George Godber, who was CMO from 1960 to 1973 and a dominating figure in the first 30 years of the NHS:

> The NHS is comprised of very many services rendered daily by physicians, nurses, dentists, pharmacists and others. The content of those services is defined, not by planners, but by essential professional knowledge and skills. Change in method and practice is brought about by intra-professional exchanges; it may be abrupt because of a scientific development such as the advent of a new drug, or it may occur gradually with experience.[20]

Policy change could thus only be an adaptive process: 'there is no initial revelation from an all-wise centre', but a gradual process of professional consensus-building. Central government might use expert committees of professionals to push along the process, but it could not instruct or command.

The emphasis in the 1950s on keeping the machinery running, on care and maintenance rather than innovation and change, also reflected the interests and ideology of our third set of actors in the health policy area: the administrators of the NHS. At the periphery, too, the creation of the NHS involved a heroic administrative undertaking. New administrative authorities – 14 Regional Hospital Boards (RHBs), 36 Boards of Governors for teaching hospitals and some 380 Hospital Management Committees (HMCs) – had to be set up. Staff had to be recruited: one new RHB started life with only a couple of clerks.[21] Information had to be collected: the new staff often did not know the hospitals in their area and lacked even basic data about the number and distribution of doctors within their administrative fief. Once appointed, the officers had to work out their style of administration. This was not easy. At every level of the NHS there were three hierarchies of officers. There were the lay administrators: descendants of the pre-NHS hospital secretaries. There were the medical administrators; and there were the finance officers. In principle, the relationship was one of equality of status, but in practice the early years of the NHS were often marked by fierce battles between the three categories of officers. In some authorities, the lay administrators sought to establish their primacy over the treasurers: the case is quoted of one Finance Officer not being allowed to see his daily post until it had been opened and perused by the Secretary. In other instances, the Senior Administrative Medical Officer sought to impose his primacy as against the lay administrator.[22] But in no case was there a simple administrative hierarchy incorporating all the disciplines.

From the start, too, the NHS's administrative structure had a characteristic which helped to shape the relationship between centre and periphery for most of its existence. This was that all officers were appointed and employed by individual authorities, whether RHBs or HMCs. Although there were national conditions of pay and service, there was nothing remotely resembling a national corps of administrators or even a national policy for recruitment and training. The values and traditions of localism were thus built into the administrative structure of the NHS from the start. Not only were most of the original staff recruited from local government or the voluntary hospitals, where the tradition had been that of loyalty to a specific authority or to a particular institution. But they also became, in their new incarnation, the servants of individual NHS authorities, sharply distinguished from the civil servants of the Ministry of Health. There was no convergence in the career paths of NHS administrators – whether lay, medical or financial – and those of the central government civil servants. If an NHS administrator wished to enhance his reputation, he would do so not by demonstrating his ability to carry out national policies, but by showing his capacity for running the affairs of his own parish smoothly and effectively. In effect, his constituency was local, not national: his occupational incentives were thus biased towards accommodating local pressures rather than implementing central government exhortations, should there be any conflict between the two.

So much for the specific political biases, administrative styles and problems of implementation in the first decade of the NHS. But, before turning to a discussion of specific policy issues that surfaced in the 1950s, it is essential also to identify some of the more general characteristics of the arena of health care policy which constrained policy-makers not only in the 1950s but subsequently as well. First, to make explicit what so far has been implicit, the NHS is an institution marked by its complexity and its heterogeneity. The NHS is complex in that its workings depend on the spontaneous interaction of a large variety of different groups with different skills, all dependent on each other: from doctors to nurses, from laboratory technicians to ward orderlies (a complexity which has increased over the years with increased occupational specialisation). It is heterogeneous in that it delivers a wide range of different services under the same organisational umbrella: from acute care to chronic care, from maternity services to mental handicap services. In both these respects, other public services – education, for example – are relatively simple administrative organisms in comparison with the NHS.[23] In both these respects, too, the NHS presents special problems which affect both policy-making and administration.

Second, compounding the problems of policy-making, the health care policy arena is characterised by the ambiguity of objectives and uncertainty about the means needed to achieve any given ends. The point about ambiguity of objectives can be simply illustrated. From one perspective, increasing patient throughput can be seen as a measure of success in terms of improving productivity and treating illness; from another perspective, though, it may be seen as an indicator of failure to prevent disease. Similarly, there is frequent uncertainty about how best to achieve any given end: what level, or mix, of skills and resources is required to provide a particular kind of service. Moreover, given the ambiguity of objectives and uncertainty about means, measures of performance which would allow the success or failure of the NHS to be assessed are difficult to devise, and it was not until the 1980s that the drive to develop such measures began. In a sense, the output of the NHS *is* the organisation. It is this which explains one of the dominant features of the assumptive world of policy-makers in the 1950s and later: dominant precisely because unargued. This is the dependence on professional judgements – that is, the judgement, primarily though not exclusively, of the medical profession – on issues of need and adequacy. Lacking independent criteria of their own, policy-makers were forced to fall back on the professional view of what services were needed and how quality should be assessed. In a sense, this dependence can in part also be seen as a legacy of the assumptions which went into the building of the NHS, discussed in the previous chapter: specifically, the assumption of the paternalistic rationalisers that the objective of a health service should be to create a world fit for experts to apply their skills to the entire population. But it was reinforced in the 1950s by political consensus which left the way clear for problems and issues to be defined within the health care arena through the perceptual lenses of the professionals.

It is against this background that we have to explore the specific policy issues that emerged in the 1950s. In what follows, this chapter will examine three policy themes which allow us to examine the way in which the problems and dilemmas inherent in the creation of the NHS worked themselves out in this period. First, what balance was struck between central and local autonomy? Second, what progress was made towards Bevan's objective of 'as nearly as possible a uniform standard of service for all'? Third, what were the consequences of institutionalising the 'voice of the expert' – that of the medical profession – in the structure of the NHS? In each case, the aim is not to provide a history of events but to analyse the dynamics of the policy process.

Centre–periphery relations: the circle refuses to be squared

In setting up the NHS the aim was to reconcile national accountability and local autonomy. Public control had, inevitably, to follow public money: the Minister of Health was accountable to Parliament for every penny spent in the NHS. In turn, Members of Parliament could and did ask questions both about broad issues of policy or expenditure and about the detailed delivery of services. In 1950, MPs asked 629 questions; in 1955, they asked 1,045.[24] The Public Accounts and Estimates Committees of the House of Commons examined, in detail, the way in which the NHS spent public money. Yet at the same time the dangers of bureaucratic over-centralisation had to be avoided: the RHBs and the HMCs had to be given, in Bevan's words, 'substantial executive powers'.

It is therefore not surprising to find, throughout the first decade of the NHS, two contrasting themes running through the debate about relations between the central government department and the peripheral health authorities. From the centre came pressure on the Ministry of Health to exercise stricter control over what was happening at the periphery.[25] Rumbling through successive reports of the Public Accounts and Estimates Committees are demands for stricter central control in the pursuit of national uniformity: demands which were, of course, fuelled by the sense of NHS expenditure being out of control. From the periphery, however, there came complaints that the Ministry of Health was interfering too much: drowning administrators in a stream of circulars. Already in March 1948, even before the NHS had formally been set up, the chairmen of the RHBs were protesting that the Ministry was not letting them get on with their job by meddling in the affairs of HMCs.[26]

The Ministry of Health's dilemma can best be illustrated by the problem posed by the challenge of bringing expenditure under control. In 1950 Bevan appointed a senior civil servant with wide experience in other departments, Sir Cyril Jones, to study the financial workings of the NHS.[27] In his report, Jones identified what he saw to be the 'fundamental incompatibility between central control and local autonomy'. This stemmed, as he saw it, from the separation of the responsibility for raising and for spending money:

> The old compulsions in favour of financial responsibility in hospital
> administration have now disappeared, viz. the limit of private gener-
> osity in the case of voluntary hospitals, whose greatest assets when
> appealing for public support were long waiting lists and bank over-
> drafts; and the odium of raising rate revenue in the case of the local
> authority hospitals. Something is needed to take their place if the
> situation is not to get completely out of hand, now that hospitals are
> administered by voluntary workers who, keen and public spirited
> though they be, bear no responsibility for providing the funds and
> cannot be called to account by those who have to pay the bill. The only
> sanction is the ultimate drastic step of dismissal which, if once invoked,
> would practically kill voluntary service in this field.

Moreover, Jones pointed out, the difficulties for the Ministry of Health were
compounded by lack of information:

> The fact is that the Ministry possesses very limited information
> regarding the financial administration of the hospitals of the country
> on the basis of which . . . the estimates are framed; has no costing
> yardsticks at its disposal by which to judge the relative efficiency or
> extravagance of administration of various hospitals, and hence no
> alternative but either to accept the estimates wholesale as submitted
> without amendment, or to apply overall cuts to the total budgets in a
> more or less indiscriminate manner.

The Jones report has been quoted for the insights it provides into the centre–
periphery relationship in the early years of the NHS. His recommendations for
action were, however, largely ignored. Chief among these was one which was to
crop up again and again during the following 30 years but never to be
implemented: this was the abolition of the regional tier of administration.
RHBs, Jones argued, 'should cease to be directly concerned with hospital
administration and become regional hospital planning bodies'. HMCs, in turn,
should become 'subject to direct control by the Ministry', to be exercised through
a system of out-posting Ministry civil servants.

A number of other recommendations which came to nothing are also worth
noting. First, Jones directly challenged 'the doctor's right to prescribe for his
patient, as he wishes'. In the case of more expensive appliances, Jones thought,
such decisions should be reviewed by the lay managers of the service. Second,
Jones argued for the exclusion of doctors from the management authorities of the
NHS: 'in any democratic organisation it is axiomatic that, while due regard must
be paid to the advice of the technical experts, if there is the slightest suspicion that
such experts may have a direct or indirect pecuniary or other self-interest in any
matters, they should not be parties to the making of decisions thereof.' In any
case, there was 'no reason in principle for according hospital medical staffs a
privileged position as compared with that of other members of the hospital staff'.

The medicine was too strong for Bevan: a reminder that radical politicians may,
in practice, be more conservative than civil servants who do not carry the political
costs of implementing change. From Bevan's point of view, the costs of changes
which threatened the position of the medical profession would be too great:
'Frankly, I do not consider the battle worthwhile.' While in principle he accepted

the idea of relegating the RHBs to an advisory role, yet he was sceptical of giving the Ministry greater direct responsibilities:

> There would have been no theoretical difficulty – there is none now – in having from the outset a tightly administered centralised service with all that would mean in the way of rigid uniformity, bureaucratic machinery and 'red tape'. But that was not the policy which we adopted when framing our legislation. While we are now – and rightly, I think – tightening up some of the elements in our system of financial control, we must remember that in framing the whole service we did deliberately come down in favour of a maximum of decentralisation to local bodies, a minimum of itemised central approval, and the exercise of financial control through global budgets, relying for economy not so much on a tight and detailed Departmental grip, but on the education of the bodies concerned by the development of comparative costing, central supply and similar gradual methods of introducing efficiency and order among the heterogeneous mass of units we took over.

In the outcome, the financial crisis of the late 1940s and early 1950s did lead to one basic change. What had started out as a bottom-up system of generating budgets – with demands coming from the local hospital authorities – became a top-down system of dividing out a fixed total: of determining capped budgets for individual authorities.[28] In effect, the dilemma of central control v. local autonomy was, in the case of expenditure, side-stepped by allowing a very large degree of discretion *within* the centrally sanctioned budgetary limits. The 'exercise of financial control through global budgets', in Bevan's words, became the guiding principle of the NHS.

Briefly, the panic about overspending did lead to more direct Ministry intervention at the periphery. In 1950 the Ministry sent out teams of experts to review the staffing establishment of hospital authorities; the exercise was designed particularly to cut administrative staff. But the lapse into interventionism was brief. From 1952 onward, responsibility for control over establishment was transferred to the RHBs. When in 1951 the Ministry launched yet another economy drive, the emphasis was on local responsibility for implementing national policy: the department underlined the 'scope for local initiative in discovering and stopping extravagance and waste'. The concept of this exercise – 'a review inspired and stimulated from the centre, but devised and applied locally'[29] – was to become the model of Ministry policy-making throughout the 1950s, and indeed much later.

Overall it is possible to see an evolving philosophy of administration in all this: a philosophy of administration which saw policy as the product of interaction, rather than as the imposition of national plans.[30] The centre provided the financial framework and advice about desirable objectives. It left the periphery free to work out the details: rationality, from this perspective, lay in recognising that the complexity and heterogeneity of the NHS made it impossible to impose uniform national standards from the centre. Nothing more was heard in the 1950s about the 'rational and effective' plans for local health services envisaged in the 1944 White Paper. The acceptance of diversity, in short, was not only a necessary concession to the principle of localism but an inevitable outcome given the nature of the NHS. The centre, quite simply, did not know best – and indeed could not know best. There was a further ingredient, however, in this philosophy of administration. Even when the centre did know best – even if governments did have clear views about what was desirable – it did not perceive itself to be in a position to command. It could educate, it could inspire and it could stimulate. To have done more would have run counter to the values both of localism and of professionalism. It would have undermined the autonomy of health authorities and challenged the right of professionals to decide the content of their work.

It is this which explains what is perhaps the hallmark of Ministry of Health policy-making in the 1950s: policy-making through exhortation.[31] Circulars poured out of the Ministry: an average of about 120 a year in the 1950s. Some half of these had to do with the implementation of Whitley Council decisions: that is, the national decisions about conditions and terms of pay and service. Others were more technical in nature: requests for information, guidance about building standards. There was also a core of circulars which gave advice about desirable patterns or standards of service provision. To the extent that these affected the practices of the professionals, however, these could only be hortatory – given the acceptance of the principle of professional autonomy. This principle of professional autonomy did not only apply to the doctors. It applied equally to other professionals, such as nurses. Thus, to take the example of an issue which has continued to be a subject of controversy throughout the history of the NHS, in 1949 the Ministry of Health asked hospital authorities to make it easier for parents to visit their children in hospital. Three years later, however, an inquiry into actual practices showed that only 300 out of the 1,300 hospitals admitting children were allowing daily visiting, while about 150 did not allow any visiting at all.[32] Those responsible for local decision-making – in this instance, primarily the nurses – had chosen largely to ignore the centre's advice.

Although, therefore, there continued to be a tension between national accountability and local autonomy throughout the 1950s – and subsequently – the balance had swung towards the latter. The local health authorities were seen not so much as agents of the Ministers but as independent bodies. 'The Minister seeks to act always by moral suasion', a departmental civil servant told the Estimates Committee. The paradox of financial stringency was that while it led to tighter control over the total budgets available to health authorities, it also weakened the centre's ability to use incentives to persuade the periphery to follow national policies: the Ministry of Health could neither command nor bribe.

The pattern of inequalities

Financial stringency had one further perverse effect. The problem of 'perpetuating a better service in the richer areas, a worse service in the poorer' – which Bevan had seen as the main argument against a local government based health service – was, in the outcome, perpetuated in the 1950s. The inherited inequalities in the geographical distribution of hospital beds – a useful though only partial indicator of the distribution of resources generally – remained virtually undisturbed. For example, in 1950 Sheffield RHB had 9.4 beds per 1,000 population, while the South-West Metropolitan RHB had 15.1. Ten years later, the equivalent figures were respectively 9.1 and 14.2.

In effect, under the pressure of financial crisis and in the absence of the information needed to make judgements about local services and needs, the

Ministry of Health settled in the 1950s for control over the inherited budgets of local health authorities as distinct from trying to devise what would be an appropriate financial allocation from first principles. Primacy was given to the issue of control, to the neglect of the issue of distribution. 'The criticism is still made, however, that the system favours most the authorities who showed the least degree of financial responsibility in the early years of the service', the Guillebaud report noted, adding, 'We agree that the main weakness of the present system of allocating revenue funds is the lack of a consistent long-term objective.' Given the overall constraints on the total NHS budget, this outcome was perhaps inevitable. The lack of substantial growth in the total budget meant that any policy designed to improve the geographical distribution of resources would, in fact, have had to be a policy of re-distribution: of actually taking funds away from the best endowed parts of the country to transfer them to the least well-equipped regions. At a time when the overriding aim of policy was to achieve stability and to avoid turbulence, this was unlikely to be appealing. In any case, given the pressures of pent-up demands everywhere, even the best off regions had no difficulty in making out a case for the inadequacy of their existing allocations. So, not surprisingly, the principle of basing allocations on historical inheritances – of giving priority to maintaining the existing service – triumphed.

In theory, the capital budget could have been used to direct new resources to the relatively deprived regions of the country: as the Guillebaud Committee noted, five per cent of the total national sum available for capital spending was reserved for the 'seven Hospital Regions needing special help'. But as the capital investment programme never topped £50 million (at 1970 prices) in the 1950s, this five per cent hardly represented a crock of gold. In any case, immediate need was the enemy of long-term planning: as one Ministry of Health civil servant saw it, 'From the beginning we gave priority to the worst off areas. But as soon as you did this, you came up against the problem of the London teaching hospitals. They were all falling down. Do you let them fall down? Or do you give more resources to London, which is already well stocked?' In the event, the decision was to shore up the existing buildings: symbolic perhaps of health policy generally in the 1950s.

The success or otherwise of improving the distribution of NHS resources cannot, of course, be measured in terms of the number of beds alone. This is, at best, only a very partial measure of access to health care. Equally important is the distribution of skilled medical manpower. In the case of general practitioner services, the NHS – as we saw in the previous chapter – introduced a system of negative controls, designed to prevent general practitioners from entering practice in the relatively well-endowed parts of the country: a policy which succeeded in reducing the proportion of patients in under-doctored areas, those where the list sizes were exceptionally large, from 51.5 per cent in 1952 to 18.6 per cent in 1958.[33] In the case of hospital consultants, however, new policies had to be devised. The history of these policies provides an illuminating case study: an example both of the rational planning precepts of the pre-NHS days being carried into effect and of their subsequent dilution under the pressure of financial, professional and administrative constraints.

In the field of specialist services, the NHS started out with two aims in 1948. The first was to increase the availability of such services by creating more consultant posts. The second was to improve their distribution, both geographically and as between different specialties. To meet both objectives, the Ministry produced in 1948 what was in effect a national plan for the specialist services.[34] This set out what was considered to be an appropriate norm of consultant posts, by different specialties, for any given population. But hardly had the circular left the Ministry than the NHS was struck by financial crisis. The expansion of the consultant posts slowed down and the targets receded into the indefinite future. Subsequently, in 1953, an Advisory Committee on Consultant Establishments was set up: a medical committee acting as agent for the Ministry. Its function was to consider all applications for the creation of new consultant posts. As in the case of general practitioners, the policy instrument for improving the distribution of consultants was negative in character. 'The committee simply advised on applications received; it could not seek them out from regions thought to be in greatest need', was the subsequent comment of Sir George Godber, the author of the 1948 plan.[35] Implicitly the hopes of introducing national standards for medical manpower had been abandoned: given financial stringency, the emphasis was on rationing rather than planning.

Overall, the creation of the NHS did increase access to specialist services. The number of consultants rose from 5,316 in 1949 to 7,031 in 1959, although as late as 1962 nearly all the specialties were below the targets proposed in the 1948 circular. A higher proportion of the increased total was, moreover, in precisely those areas of medicine which had failed to attract specialists in the pre-NHS days: for example, anaesthetics and psychiatry. So, with qualifications, this can be seen as a success story for the NHS. However, it once again illustrates the way in which the initiative passed from the centre to the periphery during the 1950s: with central government reacting to demands coming from the medical profession and the peripheral health authorities, rather than shaping the pattern of the service being provided.

Professional influence and public power

In giving an account of the role of the medical profession in the NHS during the 1950s, it is possible to present two contradictory but entirely accurate conclusions. On the one hand, it is possible to demonstrate convincingly that the NHS exploited its position as a virtual monopoly employer of medical labour to depress the incomes of doctors. On the other hand, it is possible to show equally convincingly that the medical profession permeated the decision-making machinery of the NHS at every level and achieved an effective right of veto over the policy agenda.

'The unnerving discovery every Minister of Health makes at or near the outset of his term of office is that the only subject he is ever destined to discuss with the medical profession is money', wrote Enoch Powell, in his reflections on his own period in office.[36] Indeed the politicisation of conflict over money is inherent in the nature of the NHS. Given that the NHS has a virtual monopoly of employment of medical manpower, there is no independent market for determining the appropriate income for doctors. The Ministry of Health not only determines the demand for medical manpower but also the supply (through its decisions about the appropriate number of medical school places). It is therefore not surprising that the 1950s – like subsequent decades – were marked by a series of conflicts over pay between the medical profession and the Ministry of Health, and a succession of attempts to devise a neutral machinery of arbitration. Thus the first decade of the NHS was punctuated both by regular confrontations between the medical profession and the NHS over pay and by equally regular references to neutral arbitrators. In the 1940s, the Spens Committee sought to establish a pattern of pay derived from the pre-war incomes of doctors. In 1951, Mr Justice Danckwerts adjudicated on the vexed question of how to adjust the Spens recommendations in the light of the changing value of money. In 1957, a Royal Commission on Doctors' and Dentists' Remuneration[37] was set up to examine levels of remuneration and to examine ways of regularly reviewing pay.

The report of the Royal Commission is significant for the evidence it provides of how the medical profession had fared financially during the first decade of the NHS. In the event, the Royal Commission tended to substantiate the grievances of the doctors. 'At the time of our appointment current earnings of doctors and dentists were too low', the Commission concluded. Further, it pointed out, medical salaries had continued to fall behind earnings in comparable professional occupations. General practitioners had done particularly badly. Between 1950 and 1959, the average person in Britain had become almost 20 per cent better off in real terms, while the average general practitioner had become about 20 per cent worse off. The Royal Commission not only recommended all-round increases. It also recommended the creation of a permanent review body which would regularly inquire into medical pay, mainly though not exclusively using the comparability criterion to ensure that doctors kept in line with men and women in other professions (such as accountancy and the law) where there was no government monopoly of employment.

If the power of any interest group is to be measured by its ability to secure resources for its own members, the medical profession must thus be rated as a failure in the 1950s. If the doctors saw themselves as the exploited victims of the NHS system, they were largely right. Moreover, in this respect, they did no better – or worse – than other employees of the NHS. For example, the salaries of health service administrators also fell, in real terms, by something like 20 per cent during the 1950s.[38] What this would suggest is that the power of the medical profession is in an inverse relationship to the size of the stage on which a specific health care issue is fought out. When the stage widens to bring on actors who normally play no part in the health care arena strictly defined – when the Treasury and the Cabinet become involved – then the ability of the medical profession to get its own way diminishes.[39] Once the issue is defined as that of financial control – when it is seen, in other words, as an issue revolving round national economic strategy rather than health care considerations – the medical profession simply becomes a small battalion facing heavyweight armies. Conversely, the medical profession's influence expands as the stage narrows: becoming in effect total when health care reaches the stage of a duet between doctor and patient.

The point can be illustrated by the instance of general practitioner pay. This, in the 1950s, was based on the 'pool' system. That is, a given amount of money was set aside as the pool from which all payments would be made to general practitioners: in effect, very much the same kind of 'capped' budget which was introduced for hospital authorities. The Ministry of Health's main concern thus was to contain the total size of the pool; an endeavour in which it was remarkably successful, as the earnings figures already cited indicate. However, once control over the total had been established, the Ministry was quite prepared to make concessions to the BMA about the detailed way in which capitation fees and other elements were calculated. Here the story is that of a series of concessions to the doctors.

In discussing the role, influence and power of the medical profession (or indeed of any other professional body or interest group), it is thus crucial to specify the limits of the arena in which the question is being asked. If one is prepared to draw those limits tightly enough – to put the spotlight on an area of concern so small as to be of interest only to a particular profession or interest group – then it is easy enough to conclude that the power of that profession or interest group is dominant. Thus if one were to study NHS policy on methods for making beds, then inevitably the conclusion would follow that the power of the nursing profession is absolute. What distinguished the medical profession in the 1950s, however, was the extent to which it permeated the institutional decision-making machinery of the NHS as a whole. Once an issue had been defined as belonging to the health care arena (as distinct from the wider political stage), it was the doctor who represented the voice of expertise. In the mid-1950s, the Guillebaud Committee noted, the medical membership of RHBs averaged 32 per cent: in one case it reached 42 per cent. In the case of HMCs, the proportion tended to be somewhere between 20 and 27 per cent. Similarly, the Executive Committees – responsible for general practice, among other services – had a statutory minimum of four medical representatives out of a total membership of between 20 and 40.

The Guillebaud Committee saw no objection in principle to medical membership, although it thought that the total should not go above 25 per cent. The inclusion of doctors, it argued, provided 'invaluable advice to the lay members on medical aspects of hospital management'. Of course, this is to beg the question of how to define the 'medical aspects'. Indeed it is tempting to argue that the real political battle in the health care arena is precisely a definitional one: whether or not specific problems or issues should be labelled as being essentially 'medical' in nature, and as such taboo for the non-expert. Clearly, the institutionalised medical voice within the NHS provided doctors with an opportunity to medicalise management: to define issues in terms which would ensure that they would represent legitimate, expert authority. In addition, NHS bodies were festooned with medical advisory committees, placed at every tier of the management structure.

In summary, then, the power of the medical profession – if one may be allowed to use that slippery concept – rested on two pillars in the 1950s. First, there was its ability to determine which issues were or were not put on the agenda for action: certain policy options, as we saw in the previous section, were ruled out of court because the political costs of confronting the medical profession were judged to be excessive. Second, the medical profession to a large extent succeeded in defining certain areas as out of bounds to non-professionals: its power lay, as it were, in shaping the perceptions of policy problems – of incorporating a professional bias into the assumptive worlds of the policy-makers. While it did not dominate the NHS in terms of getting what it wanted in a positive sense, it did succeed in asserting its right of veto in specific policy spheres. Above all, the medical profession had made sure that governments, whatever their ideology or ambitions, would think long and hard before seeking to change the structure of the NHS in any way which would bring the underlying concordat with the medical profession into question: from being the main opponents of the NHS, the doctors had in effect become the strongest force for the status quo.

Agenda for the future

The 1950s bequeathed a long agenda for action to the next generation of NHS policy-makers. Some of the unresolved issues have been discussed in the preceding pages. Others, however, were also clamouring for attention. Above all, there were the problems of co-ordination stemming from the division of responsibility between the hospital, the general practitioner and the local authority services. Britain, as yet, only had a national hospital service. Could this be translated into a national health service? The question perturbed the Guillebaud Committee which decided, however, that stability must come first: the shock of creation had not yet worn off, and it was premature to think of any radical reorganisation. Equally, the question perturbed nearly everyone who considered the practical problems of the NHS: the Central Health Services Council – charged with producing reports on general policy issues – gave much thought to the obstacles to co-operation between the hospital, local authority and practitioner services.[40]

The triumph of the 1950s was to make the NHS work: but the price paid for creating a consensus – for putting the emphasis on achieving financial respectability, administrative stability and professional acceptability – was to introduce a bias towards inertia. The first decade of the NHS may not have solved the policy dilemmas inherent in the creation of the NHS, discussed in the previous chapter. But it made them tolerable; furthermore, it created a powerful constituency for the status quo. Thus, ironically, one of the measures of the success of the first generation of NHS policy-makers was the difficulty faced by their successors in creating a new consensus and mobilising a new coalition for change, as the politics of consolidation gave way to the politics of movement: the theme of the next chapter.

References

1. *Hansard*, House of Commons 5th series, vol. 529, 30 July 1958.
2. Iain Macleod *et al.*, *The Future of the Welfare State*, Conservative Political Centre: London 1958.
3. The data about public and medical opinion are taken from surveys conducted by Gallup Polls. I am grateful to Gallup Polls for allowing me access to their archives.
4. Harry Eckstein, *Pressure Group Politics*, Allen & Unwin: London 1960.
5. For a discussion of corporate bias in the British system of government, see Keith Middlemas, *Politics in Industrial Society*, André Deutsch: London 1979.
6. Public Records Office, CAB 129/131, The National Health Service: Memorandum by the Minister of Health, 13 Dec. 1948.
7. Quoted in Philip M Williams, *Hugh Gaitskell*, Jonathan Cape: London 1979. For accounts of the battle between Bevan and Gaitskell over charges from the point of view of the two protagonists, see this and Michael Foot, *Aneurin Bevan, 1945–1960*, Davis-Poynter: London 1973.
8. Public Records Office, CAB 134/518, Cabinet Committee on the National Health Service: Composition and Terms of Reference, Note by the Prime Minister, 22 April 1950.

9. Committee of Enquiry into the Cost of the National Health Service, *Report*, HMSO: London 1956, Cmnd. 663. The statistical work, on which the Committee based their conclusions, was carried out by B Abel-Smith and RM Titmuss; see their *The Cost of the National Health Service in England and Wales*, Cambridge UP 1956.
10. Public Records Office, CAB 129/38, National Health Service: Control of Expenditure. Memorandum by the Minister of Health, 10 March 1950.
11. Public Records Office, CAB 128/17, p. 104.
12. All historical statistics about NHS expenditure and income are drawn from Tables E6 to E11 in: Royal Commission on the National Health Service, *Report*, HMSO: London 1979, Cmnd. 7615. Being on a constant price basis (at 1970 prices) these are not directly comparable with figures of actual spending – as given, for example, in the Guillebaud Committee.
13. Public Records Office, CAB 129/39, National Health Service: Memorandum by the Minister of Health, 30 March 1950.
14. For comparative statistics of public expenditure on different programmes, see Rudolf Klein, 'The Politics of Public Expenditure: American Theory and British Practice', *British Journal of Political Science*, Oct. 1976, pp. 401–3.
15. For the record, the Ministers were: H Marquand (Jan.–Oct. 1951); H Crookshank (Oct. 1951–May 1952); I Macleod (May 1952–Dec. 1955); R Turton (Dec. 1955–Jan. 1957); D Vosper (Jan. 1957–Sept. 1957); D Walker-Smith (Sept. 1957–July 1960).
16. This account of Macleod's ministerial career is drawn from: Nigel Fisher, *Iain Macleod*, André Deutsch: London 1973.
17. Maurice Kogan, 'Social Services: Their Whitehall Status', *New Society*, 21 August 1969.
18. Alec Spoor, *White-collar Union: 60 Years of NALGO*. Cox & Wyman: London 1967.
19. Eckstein, op. cit.
20. Sir George Godber, 'Decision-making System and Structure in the British National Health Service', *Hospital Progress*, vol. 57, no. 3, 1976.
21. Sir George Godber, *The Health Service: Past, Present and Future*, Athlone Press: London 1975.
22. Christopher Ham, *Policy-making in the National Health Service*, Macmillan: London 1981.
23. Rudolf Klein, 'Costs and Benefits of Complexity: the British National Health Service' in Richard Rose (ed.), *Challenge to Governance*, SAGE Research Series in European Politics vol. 1, Sage: London April 1980.
24. I am grateful to Dr Renuka Rajkumar for carrying out this laborious analysis.
25. By far the best study of administration in the NHS in the 1950s is the Acton Society Trust study of *Hospitals and the State*, London 1955. In what follows I draw heavily on this.
26. Public Records Office, MH 90/54, Chairmen of Regional Hospital Boards: Note of Meeting held on 16 March 1948 at the Ministry of Health.
27. Public Records Office, CAB 134/518, Cabinet Committee on the National Health Service: Enquiry into the Financial Working of the Service – Report by Sir Cyril Jones. The comments by Bevan, quoted subsequently, form an introduction to this report.
28. For a description of the system of budgeting, see Ministry of Health, *Report for the Year Ending December 1952*, HMSO: London 1953, Cmnd. 8933.
29. Ibid.
30. For a recent analysis of alternative styles of policy-making, see CE Lindblom and DK Cohen, *Usable Knowledge*, Yale UP: New Haven, Conn. 1979.
31. JAG Griffith, *Central Departments and Local Authorities*, Allen & Unwin: London 1966.
32. Ministry of Health, op. cit.
33. The discussion of medical manpower draws on Rosemary Stevens, *Medical Practice in Modern England*, Yale UP: New Haven 1966. The discussion of consultant policy also draws on this invaluable source.

34. The circular in question was RHB (48)1; its author was the future Chief Medical Officer, Sir George Godber.
35. Sir George Godber, *Change in Medicine*, Nuffield Provincial Hospitals Trust: London 1975.
36. J Enoch Powell, *Medicine and Politics*, Pitman Medical: London 1966.
37. Royal Commission on Doctors' and Dentists' Remuneration, *Report*, HMSO: London 1960, Cmnd. 939.
38. Spoor, op. cit.
39. This conclusion reflects the argument of Eckstein, op. cit.
40. Central Health Services Council, *Report on Co-operation Between Hospital, Local Authority and General Practitioner Service*, HMSO: London 1952.

Chapter 3

The politics of technocratic change

If the first decade of the NHS was the period of consolidation, the next decade and a half was a period of innovation. The financial sinner had done penitence; the years of sackcloth and ashes were over, and a new era of expansion began. The politics of administering the status quo gave way to the politics of technocratic change. At long last the paternalistic rationalisers – those who, in the years before 1946, had seen the creation of a national health service as an opportunity to apply expert knowledge to dealing with need in a planned and systematic way – came into their own.

The shift in perceptions, style and policies was both made possible and constrained by political consensus. The NHS emerged from its first decade, as noted in the previous chapter, as a national monument. Both the main political parties were in agreement about its underlying philosophy and basic structure: an agreement that only started to get frayed towards the end of the 1970s. Over-arching consensus about essentials did not, of course, rule out political skirmishes about specific issues. The Labour Party regularly raised the issue of medical charges in election campaigns rather like a mediaeval army carrying the embalmed body of a saint into battle; there were, as we shall see, other areas of disagreement. But given the continuing evidence of the popularity of the NHS – confirmed by every public opinion poll – there was no incentive to challenge the prevailing consensus. On the contrary, the NHS provides a case study of the politics of competition, as against the politics of confrontation: with both the main parties competing to establish their claim to be considered the NHS's best friend. In 1959, for example, the Conservative Party manifesto promised a 'big pro-gramme of hospital building', the development of local authority health and welfare services and a major programme to promote good health: 'We shall not only clear the slums, but also wage war on smog . . . and tackle the pollution of rivers and estuaries.' The Labour manifesto countered by pointing out that 'the Tories have completed only one new hospital', and promising that 'as a minimum we shall spend £50 million a year on hospital development'. In addition, it pledged itself to creating an occupational health service, to developing the family doctor service 'and to safeguarding the health, welfare and safety of people employed in shops and offices'. Finally, it promised to abolish all charges.[1]

In 1964, again, the language was that of rival salesmen. The Conservatives proclaimed that their hospital plan would ensure that 'every man, woman and child in the country has access to the best treatment'. It pointed out that: 'We aim to build or rebuild 300 hospitals of which over 80 are already in progress.' Community services would expand: the 'crucial work of the family doctor' would be encouraged; the law controlling the safety and quality of drugs would be improved and: 'We shall also continue our campaign against the enemies of good health, by eliminating slum environments, reducing air pollution and cleaning the rivers and beaches.' Conversely, the Labour manifesto claimed that the NHS 'has been starved of resources', and promised to remedy this situation. The 'inadequate' Tory hospital-building programme would be reviewed and given the necessary finance. The number of qualified medical staff would be greatly increased, more resources would be devoted to research and a 'new impetus' would be given to the development of community care services. It also, of course, promised 'to restore as rapidly as possible a free Health Service'. Charges apart, there is no sign here of political disagreement about policy aims: only about which party would provide the appropriate level of financial resources.

When party politics end, administrative technology comes into its own. If it is possible to characterise the health care policy arena from about 1960 to 1975 (the dates are to an extent arbitrary) as being about the politics of technocratic change, it is because the debate was about instruments rather than ideologies, about means rather than about ends. Consensus in the era of non-growth had meant making the best of the status quo. Consensus in an era of growth meant an opportunity to develop new policy tools and organisational formulas: to let the experts loose on the problems that had had to be put into cold storage during the lean years. However, consensus also imposed constraints. It meant that new policy tools and organisational fixes had to be developed in such a way as not to threaten the implicit concordat – particularly with the medical profession – that underlay the creation of the NHS. It set a boundary to the concepts of the feasible used by policy-makers: it strictly defined the limits of the possible within which change could be considered. To have crossed these boundaries, to have broken through the limits, would have risked the re-politicisation of health, and that no party wanted.

There is yet a further reason why the 1960s and the first half of the 1970s can be interpreted as the heyday of technocratic politics in the NHS. It is the emphasis on efficiency and rationality in the use of resources which marked this period. A concern about efficiency was not, of course, unique to this period. There were efficiency drives in the early 1950s, just as there were efficiency campaigns in the late 1970s. But what marks out the period in between is the development of an ideology of efficiency: the idea that policy should be directed towards squeezing the greatest possible output of health care – that elusive concept – out of an inevitably limited input of resources. Already in 1959 the Ministry of Health had set up an Advisory Committee for Management Efficiency; expenditure on 'hospital efficiency studies' rose from £18,000 in 1963–64 to £250,000 in 1966–67.[2] Economists, who did not exist as far as the Ministry of Health was concerned in the 1950s, had by the 1970s established themselves in the department as the twentieth-century equivalents of the domestic chaplains – keepers of the faith of efficiency. The translation of this ideology into practice was slow, halting and incomplete, as we shall see, but the permeation of its concepts and vocabulary into the policy debate helped to shape both the way in which problems were defined and the solutions that were considered.

In all this, the arena of health care policy accurately reflected changes in the wider political environment. The emphasis on achieving greater efficiency and rationality through planning – through the use of new techniques of government – was common to both main political parties: not for the first time did the search for national efficiency spill over into the sphere of social policy.[3] Harold Macmillan, the Conservative Prime Minister from 1957 to 1964, had earlier in his career written a book expounding the case for 'economic efficiency and rational social organisation': an aim which was to be achieved by having more planning and less competition.[4] In the early 1960s, his Chancellor of the Exchequer set up the National Economic Development Council, which introduced indicative planning to Britain.[5] In 1965, the Labour Government of Harold Wilson, which had taken office the previous year, published its National Plan[6] based on the assumptions not only that economic growth could be planned but also that planning would in turn promote growth. In 1970 one of the first actions of the Conservative administration of Edward Heath was to publish a White Paper on the reorganisation of central government:[7] the aim was to improve the 'efficiency of government', in part by strengthening the analytic capacity of the administrative machine.

New techniques of government were developed. A new machinery for controlling public expenditure – the Public Expenditure Survey Committee (PESC) system – was set up in 1961.[8] Its origins lay in the Plowden report,[9] published in the same year, which can be read as the manifesto of technocratic rationalism in government. The aim of public expenditure control, the Plowden report argued, should be to achieve stable long-term planning: 'chopping and changing in Government expenditure policy is frustrating to efficiency and economy.' There would have to be greater emphasis on the 'wider application of mathematical techniques, statistics and accountancy': for example, the Plowden report pointed out, such techniques might permit 'improvements in the method of making allocations of funds between the Regional Hospital Boards'. In turn, such a system could lead to more explicit choices and debate about priorities.

Three aspects of this new administrative rationalism, shared by both civil servants and politicians, should be noted. First, there was the faith in techniques: such as cost-benefit analysis, PPB (Planning, Programming, Budgeting) and PAR (Programme Analysis Review). Second, there was the belief that to change organisations could improve policy outputs: the 1960s saw a succession of committees charged with the reform of the civil service and local government. Third, organisational reform was largely seen in terms of giving a greater role to expertise. For example, the 1968 report of the Fulton Committee on the Civil Service[10] was much concerned with devising ways of producing a more professional corps of administrators – more managerial, more numerate and more specialised than the traditional generalist. Similarly, the 1969 report of the Redcliffe-Maud Royal Commission on Local Government was preoccupied with the problem of devising authorities large enough to employ a 'wide variety of qualified staff'.[11] All three themes – the emphasis on techniques, on organisational fixes and on creating a machinery of administration designed to give scope to experts – find an echo in the health care policy arena.

Putting a date on the introduction of this new ideology of rationality is, of course, essentially arbitrary. The start of a more expansionist and interventionist era certainly precedes 1960: perhaps the most significant symbolic event in the evolution of government policy was Macmillan's decision in 1957 to allow his Chancellor of the Exchequer to resign rather than to cut public expenditure. In the health care policy arena, 1960 can sensibly be taken as the beginning of a new era. In that year, both the political and the administrative direction of the Ministry changed. The new Minister was Enoch Powell; the new Permanent Secretary was Sir Bruce Fraser; and the new Chief Medical Officer was Sir George

Godber. Quite apart from their individual qualities, the appointment of these three was important for what they represented. The arrival of Enoch Powell marked the end of the Ministry of Health as a political backwater. Idiosyncratic, and destined to end in the political wilderness, he could not however be described as a political lightweight. His immediate successor was a future Conservative Chancellor of the Exchequer, Anthony Barber; while the amalgamation of the Ministries of Health and National Insurance into the new conglomerate Department of Health and Social Security in 1968 ensured Cabinet status for the office holder. The appointment of Sir Bruce Fraser meant that the Ministry was no longer headed by an administrator scarred by the experience of setting up the NHS. Fraser's appointment not only gave the Ministry of Health a stronger voice within Whitehall – he had previously been Third Secretary at the Treasury – it also brought into the Ministry some of the notions about long-term expenditure planning that, as already noted, were stirring within the Treasury and were embodied in the PESC system. Lastly, the promotion of Sir George Godber brought to the top of the medical hierarchy within the Ministry someone strongly committed to the ideas that had originally inspired the creation of the NHS. A radical egalitarian, the author of the 1948 plan for a rational, uniform distribution of medical specialists, he had never lost sight of Bevan's hope of universalising the best.

So the 1960s open with new men in the arena of health care policy acting in a new political environment: an essentially optimistic and expansionary environment, strong in the conviction that government action could promote economic growth. In the sections that follow, we shall examine the confrontation between new attitudes and old problems in specific policy areas. But first, as essential background to understanding the way in which individual policy issues were defined and addressed, we shall explore the apparent paradox of a growing awareness of scarcity of resources in a period of expansion.

Growing scarcity in an era of growth

The 15 years from 1960 to the mid-1970s were a period of rapid growth in public expenditure.[12] While for most of the 1950s, public spending had only slowly crept up, from 1960 onward the growth rate accelerated: a trend maintained under both Labour and Conservative governments. The NHS was one of the main beneficiaries of this trend. Between 1950 and 1958, its current budget increased by only 12.8 per cent in volume terms – that is, the input of real resources. But between 1958 and 1968, the equivalent increase was over 26 per cent. Between 1968 and 1978, the rise was almost as large again.[13] Moreover, expenditure on the NHS increased throughout these two decades proportionately faster than the growth in the national income: the NHS's share of the Gross Domestic Product rose from 3.5 to 5.6 per cent. Significantly, the growth rate of the NHS budget was not related to the political complexion of the government. Indeed, contrary to what might perhaps be expected, the NHS budget grew fastest under the 1970–74 Conservative administration; in contrast, the growth rate was marginally slower under the 1964–70 Labour Government, compelled by economic crisis to renege on its commitment to accelerate the growth of the Welfare State.

So why did increasing affluence lead to an ever more emphatic realisation of the inadequacy of the available resources and to an ever greater stress on efficiency? To answer this question it is necessary to identify the pressures and constraints faced by policy-makers during this period. Not all of them were by any means unique to this period; on the contrary, many of them simply represented a more explicit recognition of problems that had always been implicit in the structure of the NHS. In examining the debates of the 1960s and 1970s we shall often catch echoes of issues already discussed in the previous chapter. But even if many of the problems and dilemmas were in no sense novel, there is a new sharpness in the way they were perceived: they had reached the stage of what – to adapt Stendhal[14] – might be called *crystallisation* in the policy process.

One elegant explanation for the apparent paradox of financial stringency in a period of expansion was provided by Enoch Powell in his reflections on his period of office as Minister of Health, already quoted in the previous chapter:[15]

> There is virtually no limit to the amount of medical care an individual is capable of absorbing. [Further,] not only is the range of treatable conditions huge and rapidly growing. There is also a vast range of quality in the treatment of these conditions. . . . There is hardly a type of condition from the most trivial to the gravest which is not susceptible of alternative treatments under conditions affording a wide range of skill, care, comfort, privacy, efficiency, and so on. [Finally,] there is the multiplier effect of successful medical treatment. Improvement in expectation of survival results in lives that demand further medical care. The poorer (medically speaking) the quality of the lives preserved by advancing medical science, the more intense are the demands they continue to make. In short, the appetite for medical treatment *vient en mangeant*.

New advances in medical science, or drug therapy, might help to eradicate some diseases. In the late 1940s and early 1950s, tuberculosis was a case in point – though the relative contribution of drug therapy and improved social conditions is disputed.[16] In the 1960s, developments in drug therapy would raise the prospect that mental hospitals could be closed down: a hope which, however, took long to fulfill. But new techniques were creating new demands. In the 1960s, for example, there was the development of renal dialysis. In the 1970s, there was the development of hip replacement surgery. Both advances in technology were self-evidently socially desirable: renal dialysis saved lives, while hip replacement surgery made life much more tolerable for those otherwise crippled by arthritic conditions. Nevertheless, they helped to reinforce the sense of the NHS at the mercy of the technological imperative: driven by forces over which it had no control – though we shall examine below some of the attempts to contain the demands generated by the extension of the realm of the possible in medical intervention.

Then, again, there was the ageing population. In 1951 there were just under seven million men and women over the retirement age. In 1961 the equivalent figure was 7,700,000. In 1971 it had topped nine million. Moreover, within these rising totals, the proportion of over-75s was also increasing: precisely those people most likely to require health care. To the technological push, there had to be added the demographic pull. Simply coping with the changing population structure, it was reckoned, would require an extra one per cent annual increment in health spending. No wonder, then, that there was growing concern with efficiency: not only in the use of resources by the NHS, but in the way the health service was organised – given that the care of the elderly, in particular, spanned the hospital, general practitioner and local welfare services.

Lastly, although it makes sense to talk about the closed arena of health politics during the period covered by this chapter, the characteristics of the actors involved were changing. In the 1950s, as previously noted, the medical profession and other NHS employees did relatively badly in terms of income compared to the rest of the population. In the 1960s and 1970s, this began to change. One set of statistics tells the story: that of the relative price effect, which measures movements in the costs of inputs to the NHS (mainly wages and salaries) compared to movements in costs in the economy as a whole. In the 1950s, the relative price effect was negative: the NHS was buying its inputs of manpower more cheaply than other employers. Thus between 1950 and 1958, as we have seen, the volume of inputs into the NHS went up by 12.8 per cent. But the cost of those inputs went up by only 2.9 per cent. Between 1958 and 1968, however, the reverse was true. The cost of inputs rose faster than their volume: that is, the relative price effect turned against the NHS – a trend which was to continue in the 1970s.

In turn, this reflects a new mood of militancy among those working in the NHS. Denied the opportunity to exit from a service with a near-monopoly of employment for health care professionals, they engaged in voice[17] in the NHS, i.e. the politics of protest. In the case of the medical profession, as we shall see, there was increased conflict *among* doctors: general practitioners challenged the differentials between themselves and consultants, junior hospital doctors challenged the differentials between themselves and consultants, while in turn consultants rebelled against the erosion of the differentials between themselves and the rest of the profession. The established professional bodies – notably the BMA – faced increasing competition from rival groups; so undermining still further the notion of the medical profession as a monolithic entity, as it splintered into different and opposed interest groups. Others working in the NHS – organised in both professional bodies and trade unions – also became assertive. From being an oasis of industrial peace, the NHS became relatively dispute-prone. While in 1966 only two stoppages were recorded in the NHS (and an average of 0.69 days lost per 1,000 staff, as against the national figure of 100 days lost per 1,000 employees), in 1973, 18 stoppages were notched up as a result of a national strike by ancillary workers (and an average of 117.8 days lost as against a national figure of 1,104 days lost).[18] So increasingly, in the period in question, the NHS can be conceived of as a machine for generating demands, not only for more resources but also for higher rewards for the service producers.

Moreover, awareness of the perverse financial incentives built into the very conception of the NHS became sharper during the 1960s. Again, this was already implicit in the very early days of the NHS.[19] However, the 1960s are marked by the development of an intellectual debate which made these issues explicit and gradually introduced them into the language of politics. In particular the debate sharply defined the issue: was the problem one of constraining the demands made by consumers of health care or of restraining the demand generated by the producers of health care? Depending on the definition of the problem, different solutions would follow. On the one hand, the theorists of the private market argued that individuals as consumers of health services would always demand more services privately than they would supply publicly as taxpayers.[20] Given a free service with no price constraints, it was argued, there was every incentive for consumers to make unlimited demands: it was irrational to restrain demands. Yet equally, as taxpayers, they had every incentive to minimise their contribution. The solution therefore was to invoke the price mechanism: to move from State finance to private finance. On the other hand, however, it could be argued that consumer demand in effect controls itself. Even if consumers did not pay cash for medical attention, they incurred time-costs: rationing through queueing in the surgery and the waiting list. It was the producers – the doctors – who generated demands: indirectly by shaping the expectations of consumers, directly by their decisions as to what resources to apply to the treatment of any given patient.[21] From this perspective, the dilemma of policy was not how to restrain consumer demands through the price mechanism but how to reconcile the professional imperative of doctors to maximise the treatment given to any one patient with the need to maximise the health of the population at large: between an absolutist ethic of treatment and a utilitarian approach to resource use.[22] Given an absolutist ethic, it followed that every patient had to be given the best possible treatment: that the limits of treatment should be defined not by resource availability but by the current state of medical knowledge. Given a utilitarian approach, it followed that the criteria for treatment should be determined by the need to maximise the health of the population, not by the need to do everything possible for the individual patient. Indeed, following this line of reasoning, it might well be appropriate for patients to get less than optimal treatment as defined by the medical profession.

Growing awareness of the implications of financial stringency thus brought out into the open a conflict between the two main sets of actors in the health care policy arena: a conflict reflecting different values and perceptions of the aims of a health service. This was the conflict between the professional providers and the paternalistic rationalisers: between the medical profession and the policy nexus of Ministers and civil servants. Oversimplifying, the conflict was between those who saw the aim of the health service as being to provide doctors with sufficient resources to pursue the professional imperative of maximising treatment for the individual patient and those who saw the aim of the health service as being to distribute inevitably scarce funds in such a way as to reconcile the competing claims of different groups for resources. 'The doctor is primarily involved with the individual, the politician inevitably predominantly with groups of individuals', wrote Dr David Owen, a Minister of Health in the 1970s.[23]

If the underlying conflict could not be wished away, could it be eased by devising ways of raising more money for the NHS? Not surprisingly, this question came increasingly to be debated in the 1960s and 1970s. Predictably, given our analysis, the medical profession became increasingly vociferous in its demands for expanding the NHS budget. In 1967, a leading medical figure wrote:[24]

> It is the clear duty of the medical profession to present to Government and public the grim and sober truth, that without a vast increase in national expenditure on the hospitals, here and now – and far beyond anything so far envisaged even on paper and for an indefinitely receding future – they will progressively run down, and the present inadequate service will shortly give place to one that is frankly third-rate.

The same year the BMA set up a panel to look into the finances of the NHS which, in due course, came out in favour of an insurance-based system.[25]

Politicians were also preoccupied by the same question. In 1967 Douglas Houghton, Chairman of the Parliamentary Labour Party and previously the Cabinet Minister responsible for co-ordinating the social services, wrote: 'It can be contended that, judged from the standpoint of the quality and efficiency and adequacy of the services, we are now getting the worst of both worlds. The government cannot find the money out of taxation and the citizen is not allowed to pay it out of his own pocket.'[26] He proposed raising more revenue through charging. In 1969 Richard Crossman, by now Secretary of State for Social Services, gave an equally pessimistic diagnosis, not so very different from that made earlier by Enoch Powell:

> The pressure of demography, the pressure of technology, the pressure of democratic equalisation, will always together be sufficient to make the standard of social services regarded as essential to a civilised community far more expensive than that community can afford. It is a complete delusion to believe that if we had no further balance of payments difficulties social service Ministers would be able to relax and assume that a kindly Chancellor will let each one of them have all the money he wants to expand his service. The trouble is that there is no foreseeable limit on the social services which the nation can reasonably require except the limit that the Government imposes.[27]

In contrast to Houghton, Crossman rejected the policy option of charging more. In part this may have reflected his awareness of the political sensitivity of the issue: a sensitivity sharpened by the experience of the Labour Government, which had abolished prescription charges on coming into office in 1964, only to reintroduce them four years later when economic crisis compelled the Cabinet to choose between cutting NHS spending and finding new sources of income. 'The party meeting on prescription charges was the worst we have ever had', Crossman recorded in his diary.[28] Moreover, the decision to give automatic exemption from charges to broad categories of the population – like the elderly and the young – meant that, while it made them somewhat more acceptable to the Labour Party, their yield would be correspondingly low: in the outcome, 60 per cent of all prescriptions were free. Again, Crossman – like Bevan before him, and like his Conservative successor, Sir Keith Joseph – asked his officials to calculate the likely income from a boarding charge to hospital patients, but decided that the administrative and political hassle would outweigh the financial gains. Instead, he argued for greater reliance on the NHS element in the national insurance contributions.

Three aspects of this debate should be noted. First, the debate about the problems of NHS finance did not split neatly into party patterns: Labour and Conservative Ministers were agreed about the nature of the dilemma, although there was some disagreement about possible solutions. Second, debate did not lead to action. In 1964 the incoming Labour Government halved the income from charges: it fell from 5.4 per cent of the total NHS budget in 1963–64 to 2.3 per cent in 1967–68, to rise to 3.5 per cent by the end of the Labour administration's term of office. And it remained at virtually that figure throughout the Conservative administration, from 1970 to 1974. The Labour Government was prevented by economic constraints from carrying out its manifesto pledge of abolishing charges; and the Conservative Government was inhibited by problems of administration from following through its bias towards introducing more charges. Both parties were, moreover, too committed to the principle of the NHS to consider any root and branch reforms: not only conflict but policy options were constrained by consensus. Lastly, the growing acceptance by Ministers that demands would always, and inevitably, outrun resources made explicit their rationing role: the fact that central government would inescapably have to make choices between competing priorities. Once again, it is important to stress that this was not a new discovery. But in the 1960s and 1970s, the issue acquired a new salience, helping to shape the way in which specific policy problems were perceived. It is to some of these specific policy problems that we now turn.

Planning and rationing

In 1962 the Minister of Health, Enoch Powell, published a Hospital Plan for England and Wales.[29] It was the first attempt since the creation of the NHS to take a 'comprehensive view of the hospital service': to devise a national plan designed to bring about a distribution of hospital beds based not on the haphazard inherited pattern but on centrally determined criteria for matching resources to needs. Over the next decade, the Hospital Plan envisaged, work would start on building 90 new hospitals and substantially remodelling 134 existing hospitals. The total costs would be, the Plan estimated, £500 million: over three times as much as had been spent in the previous decade and a half. National norms for the appropriate number of beds for each locality were laid down: 3.3 acute beds per 1,000 population. A national pattern of hospitals would be created: District General Hospitals of 600 to 800 beds, each serving a population of 100,000 to 150,000 people. All the required medical expertise would be concentrated in these hospitals; in turn, many existing hospitals would be closed.

The production of the Hospital Plan can usefully be seen as the outcome of two trends. First, exogenous to the NHS, there were the changes in the political environment and administrative styles discussed earlier in this chapter. Second, endogenous to the NHS, there was the gradual creation of a consensus among professionals and others about the need to create a new hospital system. In 1956, as we have seen, the Guillebaud Committee drew attention to the inadequacy of the building programme. In 1959 a group of BMA consultants published a report advocating a 10-year hospital plan. A series of research studies and conferences was devoted to the subject of how many beds were needed, and just which specialties should be concentrated in the new District General Hospitals.

The Hospital Plan was thus the child of a marriage between professional aspirations and the new faith in planning: between what might be called medical expertise and administrative technology. It was designed to promote both efficiency and equity: to bring about uniform standards throughout the NHS. But, it is important to stress, the detailed recommendations of the Plan – the basic vision of what a hospital service should be like – were almost entirely determined by the medical consensus: to caricature only slightly, the vision was designed to maximise the quality of medical care being delivered. Within the Ministry the issue of determining norms and the pattern of hospitals was defined largely as a matter for the medical experts: 'a purely scientific thing, where you accept the advice of your medicos', as one of the administrators put it. There is no indication in the Hospital Plan of other possible criteria being considered, such as accessibility for patients or the effect of hospital size on staff morale or recruitment. The domination of the professional definition of the problem being tackled was all the greater for being implicit and unargued.

The point can be further illustrated by a report published in 1969 when a committee of the Central Health Services Council was asked to examine the functions of the District General Hospital (DGH) in the light of developments since the Hospital Plan.[30] Of the Committee's 18 members, under the lay chairmanship of Sir Desmond Bonham-Carter, 12 were doctors. Their main conclusion was that DGHs should be larger than envisaged in 1962. Again, the dominating criterion was the need to promote technical excellence. No consultant should ever have to work on his own; there should always be teams of two consultants, at the least, in each specialty. Similarly, the 'need for efficient organisation and staffing of supporting technical and other services' pointed in the direction of larger hospitals. So the conclusion drawn was that DGHs should serve populations of between 200,000 and 300,000, so virtually doubling the figure given in the Hospital Plan.

In the event, plans and visions were only partially fulfilled. The capital building programme of the NHS did expand rapidly after 1962: the annual rate of investment more than doubled over the next decade. But it remained vulnerable to the economic crises which punctuated these years: when Chancellors of the Exchequer insisted on cuts in public expenditure, Ministers of Health tended to accept cuts in their capital building programme in return for safeguarding their current budget. Moreover, the recommendations of the Bonham-Carter report were never accepted as official policy. The divergence between plans and achievement marks, in part, also a divergence between administrative and professional definitions of rationality, on the one hand, and political definitions of rationality, on the other. In terms of efficiency, nothing was more destructive than sudden changes in the capital investment programme: precisely the kind of 'chopping and changing' which the Plowden Committee had sought to prevent. Politically, however, cutting the capital programme was far more rational than cutting the current budget: the former meant exporting the loss of jobs into the private sector, while the latter would have meant a confrontation with the constituency of health service providers.

Similarly, politicians were more sensitive to the social costs of building large technological palaces. The argument was sharply put by Crossman:[31]

> The great case for the big hospital is first, that the expertise is gathered in one place so that all the specialists who could possibly be interested can be around the bed; and secondly, that size is now necessary for a rational use of expensive equipment. Perfectly true, perfectly true! Of course from the consultants' point of view these huge hospitals are right. But I ask myself about the social cost. . . . Nurses were often available for the small local hospital. But if you build a large hospital in the wrong place you won't draw the ladies from the six local small hospitals because they went there part-time from their villages. . . . There are all kinds of practical problems of social organisation which

seem to me to have been strangely neglected in the planning of the hospital programme.

Moreover, it was Ministers who carried the political costs of closing smaller hospitals made redundant by the development of the new DGHs. For it was Ministers who had to face the constituency protests from communities faced with the loss of their local hospitals.

The implementation of the hospital building programme presents a further puzzle. Why, 20 years after the publication of the Hospital Plan, was its vision of a country studded with modern hospitals still unfulfilled? Why did hospital building enjoy such low priority? For the politician, it might be assumed, there could be no better advertisement than a shining new hospital: a visible symbol of his or her commitment to improving the people's health. For the doctors, as already argued, new hospitals meant the opportunity to practise what the profession considered to be higher quality medicine. For the consumer, in turn, new hospitals surely meant better services with higher standards of treatment. It was Bevan who once remarked that he would rather survive in the stark impersonality of a new hospital than die in the cosy comfort of a cottage hospital. So here there would appear to be a congruence of interests which yet, in the event, was frustrated.

To explore the reasons for this seemingly perverse outcome is to illuminate also some of the special characteristics of the health care policy arena. Let us start with the politicians. If the arena of health care policy was depoliticised to a remarkable degree, one reason for this was that it offered remarkably little scope for the politician seen as a vote maximiser: *homo economicus* in the political market. Negative action, such as stopping the closure of a local hospital, might bring immediate political dividends. Positive action, except when it involved awarding higher pay to NHS employees, could rarely bring such political gains. From time to time, Ministers might announce special action to bring down waiting lists. But, over the decades, the number of people on the waiting lists hovered stubbornly around the 600,000 mark: improving the available services simply encouraged general practitioners to put more patients in the queue. The captain shouted his orders: the crew went on as before. Moreover, there was an inevitable time-lag between Ministerial intervention and outcomes: in effect, Ministers were working for the benefit of their successors. In the case of hospital building, there might be a delay of 10 years between sanctioning construction and completion. If we use a vote-maximising model to explain the behaviour of politicians, it is therefore not surprising that the NHS building programme should have received low priority.[32] However, to make this point may also suggest the limitations of such a model: to explain ministerial action – as distinct from ministerial inaction – we may have to see politicians as paternalistic rationalisers, seeking to maximise not votes but rather a certain vision of what the NHS ought to be.

Next, the medical profession did have a general commitment to, and self-interest in, building new hospitals. However, the organisations representing the medical profession, such as the BMA, had a specific and prior interest in maximising the incomes of their members. Indeed their survival as organisations depended on satisfying their members in this respect,[33] as indeed did that of other organisations – trade union and professional – representing NHS workers. They might well argue for greater public investment in the NHS: this, as we have seen, was precisely the strategy adopted by the BMA in the 1960s and it was further followed by the trade unions in the 1970s. Their immediate demands were for more money for their members. If it came to the choice between current and capital spending, then Cabinet decisions were probably an accurate reflection of the priorities of organised labour in the NHS (however much organised labour, unconstrained by the problems of revenue raising, might protest that there should be no need for such a choice).

Lastly, there were the consumers of health care. If these have so far not been discussed as actors in the health care policy arena, it is because for most of the period being discussed they were the ghosts in the NHS machinery: lacking any institutional representation until the creation of Community Health Councils in 1974 (see the concluding section of this chapter). The Regional Hospital Boards and Hospital Management Committees were agents of the Minister: they lacked all legitimacy as representatives of the local community – though some of their members were chosen after consultation with local interests. Even if they had seen their role in terms of aggregating and giving organised expression to local demands for new hospitals – which they did not – they could not have carried conviction. Indeed the history of the NHS is remarkable for the fact that not a single board or authority ever resigned en bloc in protest against inadequate funding – or, for that matter, was sacked by the Minister for incompetence. The RHBs and HMCs might lobby and nag Ministers, and they might well harness the support of their local MPs, but overt political action – in the sense of orchestrating a public campaign – was not part of the rules of the game. The NHS was designed, after all, as an organisation for controlling rather than articulating demands. If indeed there was overwhelming satisfaction with the NHS, this may have reflected the service's success in shaping public expectations rather than in being shaped by them.

The implementation of the Hospital Plan is significant from another perspective as well: that of the central–local relationship. On the face of it, the publication of the Plan might be seen as the assertion of central authority designed to bring about national standards throughout the country. In the event, however, it set the pattern for subsequent attempts in the 1970s to introduce national norms of provision: the two priority documents published in the mid-1970s (*see* Chapter 4). Its neat package of norms was subverted by the two principles, implicit in the debate about their implementation, that have haunted all attempts at national planning aimed at achieving uniformity. The first is what might be called the principle of infinite diversity: no two populations or communities are the same, no two consultants practise the same kind of medicine, and thus national norms inevitably have to be adapted to unique, local circumstances. But since no criteria are available to judge precisely how (or by what measures) local populations or consultants differ, we cannot know what divergences from national norms are acceptable or otherwise. The second is what might be called the principle of infinite indeterminacy: the future cannot be predicted, and we therefore cannot know how changes in the population structure, in the childbearing proclivities of families or in medical technology will affect the need for services. Consequently national norms had to be interpreted and adapted flexibly. Indeed national norms themselves had a disconcerting habit of changing, as more or fewer babies were born, as ideas about the number of beds required for any given population changed, as the emphasis switched from providing hospital care to enhancing community care.

Moreover it soon became apparent that the very notion of basing planning on bed norms was highly questionable. Providing beds was not, after all, the objective, only the means: the aim, presumably, was to provide services for patients. The services provided for any given population depended on the *way* in which beds were used – the numbers of medical and other staff, the technical facilities available, clinical decisions about the appropriate lengths of stay and so on – rather than on the *number* of beds available. While in theory nothing could be more concrete than norms based on bed numbers, in practice these turned out to be a somewhat metaphysical concept, as it became apparent that the relationship between means and aims was highly problematic and uncertain.

The two principles not only subverted the Plan, in the sense that what finally emerged was much less tidy than originally envisaged; they also subverted the formal relationship between the centre and the periphery. In theory, the central department could perfectly properly have instructed its agents – the RHBs and HMCs – to carry out its centrally determined plans. In practice, the command structure became a negotiated order.[34] The Department of Health and Social Security, as its civil servants told a Select Committee which inquired into the hospital building programme in 1969, simply did not know enough: 'It is not easy for us centrally . . . to form a judgment of the precise needs of each regional board.'[35] The department could 'advise', 'persuade' and 'discuss' to use the words of the civil servants giving evidence. It could dispatch the department's medical officers to the regions to discuss issues with the doctors there. But it would not dictate. If this ran counter to the constitutional fiction of Ministerial responsibility and authority, it accurately reflected the balance of knowledge in the NHS: to the extent that knowledge was defined to be experiential, judgemental and professional – too complex to be caught in crude statistics – so, inevitably, power lay at the periphery.

There remained the fact that the NHS was financed out of public money: that the Minister was accountable to Parliament for every penny spent. Hence the curious phenomenon, already noted in the 1950s, of a central government department which was often very latitudinarian on major policy issues but which behaved with nit-picking pedantry in matters of detail. If health authorities were permitted considerable freedom to interpret national plans for hospital provision or policy circulars,[36] they were given very much less freedom in interpreting departmental notes about the details of the buildings. If the DHSS could not plan a uniform national service, it is tempting to conclude from the chorus of complaints made by the RHBs to the 1969 Select Committee, it was certainly determined to impose a uniform pattern of cost control. The result was frustration at the periphery: complaints about excessive bureaucracy, about unnecessary delays while plans were repeatedly scrutinised at the centre and about the lack of expertise of a rapidly revolving cast of civil servants.

So the NHS, at the end of the 1960s, presented a spectacle of mutual frustration. The health authorities were frustrated by what they perceived to be excessive interference by central government. Yet central government Ministers felt frustrated by their inability to translate formal power into effective power. To quote Richard Crossman again, reflecting on his experience as Secretary of State at the DHSS:

> It was often said to me by Treasury officials when I was Minister, 'Of course we couldn't possibly put the Health Service under local

authorities because we wouldn't be able to control the expenditure'. And I always replied, 'But you don't control it today'. Because, of course, you don't have in the Regional Hospital Boards a number of obedient civil servants carrying out the central orders. . . . You have a number of powerful, semi-autonomous Boards whose relation to me was much more like the relations of a Persian satrap to a weak Persian Emperor. If the Emperor tried to enforce his authority too far he lost his throne or at least lost his resources or something broke down.[37]

In fact, of course, the Treasury was right: central government did control expenditure. But, similarly, Crossman was right: within the capped budgets allocated to them, the regions enjoyed a large degree of autonomy in the way they allocated their money and organised their services. To a large extent the 1974 reorganisation of the NHS – the subject of the last section of this chapter – can be seen as an attempt to devise a solution to the problem of mutual frustration.

The sense of frustrated bafflement felt by Ministers can be illustrated by the case of services for the mentally ill. From the start, everyone had agreed that these represented the slum of the NHS: as we saw in the previous chapter, Bevan in 1950 had warned his Cabinet colleagues about the likelihood of scandal breaking about poor conditions in mental hospitals. Almost every politician who succeeded Bevan as Minister of Health proclaimed the need to give priority to improving these services. Yet progress was painfully slow. There was indeed some progress: between 1948 and 1959, spending on psychiatric hospitals accounted for over a quarter of the total capital budget.[38] But achievement always lagged behind the targets set by central policy-makers: at the end of the 1960s the objectives set in the Hospital Plan and other public documents had not been met.[39] Much the same was true of other hospitals for the chronically ill, such as for the mentally handicapped. It was not surprising therefore that Crossman in 1969 seized the opportunity provided by a report revealing 'scandalous conditions' at one of these hospitals, Ely.[40] He insisted on publishing an uncensored version. He pressed the RHBs to divert funds into the chronic care sector. He exploited the chance to set up the Hospital Advisory Service (HAS): what was in all but name an inspectorate, reporting directly to the Secretary of State.[41]

The case of the services for the mentally ill, and other chronic care groups, demonstrated the limited ability of the centre to shape the pattern of services at the periphery. Equally important, it once more underlined the extent to which any organisation such as the NHS represents a pressure group for maintaining the inherited pattern. In terms of the medical profession's ladder of prestige, the specialties in the long-stay sector were at the bottom of the hierarchy – whether measured by the number of merit awards handed out or by the proportion of immigrant doctors working in them.[42] Moreover, weakness was self-reinforcing: given their lack of prestige, those working in these services were in no position to assert their claims to more resources effectively. Similarly, the consumers of these services were – by definition – those least able to articulate their demands. In contrast, the users of acute services were well placed to articulate their demands. There is thus no need to invoke a conspiracy theory of medical power to explain the strength of the constituency for the status quo in terms of the balance between the acute and the chronic sectors of the NHS. It was Crossman's Conservative successor, Sir Keith Joseph, who identified the alliance of indifference between the medical profession and the lay managers of the NHS. 'There has been no systematic demand for better standards either by the medical or lay elements', he pointed out.[43] Further, he argued, 'Doctors can be remarkably selective in choosing the ills they regard worthy of treatment. . . . No one can see better than doctors the needs of the public and the shortcomings of the service. I am not aware that there has been steady, powerful, informed medical pressure to remedy the real worst shortcomings.'

The challenge for Ministers who sought a change in this balance was therefore precisely how to create a political coalition for change: how to give more visibility to the problems of the chronic care sector and to enhance their political salience. Hence Crossman's decision to exploit scandal, despite the reluctance of some of his civil servants who were afraid of the effects on morale in the service. Hence, too, the decision to subsidise MIND (the National Association for Mental Health) – the pressure group concerned with improving conditions in mental health hospitals. This decision may seem perverse: why should Ministers use public money to finance an organisation whose aim was to embarrass them by pointing out shortcomings in the NHS? But the encouragement of this Quangig – quasi-non-governmental-interest-group – makes perfect sense once it is recognised that Ministers needed allies.

Given these problems, it is not surprising to find a move from planning towards rationing by the beginning of the 1970s: precisely the same trend evident in the case of planning for consultant manpower (*see* previous chapter). The norms of the Hospital Plan and other subsequent documents implied that there was a desirable package of provision for any given population. Further, it assumed that progress towards achieving equity in the geographical distribution of resources could best be achieved through a building programme. Both assumptions became increasingly frayed by experience. Given the principles of infinite diversity and infinite indeterminacy, were norms such a good idea? Given the stuttering progress of the capital building programme, could this be relied on as the instrument for bringing about equity?

Planning by norms was not abandoned until the 1980s (*see* Chapter 4); but it became diluted. The strategy chosen was to seek a formula for sharing out fairly the available revenue resources: essentially a rationing strategy in that, unlike the planning approach, it did not make any assumptions about the desirable *level* of provision but only about the equitable *share* of the resources to be made available to any given population. The first such attempt was made in 1970, when a new formula for allocating resources to the regions was introduced.[44] The aim of this was to achieve not equality but equity: allocations weighted by the needs of the population. Subsequently, in 1976, the distributional methodology was further refined: the formula produced by the Resource Allocation Working Party (RAWP) weighted the population primarily by age and mortality factors. Politically, the significance of this approach lay in that it gave public visibility to the existing distribution of resources: inequities which were even more glaring at the sub-regional level.[45] Some regions, notably the London ones, were clearly identified as being (relatively) over-provided. Other regions, such as Trent, were clearly identified as being (relatively) deprived. The development of new analytic methodologies thus gave new salience to the issue of distribution within the NHS: conceptually they solved the puzzle about which criteria should be used to decide who got what, but politically they intensified it.

For the future, the emphasis on greater rationality and equity in the distribution bequeathed two problems: to be discussed in subsequent chapters. First, the formulas might bring about equity in the distribution of resources. But would they bring about equity in access? Would similar bundles of resources in different areas actually mean that the populations served would get the same kind of service and have the same opportunities for treatment? Second, the formulas assumed that progress towards achieving equity could be made painlessly by a process of differential growth: the relatively under-provided regions would simply have a more rapid annual increment of growth than the relatively over-provided regions. No one would suffer. 'I can only equalise on an expanding budget', Crossman had concluded.[46] The commitment to achieving equity thus reflected optimism about the possibilities of economic growth. As that optimism ebbed away during the second half of the 1970s, so the political costs of implementing the new distributional policies increased.

National policy and medical decisions

Implicit in the structure of the NHS was a bargain between the State and the medical profession. While central government controlled the budget, doctors controlled what happened within that budget. Financial power was concentrated at the centre; clinical power was concentrated at the periphery. Politicians in Cabinet made the decisions about how much to spend; doctors made the decisions about which patient should get what kind of treatment. But this implicit bargain represented not so much a final settlement as a truce: an accommodation to what was, for both parties, a necessary rather than a desirable compromise. For central government, there was the dilemma posed by the fact that it carried ultimate responsibility for everything that happened in the NHS. If patients were not treated, Ministers were likely to get the constituency brickbats. But Ministers were in no position to do anything about what might well be the cause of overstretched services: decisions by consultants to keep patients in hospital longer than necessary.[47] All such decisions, although they had crucial implications for the use of NHS resources, belonged to the sacred realm of clinical autonomy. Similarly, the use of ineffective, inefficient or expensive methods of clinical intervention[48] had implications for the NHS as a whole: funds so spent represented opportunities forgone for improving other parts of the NHS – such as the services for the mentally ill and the chronically sick, discussed in the previous section.

The bargain was also frustrating for the medical profession. The price of preserving clinical autonomy – the right of individual doctors to do what they thought right for individual patients – was accepting the constraint of working within fixed budgetary limits. The resources of which doctors disposed were thus limited in a period when the scope for medical intervention was ever-expanding. They might have to work in out-of-date buildings. They might well not get the latest equipment. The medical imperative of maximising the input of care for the individual patient was thus at odds with the financial structure of the NHS. From the 1960s onwards, these ever-present tensions became ever more apparent. To the extent that central government became committed to promoting efficiency and rational planning, so the inhibitions imposed by clinical autonomy became more evident. To the extent that the medical profession's standards were international, so the contrast between what was affordable in a relatively poor country like Britain and in wealthier nations like the United States became more glaring: to a large degree, the frustrations of the medical profession in the 1960s, and even more in the 1970s, were accentuated by the growing gap in national incomes between Britain and its competitors among the advanced industrial nations of the West. Not only was the NHS's share of the national income lower than that of health services in these countries but, perhaps more important, Britain's national income per head was itself falling in relation to that of its competitors.[49] If the medical brain-drain was never large enough to pose a threat to the NHS – which attracted far more doctors from the poorer nations of the Indian sub-continent than it lost to the wealthier societies of North America – it symbolised the shifting economic balance.

The way in which central policy-makers reacted to this situation is significant as much for what they did not do as for what they actually did. Certain policy options were automatically ruled out by the nature of the consensus about the NHS. Thus there was no move towards controlling or even investigating the decisions of clinicians, in contrast to the United States, where an open-ended budgetary system led to a series of attempts to introduce a formalised system for reviewing clinical decisions. The doctrine of clinical autonomy continued to reign supreme; significantly, the Health Service Commissioner – whose office was set up in 1974 to deal with patient complaints – was explicitly barred from dealing with cases revolving round questions of clinical judgement. Instead, the preferred strategy was that of persuasion, education and exhortation. At a conference held to celebrate the twentieth anniversary of the foundation of the NHS, Dr Henry Yellowlees – Deputy Chief Medical Officer of the Ministry of Health – pointed out that over £2 million a year could be saved if only lengths of stay for patients with appendicitis could be reduced to the same level as that already prevailing in the US: the first of many such exhortations by ministers, civil servants and academics. But, he stressed, 'There can be no question of telling surgeons how long their patients should be in hospital'.[50] All that could be done was to put the surgeons 'in possession of the facts'.

So, consistent with the overall philosophy that developed in the 1960s, there was increasing emphasis on producing better information and on organisational solutions: given better data, given better organisation, more rational decisions would follow – or so it was assumed. A new information system was developed: Hospital Activity Analysis, which provided consultants with better information about what they were doing. A new system of medical decision-making within individual hospitals was devised: the so-called Cogwheel system. If all the consultants became aware of the effects of their individual decisions on the total use of resources, it was argued, they would themselves have an incentive to apply pressure on colleagues who used their beds wastefully: it would make it clear that one consultant's extravagance was another consultant's loss. Consultants would view beds no longer as their private property but as a common resource. It is not clear how successful this strategy was. Certainly lengths of stay fell throughout the period in question. But the chorus of exhortations to greater efficiency continued throughout the period in question, as did great variations in practice. The new information system seems to have impinged only marginally on clinical practice; the Cogwheel machinery worked somewhat creakingly.[51] More important, for the purposes of our analysis, is the fact that no other strategy was ever defined to be within the realm of the feasible.

The full complexity and subtlety of the relationship between central policy-makers and clinical decision-makers at the periphery remains to be explored, however. For the paradox is that the centre's lack of authority over clinical decisions could, in some circumstances at least, confer positive advantages on policy-makers: by absolving them from involvement in difficult decisions and by permitting them to shuffle off responsibility for providing extra resources. Two examples illustrate this point: the experience of renal dialysis and of abortion. The case of renal dialysis illustrates the way in which central government could actually control the introduction of a new technology without ever appearing to be infringing medical autonomy. Renal dialysis is an example of a technology which is both expensive and which extends lives: in short, precisely the kind of medical advance which might be expected to generate large demands for extra resources. So, when it became apparent in the early 1960s that this new technology would soon be available, the medical hierarchy of the Ministry of Health took the initiative. A series of conferences – prestigiously chaired by the President of the Royal College of Physicians, Lord Rosenheim – was called. The process of engineering a professional consensus was under way. In the outcome, medical agreement was obtained for what was in all but name a strategy of rationing scarce resources: a policy of concentrating renal dialysis facilities in a limited number of centres – a policy justified, however, not by resource constraints but by medical considerations about the desirability of concentrating expertise. Special resources were set aside for the creation of these centres, but the commitment was limited. The result was that access to renal dialysis treatment in Britain was limited. Stringent criteria of suitability for treatment arc applied: criteria which are more severe than in other countries. Thus in 1975 the number of patients being treated by dialysis (or with a functioning transplant) was 62.0 per 1,000,000 population in Britain, as against 136.1 in Switzerland, 132.4 in Denmark, 102.2 in France, 87.7 in Germany and 85.4 in Sweden.[52] In other words, people in Britain were being turned away to die who, if they lived somewhere else, would have been successfully treated. The remarkable fact that the NHS could get away with this politically – that a refusal to save lives did not raise a storm of political protest – demonstrates the positive advantages that central policy-makers can derive from the doctrine of clinical autonomy. For, of course, it is not Ministers or civil servants who decide who should be treated. It is the clinicians concerned. The definition of certain areas of decision-making as being medical – and the consequent diffusion of responsibility for the consequences – thus prevents overload at the centre. The fact that no patient under the NHS system has a legal *right* to any specific kind of treatment – that it is the clinician who determines what the patient 'needs' – means that it is possible to fragment and dissolve national policy issues into a series of local clinical decisions. Political problems are, in effect, converted into clinical problems.

The case of abortion is somewhat different, but raises some of the same issues. The starting point here is the passage of the 1967 Abortion Act: a private member's bill sympathetically encouraged by Ministers. The result was to liberalise the law and to increase the demand for what were now legal operations. However, the Act imposed no responsibility on the Ministry of Health to provide the necessary facilities, nor did it impose on individual consultants a duty to carry out the procedure. To have provided the necessary facilities would have meant finding extra resources. To have imposed a duty on consultants would have infringed the principle of clinical autonomy. The Ministry in fact did neither. As the Lane Committee pointed out in 1974, the central department gave no 'guidance to hospital authorities as to what they consider the reasonable requirement to be in the field of abortion'.[53] The result was wide variation in the facilities provided. In 1973 the Newcastle region provided abortions for nearly 90 per cent of the women living in the region who wanted them, while Birmingham recorded a figure of under 20 per cent. If the principle of clinical autonomy gave the central department a pretext for doing nothing, it was the existence of a private market which made this policy of inaction politically feasible. Demand created its own supply: in the private sector. In 1968, 35 per cent of all abortions were carried out by private clinics – some operated for profit, some run by charitable organisations. In 1971 the figure was 43.4 per cent. Central government had found yet another way of absolving itself from the necessity to command or to instruct, as well as from the need to find extra resources.

If it was thus impossible or undesirable to command, might it not have been possible to change the structure of incentives within which doctors worked? A partial answer to this question is provided by the new pay deal negotiated with the general practitioners in 1966: the so-called Family Doctor Charter.[54] The negotiations and the settlement provide an instructive case history, which illuminates both the internal political dynamics of the medical profession and the scope of the Ministry of Health for introducing change.

In 1963 the annual meeting of BMA representatives passed a motion which called for urgent action to 'upgrade the financial status of family doctors'. Implicit in this motion was not just the customary demand for more money but a demand for a change in the structure of medical earnings: the aim was to reduce the differential between general practitioners and consultants. The resentment of general practitioners at being the poor relations of the medical profession within the NHS – of being virtually excluded from the prestigious hospital world of high technology – had broken into the open. The logic of the relationship between general practitioners and consultants was essentially a commercial one: it had been forged in the nineteenth century as a way of regulating the competition between general practitioners and hospital specialists. The referral system then evolved was essentially a demarcation agreement between two crafts, of exactly the same kind that developed between different crafts in shipbuilding and other British industries. General practitioners were the gatekeepers to the whole health care system: all referrals to hospital had to come through them, and they were thus assured of patients. Similarly, once patients were past the gate, consultants took over. Both were thus assured of clients. But while the NHS removed the commercial logic behind this system, it also perpetuated it: hence the frustration of the general practitioners in the 1960s.

The militancy of the general practitioners was embarrassing for the BMA, for it exposed the fact that general practitioners and consultants did not necessarily have the same interests. Yet if the BMA was reluctant to go into battle, others were not. The Medical Practitioners' Union, a body with a long history but a small membership, took up the cause of the general practitioners. A new breakaway General Practitioners' Association was formed. Competition between the various medical organisations fanned militancy. In 1965 the proposals of the impartial review body – set up as a result of the recommendations of the Royal Commission on Doctors' and Dentists' Remuneration (discussed in the previous chapter) – were rejected. In March 1965 the BMA threatened mass resignations by general practitioners from the NHS. At the same time, the BMA published its demands in the form of a 'Charter for the Family Doctor Service'.

The details of the Charter are of no concern here, but some of the main elements should be noted. First, the general practitioners demanded an end to the 'pool' system: that is, spending on general practitioner services should be determined by the number of patients, not by a capped budget. Second, they demanded a new form of contract which would limit their responsibility for their patients to a specified working day and a five and a half day working week: the concept of professional responsibilities for patients being unlimited was to be dropped. Third, they demanded the creation of an independent corporation to provide loans for improving practice premises and equipment. Lastly, they demanded that general practitioners who did not wish to be paid on the basis of capitation fees should have a choice between salaries and item-of-service fees: that is, payment by the act.

Months of negotiations followed between the profession and the Ministry, headed by Kenneth Robinson. Interestingly the civil servant most immediately involved was Robert Armstrong, a future Cabinet Secretary – evidence perhaps of the infusion of some high-flyers into the Ministry's hierarchy. The compromise that finally emerged in 1966 was a monument to the enduring strength of the underlying consensus about the NHS. The demands of the BMA which would have undermined the basic philosophy of the NHS were effectively ignored. Nothing more was heard of item-of-service fees, although specific payments were to be paid for some general practitioner work such as night-visiting, vaccinations and immunisations. Similarly, nothing more was heard about limiting the general practitioner's total responsibility for his or her patients. But the pool was abolished. A financial corporation for encouraging investment in general practice was set up, and various modifications to the system of calculating earnings were agreed. In particular, a basic allowance – or salary element – was introduced, as were new incentives for doctors to practise in under-provided areas of the country.

The cost of the settlement to the Ministry of Health was a £24 million a year addition to the cost of general practitioner services. But, in return, the Ministry was able to give new impetus to some long-standing aims of policy. The financial provisions of the settlement were largely designed to promote better quality practice, in terms of improved surgeries, more support staff and encouragement for the formation of group practices: the 1966 settlement marks the beginning of a boom in Health Centres.[55] These, as noted in Chapter 1, had been the centrepiece of planning for general practice before the creation of the NHS. Subsequently, a combination of medical hostility and financial stringency had consigned them to a policy limbo. A combination of changes in medical attitudes and the easing of budgetary constraints had created new opportunities for central policy-makers to push a policy consistent not only with the ideological bias of the Labour Ministry of Health, but also with the efficiency bias of the technocratic rationalisers. The Family Doctor Charter negotiations thus provide a case study both of the limits on the potential for change, imposed by the prevailing consensus, and the opportunities to influence clinical practice through the use of incentives.

The history of these negotiations also underlines a trend which was to emerge increasingly strongly over the next decade: the ever-deepening divisions within the medical profession. In the 1960s, in contrast to the 1950s and again the 1970s, doctors did well for themselves financially. In 1972 the Review Body reported that 'the medical profession, taken as a whole, gained ground rather than lost it in relation to other workers' between the publication of the Royal Commission report and 1971.[56] There were, inevitably, battles between the profession and the Government, particularly when the recommendations of the Review Body ran counter to incomes policy: indeed in 1970 the Review Body resigned because of the Government's refusal to implement its recommendations fully. Pay, inevitably, could not be de-politicised in the NHS. Equally important, however, were the battles within the medical profession. In 1966 the Junior Hospital Doctors' Association was formed, successfully beginning a campaign to raise salaries which was to end by threatening the differentials between consultants and their supporting cast of doctors. Increasingly, too, the Hospital Consultants' and Specialists' Association – founded in 1948 but largely dormant until the end of the 1960s – began to challenge the right of the BMA to act as the voice of the consultants: in 1974 it unsuccessfully applied to the Industrial Relations Court for negotiating rights.[57]

These fissions helped to expose the weaknesses in the machinery of professional corporatism within the NHS. On paper, the structure was highly corporate, with the medical profession being organised in clearly defined associations and with a highly centralised negotiating structure. In practice, the associations found it difficult to deliver the goods: indeed by 1972, the BMA had become sufficiently anxious to invite a former chairman of ICI, Sir Paul Chambers, to investigate its constitution and organisation.[58] Under the veneer of disciplined corporatism, however, the reality was an anarchic syndicalism. The leaders of the medical profession – the bureaucrats of the BMA and others – faced precisely the same nagging difficulty as the paternalistic rationalisers at the Ministry of Health: how to influence, let alone control, the individualistic practitioners at the periphery. If the relationship between the professional élite and the bureaucratic élite was an intimate one,[59] it was at least in part because they shared the same problem: that of corporatist rationalisers trying to cope with a syndicalist constituency.

In search of an organisational fix

The original structure of the NHS, everyone agreed, had one fundamental, inbuilt weakness. This was the administrative separation of the hospital, general practitioner and local authority health services: a structure which reflected political expediency, not administrative logic. It is therefore not surprising that the issue of organisational reform surged back onto the political agenda in the 1960s, and that finally in 1974 a reorganised NHS emerged. Not only were these the years of faith in the ability of organisational change to promote greater efficiency and effectiveness in all spheres of government, as already noted, there was also increasing frustration within the NHS at the seeming inability of central government to implement its policies. If there was to be rational planning, then an appropriate administrative machinery had to be designed. If a further spur to action was needed, then there was the growing emphasis on co-ordinating hospital and community services in order to minimise the costs of caring for an ageing population. Once again, change was anchored in consensus. By 1968 when Kenneth Robinson, the Labour Minister of Health, published the first consultative document on reorganisation, the need for administrative reform had become part of the conventional wisdom. The agreement spanned the political parties, and reflected also the views of the medical profession: already in 1962 the report of the Porritt Committee, set up by the medical profession, had come out in favour of a unified health service based on area boards. Once again, however, consensus both made change possible and constrained its scope. For it embodied notions not only about what was desirable but also about the limits of political feasibility.

In principle, the Labour and Conservative parties were agreed that a unified health and local authority system would be the ideal solution: all the more so, since there was a great deal of complementarity and substitution between the health and welfare services, particularly for the elderly. Further, they were agreed that the best way of achieving this ideal would be to transfer the health services to local government. However, both parties were at one in accepting that such a solution was not feasible: that there was no point in even putting it on the agenda of possible policy options. In part, this was a tribute to the veto-power of the medical profession, with its tradition of entrenched hostility to local government control. While this issue was central to the medical profession, it was peripheral to the local government lobby: although local authorities were naturally in favour of taking over health services, their diffuse support would not outweigh the concentrated opposition that could be expected from the doctors. In part, too, the rejection of the local government option marked a recognition of the practical problems involved. Such a transfer of power would have required basic changes in both the money-raising capacities of local government and in its boundaries. However, it is also worth noting that another option was also ruled out of court: that of transferring local government welfare services to the NHS – an option suggested by the logic of complementarity and substitutability. If the medical profession had veto-power, so did the local government lobby. The search for an organisational solution to the NHS's problems can therefore be best understood as policy-making under constraints, where the ideal was often seen as the enemy of the feasible: the politics of the second-best.[60]

There were two further ingredients in the consensus. First, there was agreement that, since it was not possible to amalgamate health and local government services, the best available solution would be to align the boundaries of health and local authorities: the assumption being that co-habitation would lead to co-ordination. Second, there was agreement that the aim of reorganisation should be to promote better management: to give more power, as it were, to the paternalistic rationalisers, and to create more scope for the rational analysis and efficient solution of problems.

Given these shared assumptions, it is hardly surprising that the successive proposals put forward – from Kenneth Robinson's 1968 consultative document to Sir Keith Joseph's 1974 final solution – show a remarkable degree of continuity, only marginally affected by party ideology. The proposals did change in detail, but the changes were prompted as much by developments in the external environment of the NHS as by party considerations. The 'central theme' of the 1968 Green Paper was unification.[61] The new NHS was to be based on 40 to 50 Area Boards, responsible for all health services, including the general practitioner services: a number chosen because it was expected that the Royal Commission on

Local Government would recommend the creation of 40 to 50 local authorities. All other NHS authorities – including the regions – would disappear. The style of the Area Boards would be managerial. Their membership would be small; and while 'some members with broad professional knowledge of medical and related services would be needed', the representation of 'special interests' was specifically excluded. The senior officers of the Board would act as an executive directorate, with the Chief Administrator acting as Managing Director.

In 1970 Richard Crossman, now in charge of NHS reorganisation as Secretary of State for the DHSS, published yet another Green Paper.[62] The most obvious change from the 1968 document was prompted by events outside the control of the NHS: the decision to base the new system of local government not on 40 to 50 authorities but on about 90. So, given the agreement on the need for co-terminosity, this implied 90 Area Health Authorities. In turn, this raised the question of whether one central department could effectively control this number of authorities. Crossman was anxious to knock out the regional tier altogether;[63] his civil servants were less enthusiastic. In the event the Green Paper fudged the issue: it envisaged the creation of 14 Regional Health Councils with somewhat vague co-ordinating and planning roles. Crucially, however, these Councils were not to be a link in the administrative chain of command: the DHSS would deal directly with the Areas: 'The central Department will need to concern itself more closely than in the past with the expenditure and efficiency of the administration at the local level.'

The 1970 Green Paper was significant also for its attempts to meet some of the criticisms prompted by its predecessor, and its concessions to various interest groups. The managerial emphasis of the 1968 Green Paper had antagonised the medical profession, among others. For example, the *British Medical Journal* commented that 'A case for such a drastic curtailment of the participation of the public and of the profession in the management of the NHS might be made simply in the interests of efficiency. But there is a limit to the extent to which the principles of organisation and methods should be introduced into a medical service',[64] a curious echo of Morrison's protest, in the 1946 Cabinet debates, about using the efficiency argument as the determining criterion in health services organisation. Nor had local government been pleased. In response, Crossman introduced the principle of representative membership for the new health authorities: one-third of the members were to be appointed by the health profession, one-third appointed by the local authorities and one-third plus the chairman appointed by the Secretary of State. This proposal was pushed through only after a bitter battle with the Treasury, which argued that the appointment of members by interest groups was incompatible with the accountability of health authorities to Parliament. Finally, the 1970 Green Paper argued that 'there must be more, not less, local participation' in the reorganised NHS, and to this end proposed the creation of district committees 'on which people drawn from the local community and people working in the local health service can contribute to the work of running the district's services' (in ways unspecified).

The Labour Government, and Crossman with it, were voted out of office before these proposals could be implemented. In 1971 Crossman's Conservative successor at the DHSS, Sir Keith Joseph, published his Consultative Document, followed by a White Paper in 1972, legislation in 1973 and the unveiling of the new NHS in 1974. Two linked themes shaped Sir Keith's approach. First, as the Consultative

Document put it, there was the emphasis on 'effective management'[65] – harking back to the 1968 Green Paper. Second, there was the need to correct the 'imbalances and gaps', to quote the 1972 White Paper,[66] in the provision of NHS services: to redress the balance between the acute and the chronic services in favour of the latter. Effective management would be the tool used to achieve this objective. Hitherto, the White Paper argued, 'There has been no identified authority whose task it has been . . . to balance needs and priorities rationally and to plan and provide the right combination of services for the benefit of the public.' In future, the new Area Health Authorities (AHAs) would perform this role. They would identify the 'real needs' of the population, order priorities, work out plans and assess their effectiveness.

The new NHS that emerged in 1974 was different in a number of respects from that envisaged under the Labour Green Paper. First, the regional authorities re-emerged as executive agencies, the link between the DHSS and the Area Health Authorities in the chain of command: any attempt by the DHSS to control the AHAs directly – the 1972 White Paper argued, reflecting the views of the civil service – would lead to 'over-centralisation and delay'. Second, a new tier was inserted into the hierarchy of administration: larger AHAs were to be divided into districts, each run by a team of officers on a consensus basis (thus giving each member, including representatives of the local consultants and general practitioners, a right of veto over decisions). This innovation was designed to meet the problems caused by the fact that the boundaries of the AHAs were determined by the doctrine of co-terminosity and thus by decisions about the size and pattern of local government, not by decisions based on the administrative logic of the NHS. Third, every tier in the administrative hierarchy – region, AHA and district – was festooned with professional advisory committees, to ensure that decisions would be made 'in the full knowledge of expert opinion': expert opinion being defined as that of doctors, opticians, pharmacists and nurses. Lastly, the reorganised NHS included an institutional innovation: Community Health Councils (CHCs), one for each of the 200 districts. There was thus to be a division of labour: members of AHAs were intended to manage, while members of CHCs were meant to 'represent the views of the consumer'.

The 1974 reorganisation had a number of characteristics which are worth exploring further, not only for the insights they provide into the problems and dilemmas of policy-making but also for their long-term implications. Most self-evidently, it set the 'voice of the expert' into the concrete of the institutional structure even more firmly than Bevan's design had done. Not only did doctors (and nurses, for the first time) have representation on both the regional and area authorities. Not only was an elaborate multi-tiered machinery devised for articulating professional opinion. But, as we have also seen, the basic unit of management – the District Management Team – gave the representatives of the medical profession veto rights. These extensive concessions should be seen not so much as a victory for the corporate organisations of the medical profession as an acknowledgement of the reality of medical syndicalism. Since decisions at the periphery depended on the active co-operation of the doctors concerned, as the people who determined who got what, it seemed only logical to build the participation of the medical profession into the process of the decision-making machinery. Participation followed effective power.

In conceding representation to the medical profession on health authorities,

Joseph was of course only following the Labour Green Paper. Similarly, in line with the Crossman proposals, the 1974 NHS provided for representation of local government interests: a third of AHA members were nominated by local authorities. In both respects, Joseph was forced to compromise the underlying principle of his vision: managerial efficiency. His Consultative Document had firmly stated that 'it would be inappropriate for the authorities to be composed on the representational basis proposed in the 1970 Green Paper'. The main criterion for the selection of members was to be 'management ability'. But, to quote one of Joseph's civil servants, it turned out to be difficult to recruit people with business experience. 'Once you had run through his friends, you had no one else. . . . In any case you couldn't have 15 hard-faced businessmen running the AHAs.' Moreover, the medical profession and the local government lobby, backed by the Secretary of State for the Environment, were pressing for representation. So the issue was fudged. To the last the Secretary of State stressed that no one served on health authorities in a representative capacity, but the argument seemed increasingly strained as he made concessions on the methods of selection.

Paradoxically it was also the doctrine of managerial efficiency which led to the institutionalisation of the voice of the consumer, in the shape of Community Health Councils.[67] The role of members in the authorities created in 1948 had never been precisely defined: the implicit presumption was that they would combine the managerial role, as the Minister's agents, with that of articulating the interests of consumers and the local community. But what if the two roles conflicted? The report of the Ely inquiry into abuse in a hospital for the mentally handicapped, cited above, had suggested that the members of the Hospital Management Committee responsible had been more concerned to maintain staff morale than to safeguard the interests of the patients. So, given the new emphasis on the exclusively managerial role of the authority members, it seemed only logical to invent a special institution to voice consumer views: an institution which would have no managerial responsibilities. In logic, the distinction was clear; in practice, particularly given the representation of local authorities on AHAs, it often proved blurred.

Community Health Councils were notable for another feature as well. They represented a further attempt to devise a constituency for the deprived client groups in the NHS: precisely those who, as argued above, would be least able to articulate their demands. Half their members were to be appointed by local authorities; a further sixth by the Regional Health Authorities (as the Regional Hospital Boards now became). But a third were to be chosen by local voluntary bodies, with special emphasis on those representing the elderly, the mentally ill and handicapped, and other deprived groups. The constitution of CHCs is thus a good example of the paternalistic rationalisers deliberately loading the dice of representation in order to achieve a greater measure of justice as between the different client groups of the NHS.

The 1974 reorganisation is significant also for what it reveals about the changing balance of political power within the medical profession. In one crucial respect, the 1974 unification of the NHS was a fiction. General practitioner services remained an autonomous enclave. Some of the members of the new Family Practitioner Committees (FPCs), which administered general practitioner services as the successors to the Executive Councils, were indeed appointed by the AHAs. Furthermore, FPCs and AHAs shared the same administrative boundaries.

But half their members were nominated by the professions and financially they dealt directly with the DHSS. At the margins, AHAs might be able to exercise some leverage, through their control over the development of Health Centres and of nursing and other staff attached to general practice. Essentially, however, FPCs were independent bodies: the integration of hospital and primary care services remained a distant dream. In short, general practitioners had successfully asserted their right of veto: their power was measured in terms of what was not done, because it was defined to be outside the realm of the politically feasible.

In contrast, the 1974 reorganisation did mark one important step towards integration: the prestigious teaching hospitals lost their special independent status. Boards of Governors disappeared; teaching hospitals were integrated into the administrative structure of the NHS. Ministers were lobbied hard. Tory peers were strongly represented among the chairmen of the Boards of Governors; the Royal Colleges, too, added their voices to the protests. But all to no avail. The contrast between 1948 and 1974 is striking. While Bevan had had to make extensive concessions to the leaders of the specialists (*see* Chapter 1), Joseph was able virtually to ignore the special pleadings of the consultant élite. Not only had that élite been diluted by the expansion of consultant numbers; equally, it had also become more heterogeneous, as it became apparent that consultants at London teaching hospitals did not necessarily have the same interests as those at provincial district general hospitals. There could be no clearer warning against using simple-minded élite theories to explain the evolution of policy in the NHS.

So, in 1974, the network of NHS authorities set up in 1948 was swept away. In place of 700 different authorities – Regional Hospital Boards, Boards of Governors, Hospital Management Committees and Executive Councils – there was now a streamlined structure. There were 15 Regional Health Authorities, 90 Area Health Authorities each with its linked Family Practitioner Committee, and 200 District Management Teams each flanked by a Community Health Council. The change prompted two major lines of criticism. First, the new model NHS was attacked as being excessively managerialist: 'I say to the Secretary of State that his managerialism is terrifying', Crossman proclaimed in a House of Commons debate.[68] Second, the new model NHS was criticised for its excessive bureaucratic complexity. There were too many tiers of administrative authority: the DHSS, the regions, the areas and the districts. 'I am appalled by the prospect of a tremendous block of bureaucrats desiccating every original proposal and being difficult over every case', Crossman added.

In a sense the two criticisms were self-cancelling. If the design of the 1974 NHS had been inspired solely by considerations of managerial efficiency, it would not have taken the complex shape it did. Sir Keith Joseph did bring a firm of management consultants, McKinseys, into the DHSS to advise on the details of the reorganisation. But their influence is reflected chiefly in the rhetoric of reorganisation: in the jargon that clothed the proposals and in the small print of the administrative arrangements with their emphasis on functional management – chains of command based on professional expertise.[69] Some of the strongest opposition within the DHSS to the proposed reorganisation came from the business executives, whom the Prime Minister had brought into government precisely in order to promote greater managerial efficiency. From their point of view, the weakness of the NHS derived largely from the hegemony of the civil servants: as one of them put it, 'It was like pre-1914 Russia – a French-speaking élite who couldn't speak Russian'. The real need was to allow 'health service people to run the health service at the top', to end the situation 'where everyone was interfering with everyone else at different levels' and to 'de-layer' the NHS by chopping off the regions.

In the event, Sir Keith Joseph ignored the advice of these managerialists. If indeed the new model NHS emerged as an extremely complex structure, it was because he was trying to achieve a variety of policy aims, while seeking to preserve consensus and to avoid conflict. The regional tier was perpetuated partly to avoid conflict with the civil servants, and partly because the administrative boundaries of the AHAs did not provide a satisfactory basis for planning health services. In turn, the district level had to be invented because the AHAs were in many cases too large for a health service based on the concept of the District General Hospital. Finally, the elaborate cobweb of advisory committees was added in order to keep the professions happy.

Essentially, therefore, the 1974 reorganisation can be seen as a political exercise in trying to satisfy everyone and to reconcile conflicting policy aims: to promote managerial efficiency but also to satisfy the professions, to create an effective hierarchy for transmitting national policy but also to give scope to the managers at the periphery. The intention was summed up in the slogan of 'maximum delegation downward, maximum accountability upward'. The phrase summed up the nature of the policy problem; but it did not provide a solution. And the politics of disillusionment of the second half of the 1970s – the theme of the next chapter – can in part at least be understood as the natural reaction to this attempt to square the circle. As it turned out, the attempt to please everyone satisfied no one.

References

1. The source for all quotations from election manifestos is: FWS Craig (ed.), *British General Election Manifestos, 1900–1974*, Macmillan: London 1975.
2. Office of Health Economics, *Efficiency in the Hospital Service*, OHE: London 1967.
3. GR Searle, *The Quest for National Efficiency*, Blackwell: Oxford 1971.
4. Harold Macmillan, *The Middle Way*, Macmillan: London 1938.
5. For an account of economic policy during this period, see Samuel Brittan, *Steering the Economy*, Secker & Warburg: London 1969.
6. Secretary of State for Economic Affairs, *The National Plan*, HMSO: London 1965, Cmnd. 2764.
7. The Prime Minister and Minister for the Civil Service, *The Reorganisation of Central Government*, HMSO: London 1970, Cmnd. 4506.
8. For the origins of the PESC system, see Sir Richard Clarke, *Public Expenditure Management and Control*, Macmillan: London 1978.
9. Chancellor of the Exchequer, *Control of Public Expenditure*, HMSO: London 1961, Cmnd. 1432.
10. Committee on the Civil Service, *Report*, HMSO: London 1968, Cmnd. 3638.
11. Royal Commission on Local Government in England, *Report*, HMSO: London 1969, Cmnd. 4040.
12. Rudolf Klein, 'The Politics of Public Expenditure', *British Journal of Political Science*, vol. 6, pt. 4, Oct. 1976, pp. 401–32.
13. As in the previous chapter, the source for all time-series data on NHS expenditure is: Royal Commission on the National Health Service, *Report*, HMSO: London 1979, Cmnd. 7615.
14. Stendhal, *De L'Amour*, Editions de Cluny: Paris 1938, p. 43: 'Ce que j'appelle

cristallisation, c'est l'opération de l'esprit, qui tire de tout ce qui se présente la découverte que l'object aimé a de nouvelles perfection.' Translating this into the language of policy analysis, we might freely render this as: 'What I call crystallisation is the operation of the mind which draws out of the environment the discovery that there is a problem demanding attention.'

15. J Enoch Powell, *Medicine and Politics*, Pitman Medical: London 1966.
16. Thomas McKeown, *The Role of Medicine*, Nuffield Provincial Hospitals Trust: London 1976.
17. AO Hirschman, *Exit, Voice and Loyalty*, Harvard UP: Cambridge, Mass. 1970. The Hirschman model applies, of course, to consumers of services only. For the argument that, in the circumstances of the NHS, it also applies to producers, see Rudolf Klein, 'Models of Man and Models of Policy', *Health and Society*, vol. 58, no. 3, 1980, pp. 416–29.
18. Royal Commission on the National Health Service, op. cit. (see ref. 13).
19. For perhaps the earliest diagnosis of the dilemma, see F Roberts, *The Cost of Health*, Turnstile Press: London 1952. Quoted in Robert J Maxwell, *Health and Wealth*, Lexington Books: Lexington, Mass. 1981. Dr Roberts argued that: 'The expense of the health service is incurred by individuals acting singly; the bill is paid by individuals acting collectively. There is therefore a permanent conflict between the demand for greater expenditure and the demand for smaller expenditure.'
20. James M Buchanan, *The Inconsistencies of the National Health Service*, Institute of Economic Affairs: London 1965. See also Arthur Seldon, *After the NHS*, Institute of Economic Affairs: London 1968.
21. See, for example, B Abel-Smith, *Value for Money in Health Services*, Heinemann: London 1976.
22. Rudolf Klein, 'The Conflict Between Professionals, Consumers and Bureaucrats', *Journal of the Irish Colleges of Physicians and Surgeons*, vol. 6, no. 3, Jan. 1977, pp. 88–91.
23. David Owen, *In Sickness and In Health*, Quartet: London 1976.
24. Henry Miller, 'In Sickness and In Health: A Doctor's View of Medicine in Britain', *Encounter*, April 1967, pp. 10–21.
25. British Medical Association, *Health Services Financing*, BMA: London 1969. Note that the title page carries the disclaimer: 'The contents of this report do not necessarily reflect BMA policy.'
26. Douglas Houghton, *Paying for the Social Services*, Institute of Economic Affairs: London 1967.
27. Richard Crossman, *Paying for the Social Services*, Fabian Society: London 1969.
28. Richard Crossman, *The Diaries of a Cabinet Minister*, vol. 2, p. 707, Hamish Hamilton and Jonathan Cape: London 1976.
29. Minister of Health, *A Hospital Plan for England and Wales*, HMSO: London 1962, Cmnd. 1604. The evolution of this plan has been admirably analysed in David E Allen, *Hospital Planning*, Pitman Medical: Tunbridge Wells 1979, and my discussion of the document draws heavily on this source.
30. Department of Health and Social Security, *The Functions of the District General Hospital*, HMSO: London 1969.
31. Richard Crossman, *A Politician's View of Health Service Planning*, University of Glasgow: Glasgow 1972.
32. For an interesting attempt to apply this kind of model to the NHS, see Cotton M Lindsay, *National Health Issues: The British Experience*, Hoffmann-La Roche Inc: Santa Monica, CA 1980. One of the conclusions drawn in this study is that the distribution of capital expenditure can, in part, be explained by a vote-buying strategy: that is, money went disproportionately to those regions with a high proportion of marginal constituencies. But the unit of analysis, the region, seems too large and heterogeneous to put much weight on this conclusion.

33. For organisational incentives, see M Olson, *The Logic of Collective Action*, Harvard UP: Cambridge, Mass. 1965.

34. I owe this phrase to WJM Mackenzie, *Power and Responsibility in Health Care*, Oxford UP 1979.

35. Estimates Committee, *Hospital Building in Great Britain: Minutes of Evidence*, HMSO: London 1970, HC 59.

36. Rosemary Stewart and Janet Sleeman, *Continuously Under Review*, Bell: London 1967.

37. Richard Crossman, *A Politician's View*, op. cit.

38. Department of Health and Social Security, *Review of Health Capital*, DHSS: London 1979.

39. Alan Maynard and Rachel Tingle, 'The Objectives and Performance of the Mental Health Services in England and Wales in the 1960s', *Journal of Social Policy*, vol. 4, no. 2, April 1975, pp. 155–68.

40. Committee of Inquiry into Allegations of Ill-Treatment of Patients and Other Irregularities at the Ely Hospital, Cardiff, *Report*, HMSO: London 1969, Cmnd. 3975. For Crossman's own account of how he handled the report, and the subsequent setting up of the HAS, see Richard Crossman, *The Diaries of a Cabinet Minister*, vol. 3, pp. 409ff, Hamish Hamilton and Jonathan Cape: London 1977. See also Rudolf Klein, 'Policy Problems and Policy Perceptions in the National Health Service', *Policy and Politics*, vol. 2, no. 3, 1974, pp. 219–36.

41. Rudolf Klein and Phoebe Hall, *Caring for Quality in the Caring Services*, Centre for Studies in Social Policy: London 1975.

42. For distinction awards, see P Bruggen and S Bourne, 'Further Examination of the Distinction Awards System in England and Wales', *British Medical Journal*, 26 Feb. 1976, pp. 536–7. For immigrant doctors, see Royal Commission on the National Health Service, op. cit., Table 14.6. This shows, for example, overseas born doctors held 40.9 per cent of all consultant posts in geriatric medicine and 23.4 per cent in mental illness, as against 8.0 per cent in general medicine and 8.3 per cent in surgery.

43. Sir Keith Joseph, 'Marsden Lecture', reprinted as 'Sir Keith Surveys the NHS: Achievements and Failures', *British Medical Journal*, 1 Dec. 1973, pp. 561–2.

44. For an analysis of the resources allocation formulas, see Martin Buxton and Rudolf Klein, *Allocating Health Resources*, Royal Commission on the National Health Service, Research Paper no. 3, HMSO: London 1978.

45. Martin Buxton and Rudolf Klein, 'Distribution of Hospital Provision', *British Medical Journal*, 8 Feb. 1975, pp. 345–9. This analysis showed that the distribution of hospital resources by Area Health Authorities in terms of per capita income varied from 74 per cent *below* the national average to 62 per cent *above* the national average.

46. Richard Crossman, *A Politician's View*, op. cit.

47. RFL Logan, JSA Ashley, RE Klein and DM Robson, *Dynamics of Medical Care: The Liverpool Study into Use of Hospital Resources*, London School of Hygiene & Tropical Medicine Memoir no. 14: London 1972.

48. AL Cochrane, *Effectiveness and Efficiency*, Nuffield Provincial Hospitals Trust: London 1972.

49. For comparative statistics of health expenditure, see Organisation for Economic Co-operation and Development, *Public Expenditure on Health*, OECD: Paris 1977.

50. Department of Health and Social Security, *NHS Twentieth Anniversary Conference, Report*, HMSO: London 1968.

51. Gordon McLachlan (ed.), *In Low Gear?*, Oxford UP 1971.

52. Office of Health Economics, *Renal Failure*, OHE: London 1978.

53. Committee on the Working of the Abortion Act, *Report*, HMSO: London 1974, Cmnd. 5579.

54. Excellent accounts of this episode, which have been drawn upon in the text, can be found in: Rosemary Stevens, *Medical Practice in Modern England*, Yale UP: New Haven, Conn. 1966, and Gordon Forsyth, *Doctors and State Medicine*, Pitman Medical: London 1973.

55. Phoebe Hall, Hilary Land, Roy Parker and Adrian Webb, *Change, Choice and Conflict in Social Policy*, Heinemann: London 1975. See Ch. 11, 'The Development of Health Centres', by Phoebe Hall.
56. Review Body on Doctors' and Dentists' Remuneration, *Report 1972*, HMSO: London 1972, Cmnd. 5010.
57. Keith Barnard and Kenneth Lee, *Conflicts in the National Health Service*, Croom Helm: London 1977. See Ch. 2, 'Medical Autonomy: Challenge and Responses', by Mary Ann Elston.
58. Sir Paul Chambers, *Report of an Inquiry into the Association's Constitution and Organization*, reprinted in *British Medical Journal*, vol. 2, 1977, pp. 45–67.
59. Here I follow Eckstein, *Pressure Group Politics*, op. cit. For an analysis of the relationship between the two élites, see Barbara Evans, 'Corridors of Power', *World Medicine*, 10 March 1970, pp. 21–33, and Barbara Evans, 'Power Maze or Party Game', *World Medicine*, 28 Jan. 1976, pp. 17–22.
60. Rudolf Klein, 'NHS Reorganisation: The Politics of the Second Best', *The Lancet*, 26 August 1972, pp. 418–20; Rudolf Klein, 'Policy Making in the National Health Service', *Political Studies*, vol. XXII, no. 1, March 1974, pp. 1–14. This account of reorganisation draws on both sources.
61. Ministry of Health, *National Health Service: The Administrative Structure of the Medical and Related Services in England and Wales*, HMSO: London 1968.
62. Department of Health and Social Security, *National Health Service: The Future Structure of the National Health Service*, HMSO: London 1970.
63. Richard Crossman, *The Diaries of a Cabinet Minister*, vol. 3, op. cit., p. 753.
64. Cited in Klein, 1974, op. cit.
65. Department of Health and Social Security, *National Health Service Reorganisation: Consultative Document*, DHSS: London 1971.
66. Secretary of State for Social Services, *National Health Service Reorganisation: England*, HMSO: London 1972, Cmnd. 5055.
67. Rudolf Klein and Janet Lewis, *The Politics of Consumer Representation*, Centre for Studies in Social Policy: London 1976.
68. House of Commons Hansard, *Parliamentary Debates*, vol. 853, no. 86, 27 March 1973.
69. Department of Health and Social Security, *Management Arrangements for the Reorganised National Health Service*, HMSO: London 1972.

Chapter 4

The politics of disillusionment

If the start of the 1970s saw the apotheosis of paternalistic rationalism, with the 1974 reorganisation of the NHS as its monument, the second half of the decade produced the politics of disillusionment. Designed in an era of faith in problem-solving through expertise, the reorganised NHS began life at a time when technical questions increasingly became redefined as political issues. With apt symbolism, the 1980s were to begin with the demolition squads moving in to begin chipping away at the monument itself: the reorganised NHS was being reorganised yet again. Cocooned in consensus for the first 35 years of its existence, the arena of health care policy was gradually opening up as internal conflicts grew more pronounced and external pressures became more intense. If internal conflicts had previously been constrained by consensus, now these conflicts were slowly beginning to fray the consensus itself.

Two sets of factors contributed to this transformation. Within the arena of health care policy, there was the intensification of the trends noted in the previous chapter: in particular, the growing numbers, assertiveness and competitiveness of the actors involved. A stage where once the leaders of the medical profession had been able to soliloquise with little interruption had now become crowded with actors all clamouring to be heard. External to the health care arena, there was the dismaying discovery that the post-war years of economic growth were over, as Britain grappled with the twin problems of recession and inflation. In turn, the new economic situation created a new political climate reflected in the increased ideological polarisation of the Labour and Conservative parties. So demands generated from within the health care arena were increasing at precisely the time when the capacity of the governmental system to accommodate them was falling. Conversely, the ability of the health care system to adapt itself to the new economic and political environment was declining as the multiplication of veto power made the implementation of change more difficult: the snaffle was more in evidence than the horse. By the end of the 1970s, the NHS was more than ever a paradigm of British society as a whole: the stalemate society.[1]

Next, therefore, we shall examine in more detail both sides of this equation: the changes in the health care policy arena on the one hand, and those in its economic and political environment on the other. For it is precisely the relationship between the internally generated demands and the externally enforced pressures which provides the key to the politics of disillusionment.

The politics of economic crisis: the NHS in a new environment

For most of the post-war period in Britain, economic growth was the solvent of political conflict. Britain's growth rate might be slow compared to that of other advanced industrial nations. But even if the national income was rising only slowly, distributional conflicts about who should get what were blunted. The dividends of growth meant that everyone could get something: both profits and wages could rise, both consumer incomes and public expenditure on the social services could go on increasing. Competition between the Labour and Conservative parties largely revolved around the issue as to which one could successfully lay claim to being the most effective technician of economic growth.

The ever-deepening economic crisis that marked the years after 1973, as growth went into reverse gear, profoundly transformed this situation. The economics of national decline inevitably lead to the politics of conflict: a falling national income meant that competition for ever more scarce resources had become a zero-sum game. While the politics of economic growth had led to convergence between the political parties – both committed to promoting economic growth by means of technocratic planning – the politics of conflict led to an ever-increasing divergence between them. The debate about techniques (means) increasingly turned into a confrontation about ideologies (ends). By the turn of the decade, the Conservative Party, which had been returned to office in 1979, was committed to an ideology of the private market: explicitly repudiating what was perceived to have been the technocratic corporatism of the Heath administration between 1970 and 1974. Conversely, the Labour Party was convulsed by a highly charged ideological debate revolving around the question of what Socialist principles were and how best to implement them: a debate marked by the attacks on the managerial corporatism of the 1974 to 1979 Labour administration. The differences between the two parties had crystallised (to exaggerate only a little) into a confrontation between the values of individualism and those of collectivism.

One casualty of the new politics was the faith in technocracy that had marked the 1960s and early 1970s: the re-politicisation of issues which had once been defined as belonging properly to the realm of the expert. If the techniques derived from Keynesian economics could no longer be relied upon to produce growth, then inevitably politicians had to handle the conflicts generated by distributional issues. Moreover, the challenge to expertise was reinforced by a further trend, whose roots lay in the 1960s but which emerged with ever-increasing visibility in the course of the 1970S.[2] This was the emphasis on the values of participatory democracy: a revolt against centralised bureaucracy. Just as successive governments were reorganising the civil service, local government and the health service on criteria based on the values of efficiency (*see* previous chapter), so a groundswell of opposition to these values was making itself felt. Already in 1968, the publication of the Skeffington report[3] had reflected the demands for citizen involvement in the processes of town planning. In the 1970s, the demands increasingly spread to other policy areas.

The change was reflected in the currency of political rhetoric. Already in 1974 the Labour manifesto proclaimed that 'we want to give a much bigger say to citizens in all their various capacities – as tenants, shoppers, patients, voters. Or as residents or workers in areas where development proposals make them feel more planned against than planned for.' The Conservative manifesto made much of worker participation in industry and parent participation in the running of schools.[4] The rhetoric may not have been translated into action but it was significant as a recognition of a new mood. While the Right was suspicious of bureaucratic technocracy because of its belief in individualism, the Left was suspicious because of its commitment to wider participation in decision-making.

The second half of the 1970s therefore represent a retreat, begun under the Labour Government and accelerated under the Conservatives, from big government. While political scientists launched the concept of governmental overload[5] – of an imbalance between the demands on governments and their capacity to respond – economists identified rising public expenditure as the source of Britain's economic ills.[6] Intellectual arguments apart, in any case, governments had a more direct political incentive to try to restrain public spending: in a period of nil growth, rising public spending meant increasing taxation. Economic crisis compelled a choice between continuing to expand the public sector and maintaining disposable consumer incomes. By 1976 the Labour Government had made its choice. Between 1971–72 and 1975–76, the ratio of public expenditure to national income had risen from 50 to 60 per cent, the 1976 Public Expenditure White Paper pointed out.[7] Now the intention was to reverse this trend, and public expenditure plans were cut accordingly. It was the first of a succession of such attempts to hold back the momentum of the inherited public expenditure policies: attempts which reflected a reluctant concession to economic and political pressures by the Labour Government and an enthusiastic ideological commitment by the Conservative administration.

This, then, was the NHS's new economic, political and intellectual environment in the second half of the 1970s. All the factors identified – the increasing ideological polarisation of politics, the revolt against the values of expertise, the interest in participatory democracy and, above all, the commitment to reducing public expenditure – were to have an influence on the politics of the health care arena, as we shall see. Indeed the internal politics of the health care arena are incomprehensible unless account is taken of these new environmental forces. But, equally, it is important to stress, the process of change was gradual: there was no frontal assault, only a dawning realisation that the perceptions and assumptions which had for so long shaped health care policies required adapting to the new environment.

To a remarkable degree, the NHS remained sheltered, if not insulated, from the harsh new economic and political environment in which it was operating. It was protected, as always, by its continuing popularity. The political consensus – although frayed by ideological battles (*see* below) – held. In the 1979 election, both parties committed themselves to giving financial priority to the NHS, just as both committed themselves to simplifying its structure. Despite the annual ritual of public expenditure cuts, spending on the NHS was not reduced. In the financial year 1980–81 the current budget of the NHS was £644 million higher in volume terms (measuring the input of real resources) than it had been in 1975–76: a rise of 9.3 per cent over the period.[8] As in the past, and in line with the analysis offered in the previous chapter, successive Secretaries of State traded in reductions in the NHS's investment programme in return for safeguarding the current budget against cuts: capital spending declined throughout the period. In contrast, spending on both education and housing – both programmes which in the 1950s and later had taken precedence over the NHS – actually fell during the same period, substantially so in the case of housing. Clearly, the NHS had moved to the top of the queue in terms of the political priorities in the allocation of resources: its share of the national income was rising (a fact which reflected as much the decline in the national income itself as the increase in the NHS budget).

If the reality was a rising budget, the perception within the NHS was of increasing financial stringency. The rhetoric of financial crisis rose to a crescendo in the second half of the 1970s, and provides the background music to the specific policy issues explored subsequently in this chapter. This is a phenomenon already encountered and explored previously in the context of the 1960s, and many of the factors which explained the perception of inadequacy in a period of expanding budgets in the 1960s continued to be relevant in the 1970s. The demands generated by demographic changes and technological developments continued to assert themselves. Moreover, the gap between what could be done within the budgetary limits of the NHS and what could be done in the health services of wealthier nations widened, if anything, as Britain's national income fell ever further behind that of Sweden, Germany and other advanced industrialised nations.

There were other, more specific reasons. The opening years of the decade had seen an exceptionally fast rate of growth in the NHS budget: an average annual rate of increase of 4.3 per cent under the 1970–74 Conservative Government. In contrast, the equivalent figure under the 1974–79 Labour Government was only 1.5 per cent: the Labour Government's ideological commitment to the NHS having been eroded by the waves of economic crisis.[9] The figure was maintained at the lower level by the incoming Conservative Government in 1979. So, the NHS was a case of relative deprivation over time. Moreover, the perception of stringency was reinforced by growing uncertainty and unpredictability. In 1976 the Treasury introduced a new system for controlling public expenditure: the so-called cash limits system. This meant that if the costs of providing any particular level of public provision rose faster than assumed by the Treasury – particularly if wages and salaries, which accounted for about 70 per cent of the NHS's total budget, increased faster than predicted – there would be no automatic supplementation as in the past. Instead, there would have to be a compensatory cut in the input of real resources. In both 1976–77 and 1979–80, the NHS suffered from a severe cash limits squeeze;[10] all budgetary commitments had to be hurriedly revised during the course of the financial year. In the latter year, there was virtually no growth in the NHS's budget in terms of real resources. The figures of average annual increases thus tend to present a somewhat misleading picture of the NHS's financial position, in so far as they iron out the disconcerting year-by-year fluctuations.

More important still, financial turbulence threatened to make nonsense of the principles on which the 1974 NHS was designed. The philosophy of reorganisation was, as we have seen, to create an NHS which could carry out rational planning. Reorganisation was followed by a flurry of planning initiatives. In 1976 the DHSS unveiled its planning system: a system whereby the health authorities were intended to produce strategic plans, reflecting DHSS guidelines and national priorities.[11] The same year the DHSS published a priorities document,[12] setting out its objectives for different services: objectives expressed partly in terms of norms of provision and partly in terms of expenditure allocations. At the same time, the department was pursuing its policies for redressing inequities in the geographical distribution of resources by means of differential growth rates in the allocation of funds to the regions. All these strategies assumed not only growth but some degree of predictability: in other words, the NHS found itself committed to a whole range of policy objectives, forged in the era of optimism about economic prospects, and about the consequent scope for rational long-term planning – just as it entered the era of economic pessimism.

Symbolic of its dilemmas, the NHS found itself increasingly embarrassed by the completion of the hospitals designed and approved in the days of optimism. These had been built on the assumption that future generations would inevitably be better able to afford higher standards than their predecessors; accordingly, their running costs were much higher than those of the buildings they were to replace. Economic crisis had shattered the underlying assumption, but the financial commitments embodied in the new hospitals remained. So the great success story of NHS planning in the 1960s became, ironically enough, one of the causes of financial stringency by the end of the 1970s. It is therefore not surprising (*see* below) that the faith in planning was, in turn, to become a casualty in the new political and economic environment. Compounding these problems of the NHS, there were the changes within the arena of health care policy: changes which were in part specific to the NHS but which also reflected the wider environmental forces discussed above. It is to an analysis of these that we now turn.

The exploding health care policy arena

If the 1960s gave birth to a new spirit of militancy among those working in the NHS, as noted in the previous chapter, by the mid-1970s the infant had grown into a large, aggressive adult. The phenomenon marked the convergence of two trends. While the trade unions began increasingly to demonstrate the kind of obstreperous assertiveness which had once been the monopoly of the medical profession, the medical profession in turn began to use the weapons of industrial warfare which had once been the monopoly of the trade unions. Implicit in this was a shift in the balance of power. For the trade unions – and other organisations representing the non-medical professions in the NHS – militancy was a sign of a growing awareness of their muscle, of their ability to exert pressure by threatening to withdraw their labour. This was a threat which was all the more persuasive given the complex nature of the NHS, and its dependence on the spontaneous co-operation of people with a large variety of skills. In the case of the medical profession, however, militancy reflected a collective sense that power was slipping away from the doctors and towards the other participants in the NHS policy arena: gone were the days when the medical profession could assume that it could get its way without indulging in such unprofessional conduct as taking industrial action.

The growing militancy of the trade unions can be explained partly by reasons specific to the NHS, partly by more general societal factors. For the trade unions, the NHS provided a tempting game reserve for recruitment. Between 1948 and 1974, the proportion of NHS workers belonging to trade unions rose from 40 to 60 per cent, with most of the increase coming in the second half of the period.[13] By the standards of the public sector, even 60 per cent represented a low degree of unionisation: in central and local government, the proportion was nearly 90 per cent. So here there was a direct incentive to the trade unions to show their muscle: to advertise the advantages of membership by pressing for higher wages and salaries. The 1973 strike of ancillary workers had not only brought results; it had also destroyed the traditional assumption that people working in the NHS simply did not take industrial action – that their responsibilities to the patients necessarily imposed a self-denying ordinance on them.

Further compounding militancy was the fact the trade unions were competing against each other for members. There were, for example, no clear demarcation lines between the Confederation of Health Service Employees (COHSE) and the National Union of Public Employees (NUPE). The former tended to recruit chiefly among those with the least prestigious professional qualifications, such as the less skilled nurses working in mental care and other long-stay hospitals. The latter tended to recruit chiefly among ancillary workers: hospital porters, ward orderlies and cooks. But there was a considerable degree of overlap between them. Lastly, the trade unions were not only competing against each other but also against professional organisations: in particular, they increasingly challenged the Royal College of Nursing's role of acting both as a professional organisation and as a trade union. Militancy was further encouraged, if only inadvertently, by national policies in the 1970s. It was the National Board for Prices and Incomes which encouraged the introduction of local productivity deals in the NHS, in the hope that pay settlements could become self-financing.[14] Negotiating such deals gave greater salience to the role of the trade unions: an unexpected by-product of the drive for greater national efficiency. Equally important was the recurrent introduction of incomes policies by successive Labour and Conservative governments. These tended to distort traditional patterns of differentials so creating, in time, pressures to restore the inherited wage and salary contours: paradoxically a conservative attachment to inherited patterns thus became a source of radicalism.

The new assertiveness of the NHS workers paid dividends. If the real input of resources into the NHS increased only slowly, the input of money soared up: between 1974 and 1976 alone, there was a rise of 25 per cent in the cost of the NHS (in constant price terms) – reflecting largely a series of expensive pay settlements. Indeed NHS workers did better than the population as a whole.[15] Between 1970 and 1975, the average earnings of British workers rose by 107.8 per cent. The equivalent figure for ancillary workers in the NHS, however, was 134 per cent, while that for nurses was 143 per cent. Only doctors were lagging behind: the equivalent figure for them was 84 per cent.[16]

It is therefore not surprising that the second half of the 1970s was a period of medical militancy, as well as of trade union militancy: of a gradual convergence in the tactics of the trade unions and the professional medical organisations. Medical salaries were particularly affected by income policies designed to favour lower-paid workers: not only were differentials between doctors and other NHS workers being squeezed, so were differentials within the medical profession. Above all, the medical profession was losing out on the comparability criterion put forward by the 1959 Royal Commission: its earnings were falling behind the comparable professions. The 1976 Review Body report drew attention to the 'anomalies and injustices' created by incomes policies.[17] The 1977 report concluded that the living standards of the average general practitioner or consultant had fallen by 20 per cent between 1975 and 1977.[18] The 1978 report underlined 'the need to reverse the serious decline in morale that has accompanied the decline in pay and standards of living relative to others in comparable walks of life since 1975'.[19] It was not until 1980 that the medical profession collectively managed to re-establish its traditional place in the hierarchy of rewards:[20] a place which was perhaps all the more strongly defended because it reflected the arbitrary accidents of history rather than being based on any rational or objective criteria.

So, for the first time in the history of the NHS, doctors took industrial action. The medical profession collectively had threatened to refuse to co-operate with the Government in both 1911 and 1946. But now, breaking with all precedent, they actually withdrew their labour without withdrawing from the NHS. In October 1975, junior hospital doctors in Leicestershire took industrial action over pay, which subsequently spread to the rest of the country. The details of the dispute are of no concern here.[21] But two aspects of it should be noted. First, contributing to the militancy, there was the competition between the BMA and the Medical Practitioners' Union (which had merged with a trade union, the Association of Scientific, Technical and Managerial Staffs, in 1970): the tactics of the junior doctors largely represented a grassroots revolt against the leadership of the BMA. Second, the outcome of the dispute was the introduction of an industrial-type contract for the junior hospital doctors, with overtime payments for virtually all hours worked over and above the basic 40-hour week: the notion of the professional being someone who looks after his patients at all times of the day and night had taken another knock. In turn, this system of overtime payments led to the erosion of differentials between senior registrars and consultants. The 1977 Review Body report specifically highlighted the conse-quent 'sense of injustice' felt by consultants.

In any case, the consultants were already embroiled in a battle with the Government over their contracts and private practice (*see* below). They, too, were adopting militant tactics: their 'sanctions' consisting of threats, only sporadically carried out, to limit their NHS working commitments to care for emergencies only.[22] The threat, made in 1974, split the medical profession. It was publicly criticised by the heads of the Royal Colleges. Even the *British Medical Journal* pointed out that the use of industrial sanctions 'represents a regrettable decline in professional self-esteem which could permanently damage relations between doctors and the public'.[23] The adoption of industrial sanctions would seem to be significant of a profoundly important shift in the position of the medical profession. It eroded the assumption that doctors were somehow different from other workers in the NHS: that their power reflected the legitimate deference paid to a profession with a calling to serve the public – a calling which imposed special responsibilities and inhibitions on them. Sir Theodore Fox, a former editor of *The Lancet* and a much respected medical figure, pointed out that the 'conversion of junior hospital doctors to the methods of militant trade unionism' suggested that 'they are beginning to see themselves as workers in an industry rather than members of a profession – as technologists rather than doctors'.[24]

The divisions within the medical profession ran deep, and in 1977 a special working party representing both the Royal Colleges and the BMA produced a discussion document on the ethical responsibilities of doctors.[25] The report offers an interesting view of how the doctors viewed the implicit concordat between the profession and the Government established in 1946. Doctors, the report con-ceded, had an ethical responsibility to their patients, but:

> Those who maintain that it is always unethical for a professional man to withdraw his services – which in the view of many is the only effective weapon available to him when persuasion fails – are in danger of accepting for doctors a position of subservience to their employers that would preclude them from maintaining their stan-dards. The desire not to harm patients by direct action may then result in harming them by doing nothing. It is unreasonable to expect a profession to remain passive in the face of declining standards, inadequate resources, and lay intervention in the doctor–patient relationship.

It was therefore essential, the report concluded, for:

> both sides to avoid causes of conflict to a point at which some withdrawal of services becomes the only remedy for doctors to preserve their professional standards and protect the long-term inter-ests of their patients. Government has a special responsibility not to create such conflict by pursuing purely political ends. The profession has a special responsibility not to create such conflict purely to further the advantage of its own members.

The report has been quoted at some length because it shows the nature of the dilemma faced by both government and the medical profession. Mutual depend-ence indicated conflict-avoidance strategies: if achieving change in the NHS was difficult, it was because of the inbuilt incentives to seek compromise – and to avoid action on those issues where conflict was inevitable. But since it was the medical profession which determined which policies were being pursued for 'purely political ends', the desire to avoid conflict inevitably tended to reinforce the veto power of the doctors over what appeared on the agenda for discussion.

The report also brings out into the open some of the tensions that were becoming apparent in the health care policy arena in the second half of the 1970s. 'The profession may justifiably think that it has an ethical responsibility to provide the best available treatment', the report argued, 'while the State may regard itself as being responsible to the community to limit the resources available to the National Health Service on criteria other than the needs of the patient.' This conflict was, as previously argued, always implicit in the structure of the NHS, but economic crisis inevitably meant that the other criteria would have greater force. Again, the report's complaint about 'lay intervention in the doctor–patient relationship' reflects the changes that were taking place. For the militancy of the trade unions did not find expression only in battles over pay. At the national level, it led them into a direct conflict with the medical profession over the issue of private beds in NHS hospitals, further discussed below: a direct challenge, as the doctors saw it, to what had hitherto been the medical domain of policy-making. At the local level, trade union members began to assert their right to share in decisions about hospital policy and, more threateningly still, to question clinical judgements. Significantly, it was the trade unions represented in the mental illness and chronic care sector – especially COHSE – which took the lead:

this was an area of the NHS where doctors were thin on the ground and where nurses traditionally had played a greater role. In a number of cases, the trade unions challenged medical decisions to admit patients. 'Who was responsible for patients – the consultant or the shop steward?', asked one indignant doctor.[26] In the case of Brookwood Hospital, staff announced the formation of a workers' council to run the 900-bed mental hospital: a significant, albeit temporary, assertion of worker syndicalism in rivalry to medical syndicalism.[27]

Adding to the medical profession's sense of losing control was the growing assertiveness of groups representing NHS consumers. The 1974 reorganisation institutionalised the voice of the consumer, as we have seen, in the shape of Community Health Councils, though their composition betrayed a basic ambiguity as to whether they were supposed to represent the local community as *consumers* of health services or as *citizens*. They were a compromise, as it were, between the demands of consumerism and the demands for participation: the former being essentially a market ideology concerned to maximise value for money and services, the latter being a political ideology concerned to maximise opportunities to influence policy. CHCs varied greatly in their style and their activities.[28] But they not only had the right to demand information; they also had the right to be consulted over decisions to close hospitals and other changes: any decisions not approved by CHCs had to be referred to the DHSS. Their power consisted, as it were, in the ability to throw grit into the normal machinery of NHS decision-making: to impose delays. While CHCs might in some circumstances be seen as allies by the medical profession – as platforms for publicising shortcomings in the service and so reinforcing their demands for more resources – they could also be perceived as a threat: a prime example of 'lay intervention'.

Others, too, were crowding into the health care policy arena. By 1979 a Directory of Organisations for Patients and Disabled People could list over 230 such bodies.[29] Some existed to provide services for deprived groups, to encourage research or to provide information. For example, the aims of the British Migraine Association were to encourage migraine sufferers to support research and to diffuse information about treatment, while the Sole Mates Club (*sic*) served to help 'people with odd shoe sizes to exchange shoes'. Others existed to provide a platform or forum for particular groups of patients or for people with special needs. For example, the Down's Children's Association sought to 'provide a forum for parents', among other objectives, while the Society To Support Home Confinements aimed 'to support, advise and assist women who want a home confinement but meet with difficulties when trying to make the necessary arrangements'. Only a minority of the organisations explicitly gave their aim as being to influence policy in the NHS, and thus can be classified as pressure groups in the traditional sense of that versatile phrase. For example, MIND gave its aim as being 'to campaign for the needs and rights of mentally ill and mentally handicapped people', while the British Kidney Patient Association sought to 'lobby for more facilities'.

Simply to list some of these organisations is, however, to suggest that even where their aim was not explicitly to exert influence, their mere existence served to introduce a new factor into the policy-making processes, both nationally and locally. Where previously decisions about maternity care policy were taken by the experts, in the light of their desire to minimise risks and maximise the medical technology available by concentrating all births in specialised hospital centres, now a group existed to articulate the desire of some women to have their babies at home, risks and all. The mere existence of an organisational focus for a particular group of patients was likely to give visibility to their demands. In short, the growth of such organisations multiplied the demands being made on the NHS: demands which involved calling for the investment of extra resources or which challenged existing clinical and other practices. It is important not to exaggerate. The growth of special interest groups and lobbies should not be interpreted as evidence of a general desire for public involvement in the health care policy arena. For the main characteristics of these groups and lobbies were that they were organised around very specific issues and were run by middle-class activists. Their strength lay precisely in the fact that they were unrepresentative of NHS consumers or citizens at large: that they were exceptionally articulate in putting forward the case for particular interests. But their mere existence represented a question mark against the traditional assumption that health care policies could be determined according to criteria of need and technical excellence, as defined by the experts, as against criteria based on consumer demands. The major battles were still fought by the big battalions of the health service producers: the theme of the next section. However, the political landscape against which these battles were fought had changed, if only marginally and subtly.

The politics of ideological confrontation: a case study

New forces operating in a new environment inevitably introduced a new kind of politics into the health care policy arena: the politics of ideological confrontation. Between 1974 and 1976 the Labour Government and the medical profession were locked into what was the most bitter political struggle since the inception of the NHS: the battle over private beds. It was not, of course, the first occasion on which the government and the doctors had come into conflict: conflict over pay, as noted in earlier chapters, provides a recurrent theme running through the entire history of the NHS. The battle over private beds was, however, different in that it threatened the very consensus which in the past had contained conflict. It therefore provides a case study of the impact of the changes in the arena of health care policy, and in its political environment, discussed in the previous section.[30]

The existence of pay beds in NHS hospitals, to which consultants could admit their private fee-paying patients, was a legacy of Bevan's 1946 compromise with the medical profession. They represented a concession to the consultants made in return for their support of the principle of the NHS. In 1974, when the crisis broke, there were 4,500 such pay beds, handling some 120,000 patients a year: they represented just over one per cent of all NHS beds and the private patients treated in them represented two per cent of all non-psychiatric cases handled in the NHS. If pay beds were relatively insignificant in terms of their numbers, however, their symbolic significance to the Labour Party was great. They represented a flaw in the pure crystal of the NHS's underlying conception: the idea that the treatment of patients should be determined exclusively by criteria of need, as distinct from the ability to pay. In theory, pay beds did not affront this principle. Private patients were buying not the right to treatment, only the right to be treated by a consultant of their own choice in a room of their own. But in practice, it was argued, pay beds allowed patients to jump the queue for treatment: there was at least some evidence to suggest that consultants would admit their private patients ahead of other people on the waiting list. The existence of private beds therefore introduced a dual system of standards into the NHS.

The issue was clearly defined by Barbara Castle, who became Secretary of State for the Social Services in the incoming Labour Government of 1974, and who led the attack on private beds. 'The issue before us is whether the facilities of the NHS, which are supposed to be available only on the principle of medical priority, should contain facilities that are available on the different principle of ability to pay. We say that those two principles are incompatible in the NHS', she told Parliament in 1974. In other words, the issue was central to Labour's vision of itself as a crusader for social justice. The religious metaphor is apt, as Mrs Castle was to point out on a subsequent occasion: 'Intrinsically the National Health Service is a church. It is the nearest thing to the embodiment of the Good Samaritan that we have in any respect of our public policy. What would we say of a person who argued that he could only serve God properly if he had pay pews in his church?'

Given this fundamental incompatibility between Labour's vision of the NHS and the existence of private beds, the decision to tackle this issue may seem the inevitable outcome of a long-standing ideological commitment. Barbara Castle was simply paying an overdue political debt to the party's ideals. But this still leaves an unexplained puzzle. Labour's hostility to private beds was long-standing. But the previous Labour Government, in office from 1964 to 1970, had done nothing about them. Kenneth Robinson, the Labour Minister of Health, had reduced the number of pay beds, not on ideological grounds but because they were much under-utilised: he did so in agreement with the medical profession, in return for lifting the limits on the fees that could be charged by consultants. So why did the 1974 Labour Government act, while its predecessor had resolutely ignored the issue?

One explanation lies in the increasing salience of the issue within the Labour Party. In 1971 the Labour majority on the Employment and Social Services Sub-Committee of the Parliamentary Expenditure Committee exploited an inquiry into NHS facilities for private patients to direct attention to the abuse (as they saw it) of these facilities. Their report argued that the system of pay beds permitted 'queue jumping for non-medical reasons', that it was unfair on junior hospital doctors, nurses and technicians 'used for private purposes and without willing consent', and that it encouraged consultants to congregate in those parts of the country where there was greatest scope for private practice. The report was based on thin evidence, but its conclusions had resonance within the Labour Party. The Party's latent sensitivity on this issue was activated. The 1974 Labour manifesto pledged the Party to 'phase out private practice from the hospital service'. The manifesto also pledged the Labour Party to carry out another long-standing ideological commitment: to 'abolish prescription charges'. This, however, remained a dead-letter throughout the Labour Government's period in office. So the implementation of the pledge to phase out private beds cannot be seen as the inevitable consequence of the manifesto commitment. There was nothing automatic about the implementation of such pledges, particularly if they cost money. Barbara Castle's decision to act on the issue of pay beds reflected the changing balance of power both within the health care policy arena and in its environment. The political costs of doing nothing had become greater than the political costs of action.

No sooner was Barbara Castle installed in office, than her hand was forced. At Charing Cross Hospital – one of London's major teaching hospitals, strategically situated for attracting the attention of the media – members of NUPE took strike action in an attempt to force the closure of the private wing. Sporadically, similar action followed in other hospitals throughout the country: action which perhaps reflected as much hostility to the special privileges enjoyed by private patients, and the extra income derived by consultants, as ideological commitment. Barbara Castle tried to enlist the support of the trade union leaders to head off this attempt to take direct action. But as Len Murray, the Secretary-General of the Trades Union Congress told her, 'Congress is in favour of getting rid of private practice'.[31] Although the leaders of the health service trade unions had not instigated the industrial action – 'we didn't spark off the campaign . . . the issue blew up fortuitously', one of them remarked – the strikes had given political visibility to their own, long-standing commitment to closing private beds. Even if they had wanted to do so, they could not now consign this commitment to the limbo of pledges made in the confident belief that they would never have to be implemented. Nor could the Labour Government, dependent as it was on the co-operation of the trade unions for the success of its economic policies. While it might have been able to ride out the protests of the grassroots movement, it could not afford to ignore the demands of organised labour: private beds would be phased out.

The attack on private beds was essentially ideological: an attack on visible symbols of privilege. But the more general issue of private practice also raised some non-ideological issues. If private practice was obnoxious in principle to the Labour Party, it was irritating in practice to those committed to introducing more rational planning into the NHS. By the mid-1970s, the proportion of consultants holding part-time contracts – that is, ones permitting them to engage in private practice – had fallen to below 50 per cent. But the very existence of the system introduced some perverse incentives into the NHS. While the aim of public policy was to encourage the development of the mental illness, geriatric and chronic care services, part-time contracts gave doctors an incentive to move into those specialties where the opportunities for private practice were greatest. Thus 94 per cent of all consultants in geriatric medicine had whole-time contracts, as against less than 15 per cent in general surgery. Similarly, while the aim of public policy was to achieve a better geographical distribution of specialists and other doctors, part-time contracts gave doctors an incentive (as the Expenditure Committee had noted) to move into those parts of the country where opportunities for private practice were greatest, notably London and other well-provided regions.

At the same time that Barbara Castle was pursuing the issue of pay beds, the Minister of Health – Dr David Owen, who could by no stretch of the imagination be described as a left-wing ideologue – was therefore trying to negotiate a new contract with the consultants. These negotiations had begun in 1972: the consultants, fired by the success of the general practitioners and junior hospital doctors, were themselves anxious to negotiate a new form of contract. In particular, they wanted to secure a contract where payments would be more directly related to the amount of work done: where their commitments to the NHS would no longer be open-ended and where, consequently, they would have a chance to supplement their basic salaries by overtime and other payments. But the Labour Government introduced a new element into the negotiations. It sought to introduce financial incentives designed to encourage full-time practice in the NHS. Extra rewards were to go to those consultants who committed themselves wholly to the NHS; the merit award system, which tended to be biased towards the most prestigious specialties where private practice flourished, was to be replaced by payments for particularly valuable contributions to the running of the service – payments available only to whole-timers, moreover.

The combination of the Labour Government's commitment to phasing out pay beds from the NHS and of the new proposals for loading the consultant contract in favour of full-time consultants turned out to be explosive. For the medical profession, these steps represented a repudiation of the 1946 concordat: an attempt by the Labour administration to abolish the right of doctors to engage in private practice. No matter that Barbara Castle assured them that she merely wanted to separate private practice from the NHS, not to abolish it; the suspicions of the doctors were reinforced by the 1975 Labour Party Conference which voted, much to Barbara Castle's dismay, in favour of the outright abolition of all private medicine. No matter that a majority of consultants, the full-timers, would actually benefit from the proposed changes in the contract: even if the leaders of the profession had been disposed to compromise, the rivalry between the BMA and the Hospital Consultants' and Specialists' Association meant that they were engaged in a competition in militancy.

For the medical profession, as for the Labour Party, the issue of private practice was symbolic. Self-interest was, of course, involved. Private practice added on average something like 20 per cent to the incomes of those NHS consultants who engaged in it. Moreover, a minority of consultants could make much more: one indignant consultant, appalled at the prospect of losing his pay beds, pointed out that he could double his NHS income simply by carrying out 24 private operations a year.[32] More centrally, any threat to private practice aroused the medical profession's fear of total dependency on the State. If many consultants and other doctors who did not benefit personally from private practice yet fought to preserve it, the reason was that it was a symbol of professional independence. It was, in truth, a fragile symbol. The reality was that doctors did depend financially on the State, and that private practice represented not an alternative to their incomes from the NHS but icing on the cake. But perhaps it was the very fragility of the symbol that made doctors all the more sensitive to perceived threats. The confrontation that followed between Ministers and the medical profession was more bitter than any in the history of the NHS. Nothing like it had been seen since the days when Bevan was embattled with the general practitioners. Meetings between Ministers and the medical profession inevitably ended in acrimony, as Mrs Castle faithfully recorded in her diaries. Finally, the medical profession, as noted in the previous section, mobilised for battle: its ultimate deterrent – sanctions – was wheeled on stage.

Like other ultimate deterrents, that of the medical profession was more for show than use. In any case, as we have already seen, doctors were by no means unanimous in supporting such a weapon. Similarly, the Government did not want to risk an all-out battle with the medical profession. 'This Cabinet had no fire in its belly for this particular fight', Barbara Castle noted at one point in the negotiations.[33] Moreover, within the DHSS, civil servants were unenthusiastic in their support for their minister's policies. From their point of view, the long-term political costs of a confrontation with the medical profession over the issue of private practice outweighed any possible benefits. If Barbara Castle was dependent on the support of her political constituency in the Labour Party and the trade unions, her civil servants were dependent on the organisational constituency of the NHS. Phasing out private beds might well be desirable; negotiating a new contract might well be advantageous. But maintaining a working relationship with the medical profession was essential if other desirable or advantageous aims of policy were to be achieved in future. There was no point in exhausting the capital of goodwill over a largely symbolic issue. Not surprisingly, therefore, moves to devise a compromise soon followed. In 1975 Harold Wilson, the Prime Minister, intervened. He brought into action Lord Goodman, an experienced mediator, to act as go-between between Barbara Castle and the medical profession over the issue of pay beds. He also set up a Royal Commission to examine the state of the NHS: so responding to the demands of the doctors for an inquiry into the whole basis, financial as well as organisational, of the NHS.

The Goodman compromise, translated into legislation in 1976 with virtually no changes, was based on two principles. First, it was agreed that private beds and facilities should be separated from the NHS. Second, the Government formally recognised that private practice should be maintained in Britain, and that doctors should be entitled to work both privately and in NHS establishments. All this was in line with Mrs Castle's own Consultative Document on Private Practice published in 1975.[34] But the Goodman formula included other features designed to reassure the medical profession. Only 1,000 of the pay beds were to be phased out immediately. Decisions about phasing out the rest were to be taken not by the Secretary of State but by an independent board with half its four members drawn from the medical profession and the rest appointed after consultations with the trade unions and other interested parties; an independent chairman would have the casting vote. The board, to quote the Secretary of State, would be guided by the following criteria in phasing out pay beds: 'That there should be a reasonable demand for private medicine in the area of the country served by a particular hospital; that sufficient accommodation and facilities existed in the area for the reasonable operation of private medicine; and that all reasonable steps had been or were being taken to provide those alternative beds and facilities.' In contrast to the Consultative Document, which had proposed that the total size of the private sector should be frozen, no such limit was set under the Goodman formula. Similarly, no date was set for the completion of the phasing out operation. In 1980 – when the Health Services Board, set up to implement these policies, was wound up by the Conservative Government – the number of pay beds in England had been reduced from 3,444 to 2,533.[35]

The negotiations over the consultant contract dragged on for the remainder of the Labour Government's term of office. Again, the outcome was a compromise. The profession secured changes designed to 'relate remuneration more closely to the work done':[36] in other words, consultants were to share in the opportunities, already enjoyed by their juniors, to get overtime payments. In exchange the DHSS obtained changes which slightly tilted the financial advantage towards full-time consultants. The proposal to abolish the merit award system was dropped; in return, though, it also was to be amended to favour full-timers. However, the 1979 contract never came into force. Disagreement about its pricing – not about its principles – prevented its implementation. It was left to the incoming Conservative Government to introduce a new contract (*see* below).

In the end, therefore, the consensus about the NHS emerged from the post-1974 crisis battered and frayed but still basically intact. Conflict had, after all, been constrained by consensus. In retrospect the bitterness aroused by the issues involved seemed disproportionate to their importance. As the Royal Commission put it in its 1979 report, 'We have reached no conclusions about the overall balance of advantage or disadvantage of the existence of a private sector . . . but it is clear that whichever way it lies it is small as matters now stand'. Moreover, it pointed out, 'From the point of view of the NHS the main importance of pay beds lies in the passions aroused'.[37]

If the drama of these years did little to change the nature of the NHS, it did, however, illuminate the changed nature of the health care policy arena itself. Not only did the issue of pay beds represent a threat to the existing order – the intrusion of political ideology into the NHS's organisational ideology, with its emphasis on incremental change achieved through consensus-engineering – but it also revealed powerful new actors on stage: the trade unions. It showed that, in the last resort, the medical profession could only respond to the challenge of these new forces by adopting their tactics and by conceding openly that its own power rested not on its professional status but on its ability to use its industrial muscle.

The politics of organisational stasis

The confrontation between the medical profession and the Government, the growing assertiveness of the trade unions and the gradual tightening of the NHS's budget all contributed to the sense of crisis which marked the second half of the 1970s. 'We were appointed at a time when there was widespread concern about the NHS', the Royal Commission commented in its 1979 report. Not for the first time the NHS offered the seemingly paradoxical spectacle of contented consumers and disgruntled producers. While the consumers were continuing to show overwhelming satisfaction with the services provided by the NHS, as shown by surveys carried out on behalf of the Royal Commission,[38] the producers were protesting about falling standards. If there was a revolution of frustrated expectations, it was among the producers not among the consumers.

To an extent the discontent of the producers – doctors, nurses and others – reflected a special characteristic of the NHS discussed earlier: the fact that producers had a direct incentive to emphasise the shortcomings of the NHS in order to dramatise their own case for better pay and conditions of work. But compounding this endemic discontent was the dry rot of disillusionment with the new structure of the NHS created by the 1974 reorganisation. This disillusionment was, to a large extent perhaps, merely the rationalisation of a general sense of frustration reflecting the gap between the hopes aroused in the years of optimism and the financial reality of the years of economic crisis. But it also reflected the fact that the reorganised NHS was not delivering the goods: that the vision of a rationally planned health service was not being translated into reality. On the contrary, the reorganised NHS appeared to have introduced new obstacles in the way of implementing change.

Hardly had the new NHS been inaugurated, than the critics of Sir Keith Joseph's architecture appeared to have been justified. The new structure, it was widely agreed, was indeed too complex. Designed to please everyone, the structure satisfied no one. By 1977 a survey of 482 administrators and others working in the NHS[39] showed overwhelming dissatisfaction with the structure. Four-fifths of those interviewed favoured some change to reduce the number of tiers. Moreover, structural complexity did lead to greater bureaucracy – at least as measured by the number of administrators employed. The number of administrative and clerical staff rose from 87,000 in 1973 to 113,000 in 1976, when the DHSS launched a drive to cut the costs of management. Nor, on the face of it, had the new NHS solved the problems which it was designed to tackle. Implicit in the reorganisation was a clear separation in the functions of central government and the peripheral health authorities, encapsulated in the gnomic phrase (quoted in Chapter 3) of 'maximum delegation downward, maximum accountability upward'. The centre would lay down policy objectives; the periphery would implement them. In practice reorganisation did little to resolve the tensions between centre and periphery, inherent in the concept of the NHS as a national service financed out of public funds.

For how could the DHSS delegate, while it remained accountable to Parliament for every penny spent? Not surprisingly, the complaints about excessive interference by the centre that followed reorganisation were remarkably similar to those already encountered in the pre-reorganisation days. In 1976 a report produced by the chairmen of the regional authorities[40] rehearsed a familiar litany of grievances. The DHSS was exercising an excessive degree of control over building: 'Rather than promote the economic and effective use of capital, the system of detailed checking produces interference in minutiae and certainly results in duplication of staff and effort; there is often argument over petty design detail, and above all lengthy delay.' Moreover, the department – in the view of the regional chairmen – spent an excessive amount of time following up the 3,000 parliamentary questions that were asked every year by MPs: the DHSS should leave it to the field authorities to deal with these questions and resist the temptation 'to interpret or check the results'. Overall, those working in the NHS were baffled by the complexity of the DHSS's internal structure, frustrated by the department's habit of 'proffering advice on unattainable objectives which cannot be funded' and resentful of the rigidity imposed by national agreements about numbers of staff and levels of pay: 'Too often in the NHS, authorities are forced under existing regulations to employ staff of inadequate calibre, where fewer – but better – people would produce much more effective results.' And the report concluded by calling for 'a reduction in the functions performed by the DHSS and a consequent reduction in size'. The department's chief function should be to act 'as the midwife of ideas' – leaving detailed implementation to the administrators and professionals at the periphery who, in any case, were better informed and better equipped to take decisions than the rotating cast of civil servants at the centre.

Yet while those at the periphery were voicing their resentment of central control, Parliament was voicing its dissatisfaction at the lack of effective accountability. The Committee of Public Accounts was pressing the DHSS to tighten up financial control: 'We remain disturbed about the effectiveness of the financial control exercised by some health authorities, and we recommend that urgent considerations should continue to be given to means of improving financial control and accountability within the present structure', it reported in 1977.[41] The Social Services Sub-Committee of the Expenditure Committee was urging the DHSS to devise more effective tools for monitoring what was happening in the NHS. Expenditure statistics, it argued in 1977, should be complemented by information about 'the adequacy or otherwise of the services provided, in terms either of the availability of facilities for treatment or of standards of care'.[42] The theme was to recur, again and again, in the reports of the Expenditure Committee's successor, the Social Services Committee. Its 1980 report, for example, stressed the need to develop 'a comprehensive information system which would permit this Committee and the public to assess the effects of changes in expenditure levels or patterns on the quality and scope of services provided'.[43]

The DHSS's dilemma – caught in a crossfire of criticism from both the NHS authorities and Parliament – further underlines a fundamental weakness in the whole concept of rational planning which underlay reorganisation. The rhetoric was all about accountability and monitoring. But what was the currency of accountability and where were the tools of monitoring? It was easy enough to establish a machinery of financial accountability and an administrative hierarchy responsible for monitoring. But it was much more difficult to answer questions about what the money was buying in terms of services provided to patients or about the quality of the care being offered. The required instruments of measurement simply did not exist. Indeed the available information was dangerously ambiguous. The DHSS might well have figures of the unit costs of treating patients in acute beds or patients in hospitals for the mentally handicapped. The general presumption was that it was desirable to lower the unit costs of treating each acute patient (since it was a sign of increased efficiency) and to increase the unit costs of caring for long-stay patients (since this was a sign of improved quality as measured by the input of staff). This, indeed, was the aim of DHSS policy, and by the end of the 1970s, it was succeeding.[44] But there remained some nagging questions. What if lower unit costs in acute beds reflected, as the doctors were inclined to claim, not increased efficiency but lower quality? What if higher unit costs in the chronic care sector reflected not better quality care for patients but more leisure for staff?

In the attempt to answer such questions, the DHSS inevitably was drawn into taking a close interest in the implementation of policy. The only information available was qualitative, DHSS witnesses repeatedly told the Social Services Committee: the impressions of the department's professionals. Only professionals, in other words, could assess the work of other professionals. Judgements of adequacy or quality could not be derived from statistics but had to be based on expert opinion. Much the same was true of planning. The DHSS might publish priorities documents setting out desirable objectives expressed in norms of inputs (whether beds or nurses) for particular client groups such as the mentally handicapped or the elderly. Similarly, the department might publish a programme budget showing the desired shifts in expenditure patterns as between different client groups. But, given the principle of infinite diversity the department could not impose such norms irrespective of local circumstances. On closer inspection, the DHSS's apparently solid policy targets dissolved under the acid of reservations. 'Local priorities will naturally be affected by a range of factors – demographic, social and practical – peculiar to individual areas; and it is accepted that local plans will often not correspond to the order of national priorities proposed here', the DHSS's 1976 Priorities Document admitted. And its 1977 successor made it clear that the expenditure objectives – envisaging a shift of resources to favour the elderly and other deprived groups, and from the hospital to the community services – were 'not specific targets to be reached by declared dates in any locality'.[45] In practice the language of norms and objectives turned out to be merely a vocabulary of exhortation.

No wonder that studies of policy-making within individual health authorities unanimously came to the conclusion that national priorities impinged at best marginally on local decision-making: that decisions were shaped, unsurprisingly, by the constraints of inherited commitments and the balance of power within the arena of local health care policy.[46] Exhortation could help to nudge such decisions in the direction desired by the central department; for example, between 1975–76 and 1979–80 the average annual expenditure on geriatric services rose by 2.3 per cent, as against only 1.1 per cent for acute services, while spending on community services rose marginally faster than that on hospital services.[47] The price to be paid for such success was, once again, continued pressure and intervention by the DHSS. If planning could not be carried out in terms of imposing centrally determined norms and standards on the periphery, then it inevitably became a process of negotiation between the two sides. If rationality could not be found in *techniques* – by devising formulas for priorities and standards on the basis of consulting the entrails of epidemiological statistics or the application of other scientific methods – then it had to be sought in *process*: in institutionalising dialogue between centre and periphery. In short, the experience of attempting to plan rationally not only led to greater scepticism about the concept itself, as awareness of the technical problems involved grew,[48] but also perpetuated the dominating role of the DHSS. If the rationality of any policy had to be tested by the way in which it was implemented locally, then the DHSS could not disinterest itself. Contrary to the hopeful assumptions made before 1974, the line between policy-making and implementation was far too blurred to permit a neat separation of central and local functions.

The years following 1974 also undermined some of the other assumptions underlying the 1974 reorganisation. The justification for introducing an area tier into the administration structure of the NHS was, it will be recalled, that co-terminosity between health and local authorities would lead to co-operation. Experience suggested otherwise,[49] even though in 1976 the DHSS introduced financial incentives designed to encourage collaboration: earmarked grants for schemes jointly worked out between health and local authorities. Predictably the incentives built into the very structure of the two services turned out to be stronger: each of the two services had an incentive to offload problems on to the other, each tended to define issues in terms of the rather different perspectives of its own professionals. Moreover, government policies – while extolling the virtues of co-operation at the local level – were themselves notably lacking in co-ordination at the national level. If the DHSS was anxious to encourage the development of community services, the Treasury was even more anxious to cut back the growth of local government spending. Even while the DHSS was planning on the assumption of expansions in such local government services, the Treasury was making it impossible. From 1979 onward the Government was putting pressure on local authorities to cut spending on the personal social services.[50]

Again, the architects of the 1974 reorganisation had assumed that defining the roles of the members of the new Area Health Authorities more tightly would produce more effective management. Not only would members of AHAs be collectively accountable for implementing national policy, but they, in turn, would also ensure that their officers were accountable to them. In practice, AHA members turned out to be a weak link in the chain of accountability. On the one hand, according to a 1977 survey,[51] they 'found it difficult because of lack of time as much as of knowledge to come to grips with so complex a system'. On the other hand, the consensus system of decision-making in officer teams meant that AHA members tended to be offered agreed solutions, not alternative proposals, so giving them little scope to influence policy. The gap between the role accorded to AHAs in the philosophy of reorganisation and their actual performance, between the doctrine and the practice of accountability, is admirably illustrated by the example of the Normansfield Hospital Inquiry:[52] a case study which also illustrates some of the other themes developed in this chapter. The inquiry was held in 1978, nine years after the similar inquiry into conditions at Ely (*see* previous chapter), which had illustrated many of the weaknesses in the pre-reorganisation NHS and reinforced the case for changes. Like Ely, Normansfield was a hospital for the mentally handicapped. Like the Ely inquiry, the Normansfield inquiry revealed some scandalous conditions.

Perhaps the most significant aspect of the Normansfield affair – as revealed in the inquiry – was that everyone had known about the problems that afflicted the hospital. Everybody, at all levels, was well aware that 'the standard of nursing care was extremely low and the quality of life of many of the patients suffered accordingly'. Everybody, too, knew the main cause: the personal eccentricities and conduct of the consultant psychiatrist whose running battle with nursing staff and medical colleagues turned the familiar problems of hospitals for the mentally handicapped, decaying buildings and staff shortages, into what one visitor described as a 'time-bomb'. The CHC had done its duty by protesting about conditions at Normansfield. A succession of visitors – from the DHSS, from the region and from the AHA – agreed that the situation was appalling. But nothing was done until a strike by the nurses compelled the setting up of the inquiry, which in turn eventually led to the retirement of the consultant.

The case of Normansfield was significant for a number of reasons. First, it once again showed the new militancy of NHS workers. Second, it demonstrated the limits to CHC influence: CHCs could protest, but they could not compel action. Third, it underlined the ineffectiveness of AHA members. 'The conditions we saw during our four days of visiting', the inquiry report commented, 'gave every appearance of being of some duration and were such as to make us wonder how sensitive, caring members of the Authority could have tolerated them without vigorous protest leading to concerted action by officials of the Authority.' Fourth, it suggested that both the central department and the regional authority were prepared to invoke the doctrine of delegation of responsibility in order to avoid being drawn into a messy imbroglio. Lastly, and perhaps most important, it demonstrated the importance of the inertia factor in the NHS as a whole: the difficulty of introducing change – in particular when change involved dealing with a consultant.

The paradox of the reorganised NHS was that it strengthened the inertia factor at precisely the point – as argued at the beginning of this chapter – in the history of the service when external pressures and internal demands were reinforcing the need for change. If new priorities to favour the deprived groups of patients were to be implemented in a period of only marginal growth in the total NHS budget, then this could only be achieved by shifting resources from existing services. If geographical equity in the distribution of resources was to be achieved, then once again resources would have to be shifted from the well-endowed to the poorly endowed parts of the country. The latter problem was particularly acute at the sub-regional level. The national formula for allocating resources to the regions – the RAWP formula – did not involve cutting the funds of any region. If the rate of differential growth slowed down, and the date for achieving equity kept on being postponed, at least all the regions could count on getting at least a marginal increment every year. But within the regions things were different, particularly in the case of London. In the national context, the London regions were relatively over-provided. But within them, many of the areas were under-provided. While the population of London was mobile, hospitals were not; while the population moved into the suburbs, and beyond, inner London was left with an embarrassing surplus of hospitals. The demands of the outer London areas could only be satisfied by cutting hospital provision in inner London: demands which were all the more insistent since the creation of AHAs had given political visibility to the distribution of resources below the regional level.[53]

Reorganisation had, however, increased the costs of such adaptation by institutionalising the right to oppose change. The ability to veto change – or, at the very least, to resist it it by imposing delays – had been diffused. Within the NHS, any decision had to go through the elaborate system of advisory committees which had been set up in 1974. Outside the NHS, a variety of other bodies also had to be consulted: the emphasis on co-ordinating health and local authority services inevitably led to the perfectly logical conclusion that NHS planning should no longer be an introspective process. Thus the DHSS handbook on planning instructed AHAs to consult: CHCs, local authorities, the Family Practitioner Committee, the various Area Advisory Committees and the Joint Staff Consultative Committee. In addition to the formal mechanisms introduced by the 1974 reorganisation, however, the expansion of the health care policy arena reinforced the opposition to change. No sooner was a hospital threatened by closure than informal action committees sprang up: coalitions of workers whose jobs were threatened and groups of citizens whose access to their local health facilities was in danger. If national policy was designed to bring about equity, local interests had an interest in perpetuating inequity where the existing distribution of resources favoured them.

The point is well illustrated by a case history drawn from the research evidence submitted to the Royal Commission:[54] the closure of Poplar Hospital – a small institution, built in 1855, in the East End of London. The dispute over the closure started in 1972; the doors of the hospital did not actually close until the end of 1975. It is a reminder therefore that while the reorganisation of the NHS may have exacerbated the problems of change, the new structure cannot be blamed for all the difficulties. The most significant aspect of the long-drawn-out process was the militancy and numbers of the local opposition groups. Just taking this one local health care policy arena, the actors included: consultants, the Hospital's League of Friends, local MPs, the local Labour Party, a specially formed Save Poplar Campaign, NUPE, local councillors and the Transport and General Workers' Union. The strategy of delay included both a local press campaign and appeals to the Secretary of State. The issue moved repeatedly up and down the decision-making hierarchy: from the District Management Team to the Area, from the Area to the Region, from the Region to the DHSS, and so da capo. The wonder is not that it took three years to close Poplar Hospital but that it was ever closed at all.

To describe the delays and administrative costs involved in implementing change may, however, understate the full effect of the growing capacity of an increasing number of actors to throw grit into the machinery: to introduce politics into the self-contained world of the NHS and to challenge the monopoly of technical expertise in decision-making. This could only be measured in terms of the decisions that were not even contemplated for fear of the consequences: the way in which the new political and organisational factors constrained the sense of what was feasible. If the emphasis on decision-making through agreement – the hallmark of the 1974 reorganisation – had started out as a strategy for mobilising consent to change, it had ended up as a strategy for encouraging the mobilisation of opposition to change. The perverse irony, it turned out, was that public interest in health care policy seemed to be a function of opposition to national policies. Once again we recognise a familiar phenomenon in health care politics: while national constituencies for change are diffuse, local constituencies representing the status quo are concentrated and organised. It was a phenomenon which contributed in no small measure to the sense of disillusionment with the possibilities for using the NHS as an instrument of rational social engineering that characterised the late 1970s.

Back to the drawing board: the consensus under challenge

The report of the Royal Commission on the NHS, published in 1979, both reflected the growing disillusionment and represented an attempt to maintain the consensus. It accepted the need for a simplification in the structure of the NHS: thus adding its seal of approval to the new conventional wisdom that there was one tier too many. But it reaffirmed the basic philosophy of the NHS. Like the 1956 Guillebaud report, it argued that there was no way of settling the argument as to what the appropriate level of financing for the NHS was: the 'right' level of spending was essentially a metaphysical concept. Moreover, it pointed out that 'international comparisons do not suggest that greater expenditure automatically leads to better health . . . and it is at least arguable that the improvement in the health of the nation would be greater if extra resources were, for example, devoted to better housing'. The Royal Commission therefore rejected the notion that a change in the method of financing health services, such as adopting an insurance-based system, would solve the problems of the NHS. Like the Guillebaud Committee, too, the Royal Commission conceded the attractions in principle of transferring responsibility for health services to local government, but rejected it on grounds of feasibility – not least because such a solution would be unacceptable to the NHS producers, the trade unions among them.

This is not to suggest that the Royal Commission's report simply represented a blessing of the status quo. In all, its report made 117 recommendations. Some indeed were radical. For example, it proposed that Family Practitioner Committees should be abolished and their functions assumed by health authorities, in order to incorporate general practice into the mainstream of the NHS. Again, in an attempt to resolve the conflict between centre and periphery, it proposed that the regional health authorities should be directly accountable to Parliament for the delivery of services, while the DHSS would only be accountable for national policies. But, overall, its report was an overwhelming – though not uncritical – endorsement of the NHS's achievements. In this respect it again resembled the Guillebaud report. But while the Guillebaud report virtually silenced political argument about the NHS for 10 years, that of the Royal Commission marked on the contrary the beginning of a new debate. For while the Royal Commission had been set up by a Labour Government to reassure medical and public opinion, in the hope that it would defend the consensus against criticism, its report was published only three months before the installation of a Conservative Government in office. If the incoming Labour Government of 1974 had brought its own ideological commitments in its luggage, so did the incoming Conservative administration of 1979. The 1979 Conservative administration, in strong contrast to its 1970 predecessor, was not committed to the ideology of rational planning. On the contrary, as noted at the beginning of this chapter, it explicitly repudiated this ideology. Instead, it invoked the virtues of minimal government and the market economy.

Inevitably these themes were reflected – if only in a subdued, minor key – in its policies for the NHS. 'We will simplify and decentralise the service and cut back bureaucracy', the Party's 1979 manifesto proclaimed. While the rhetoric of decentralisation and hostility to bureaucracy were by 1979 the common language of political debate about the NHS, reflecting general disillusionment with the paternalistic rationalisers, the Conservative manifesto also promised to end 'Labour's vendetta against the private health sector'. Lastly, the manifesto raised the possibility, no more, of long-term changes in the methods of funding the NHS.

In the event, Patrick Jenkin, the new Conservative Secretary of State, carried out the manifesto's specific commitments.[55] Labour's policies towards private practice were smartly reversed: an act of ideological restitution, as it were. The policy of phasing out pay beds was abandoned; the Health Services Board was scrapped. Tax relief on medical insurance schemes operated by employers was restored. Finally, a new contract was quickly negotiated with the consultants. This permitted all consultants to engage in some private practice without loss of earnings, while the differentials between part-timers and full-timers were narrowed. In this respect, tactical considerations reinforced ideological bias. Given that demands for extra resources for the NHS tend to come from concentrated and organised labour within the service rather than from diffuse and unorganised patients outside it, then a Government concerned to limit public spending (as the 1979 Conservative administration was) may find it cheaper to buy off the producers than to try to satisfy the consumers. Investment in silencing consultants, and other interest groups within the NHS, may thus be seen as an alternative strategy to expanding the service as a whole. In return for the new contract the consultants further agreed to self-policed guidelines designed to prevent queue jumping by their private patients.

Similarly, if less controversially, the new Conservative Ministers carried out their manifesto pledge to decentralise the NHS. Their proposals faithfully reflected the change in opinion that had taken place since 1974, which is well caught in the following two quotations:

> In the reorganised service, there will be a more systematic and comprehensive planning process than now exists. The Department

will annually prepare guidance on national policy objectives for AHAs and RHAs who will then draw up their plans for the development of their services to meet these objectives together with their own local priorities . . . The reorganisation of the Department will provide for it to have close and more regular contact than in the past with the health authorities . . .

We are determined to see that as many decisions as possible are taken at the local level – in the hospital and in the community. We are determined to have more local health authorities, whose members will be encouraged to manage the Service, with the minimum of inter-ference by any central authority, whether at region or in central government departments.

The first quotation comes from the 1972 White Paper on reorganisation published by the then Conservative Secretary of State, Sir Keith Joseph. The second quotation comes from the Consultative Document on reorganisation, *Patients First*, published by Patrick Jenkin in December 1979,[56] and subsequently incorp-orated, with only minor modifications, in the legislation and consequential regulations which shaped the new NHS unveiled in 1982.

The central feature of the 1982 model NHS was the simplification of the NHS structure: the central tier – the AHAs – disappeared. These were replaced by District Health Authorities (DHAs). As in the years leading up to 1948, and again up to 1974, there was some debate about the role of the regional authorities. But, in the outcome, the regions were reprieved. While the Government rejected outright the proposal of the Royal Commission for a strengthened regional role – on the grounds that direct regional accountability to Parliament would be incompatible with the Secretary of State's responsibilities for the NHS as a whole – a review of the RHAs was relegated to the indefinite future. If anything the logic of replacing 90 AHAs by some 200 DHAs, a change which inevitably compounded the problems of control by the DHSS, suggested a strengthened regional role in future.

The central role of the new District Health Authorities in the new model NHS reflected the change in the 'public philosophy' that had taken place during the 1970s and that was complete by the 1980s. Where the 1974 reorganisation emphasised the values of efficiency and rationality (*see* the quotation from Sir Keith Joseph's White Paper, above), the 1982 reorganisation stressed the virtues of localism and small size. 'The thrust of our policy', one of the DHSS Ministers, Sir George Younger, told Parliament, 'is to have decisions taken as near to the point of delivery of services as is possible'. The DHAs should be established, a government circular laid down,[57] 'for the smallest possible geographical areas within which it is possible to carry out the integrated planning, provision and development' of health services. Only in the most exceptional cases would Ministers permit DHAs to have a population of more than 500,000 or less than 150,000. In the event, these instructions were carried out somewhat flexibly, influenced seemingly by local political pressures;[58] one DHA had a population of over 800,000, while a handful had populations below 100,000.

One criticism made of the change was that it would dilute the scarce resources of technical expertise available in the NHS. Before 1974 the relevant specialists in community medicine, statistics and planning were concentrated at the AHA level, and even so were in short supply. Now, in the remodelled NHS, they were scattered more thinly still, with the DHAs under pressure to cut the costs of management. But this criticism misses the whole point of the 1982 reorganisation, in so far as it represented a revolt against expertise. Given the underlying assumption that local people know best, there was inevitably less scope for the expert. Appropriately enough, Conservative Ministers repudiated the great technological dream of the 1960s – the giant District General Hospital – at the same time as they were remodelling the NHS. In 1980 the concept was officially buried.[59] In future, the Government laid down, the maximum size for a DGH would normally be 600 beds, stressing at the same time the value of small, local hospitals. It was a decision which at one and the same time reflected the new philosophy of 'small is beautiful', rationalised the cuts in the capital investment programme, and satisfied local political demands for accessible community hospitals.

The new emphasis on localism, and the reaction against expertise, was further reflected in a new permissiveness in planning. The document setting out the Conservative Government's priorities for the NHS published in 1981[60] marked a significant change from its predecessors published during the 1970s. The priorities themselves remained substantially unchanged, although there were some new themes such as the importance of co-operation between the NHS and the private sector. Like its predecessors the document – *Care in Action* – gave priority to the services for the elderly, mentally handicapped and other deprived groups. But if there was continuity in policy aims, there was a sharp break in the policy means. Unlike its predecessors, the 1981 document no longer expressed its priorities in terms of norms or financial targets: a reflection, in part, of the disillusionment with planning discussed in the previous section. Nor did it suggest how extra resources could be found for the priority services at a time of severe budgetary constraints, apart from the ritualistic invocation of the scope for greater efficiency. If the implementation of the priorities implied even tighter rationing in other service sectors, the responsibility was firmly delegated to the peripheral authorities. The Government, clearly, did not want to know. The only echo of the language of rational planning was the insistence on the importance of developing improved tools of analysis and information systems designed to assess the quality and efficiency of the services being provided.

In putting the stress on simplification and decentralisation as against central planning, the Conservative Government was largely acting within the new consensus that had developed in the second half of the 1970s. On one point, though, there was sharp disagreement: the constitution of the health authorities. While the 1974–79 Labour Government had, reluctantly, accepted the organisational framework created by Sir Keith Joseph, it had made one change: minor in its impact, but richly symbolic. The new authorities set up in 1974, the Labour Party argued, were undemocratic because appointive. So in 1975 the constitution of the AHAs was changed to strengthen the representation of local authorities:[61] at least a third of all members were to be drawn from local government – on the principle, seemingly, that someone annointed with the holy oil of election for one purpose automatically became sanctified as an all-purpose democratic representative. At the same time, the Labour Government proposed that two further members in each AHA should be 'drawn from amongst those working in the NHS': so extending representation from doctors and nurses to other NHS workers.

This proposal came to nothing because of disagreement among the trade unions, and between the trade unions and professional organisations, as to how these two worker representatives should be chosen.

On both counts, the 1982 model marked the rejection of Labour policies. The representation of local authorities on the DHAs was reduced to a quarter of the total membership, and the idea of worker representation was abandoned – although one member was appointed on the recommendation of the trade unions. However, the 'voice of the expert' remained represented, each DHA contained a consultant, a general practitioner and a nurse. If medical domination of the health authorities was numerically less visible than in the original NHS created by Bevan (*see* Chapter 2), medical representation continued to be institutionalised.

Like the original 1948 NHS and like the reorganised 1974 service, the 1982 NHS represented a compromise between competing ends and values. In order to achieve simplification, a price had to be paid: once again it proved impossible to reconcile the various desirable policy aims. The disappearance of AHAs meant the abandonment of shared boundaries between health and local authorities: if co-terminosity had not automatically led to greater collaboration, the new arrangement inevitably introduced new administrative complexities into the search for co-operation. Similarly, the disappearance of AHAs signalled the abandonment of any hope of integrating the administration of general practice more closely into health service planning. Under the new system, Family Practitioner Committees – like the original 1948 Executive Committees – once again became free-floating bodies. Both their boundaries and their finances were entirely independent of the DHAs. This not only represented a recognition of defeat in the past – the fact that FPCs had remained stubbornly independent of AHAs; it also represented the acceptance of the fact that an attempt to integrate general practice into the NHS by abolishing the FPCs, as recommended by the Royal Commission, would carry excessive political costs by leading to a confrontation with general practitioners. Once again the medical profession had been able to veto change, not by opposing it explicitly but by constraining the concept of feasibility held by policy-makers.

Above all, the 1982 model left unresolved the basic dilemma of the relationship between the centre and the periphery: a dilemma which had haunted the NHS since its inception and which featured so prominently in the Cabinet debates of 1946 (*see* Chapter 1). Everybody paid verbal homage to the principle of decentralisation, but how was this going to be achieved in a nationally financed service? 'I remain firmly convinced that the National Health Service is a noble concept but we can make it work a great deal better', Patrick Jenkin pronounced. 'First and foremost, I believe that we must see the NHS, not as a single national organisation, but as it is perceived by those who use it and those who work in it at the local level – as a series of local services run by local management, responsible to local needs and with a strong involvement from the local community.' The Secretary of State also recognised, however, the problem of squaring central accountability and local autonomy: 'This is difficult in a service where virtually the entire finance comes from the centre – from the Exchequer. That is why in the longer term I think it right that we should examine whether it is not possible for more of the finance for the Health Service to be generated locally as they do in so many other countries.' So, inevitably, the attempt to solve organisational problems – to translate a new political ideology of disengagement into practice – led to the questioning of the financial basis of the NHS. The Conservative ideology in any case predisposed Ministers to search for alternatives to the inherited system of financing health care, with a strong bias (as we have seen) towards the private market. But this predisposition was further reinforced by the realisation that organisation and finance were the two sides of the same coin: political disengagement by central government could only follow financial disengagement.

Unsurprisingly, therefore, the Conservative Ministers embarked on a search for new methods of financing health services. But the only actual change introduced – apart from the familiar step of increasing the revenue from prescriptions and other charges – was to permit and encourage DHAs to engage in local fund-raising activities. Although denounced by the Labour Opposition as a return to the pre-1948 days, when voluntary hospitals had to generate funds by flag-days and bazaars, the significance of this change turned out to be largely symbolic. The yield of subsequent fund-raising activities never represented more than the small change of the NHS's revenue. However, the change provided further evidence of a shift in the Government's ideology. For it implied once again a shift from national uniformity as the overriding policy objective for the NHS to the accept-ance of a great degree of diversity, since the fund-raising capacity of DHAs was bound to vary. If hypocrisy is the tribute vice pays to virtue, symbolic action is the tribute political necessity pays to party ideology. Just as the Labour Ministers in 1974 felt compelled to take action on pay beds by the need to satisfy their political constituency, so the Conservative Ministers in 1979 were forced to make a show of their commitment to their party's new ideology. In both cases it proved more expedient to make changes which were ideologically resonant rather than financially or politically costly.

Overall, then, the real significance of the policy innovations and changes that marked the start of the 1980s did not lie primarily in their direct effect on the structure, organisation and financing of the NHS. These were marginal. It lay in the insights they provided into the changing nature of the health care policy arena. To summarise the arguments of this chapter, these are as follows. First, the arena became more crowded with increasingly assertive actors. Second, the prevailing consensus came under strain as political ideology grew, reflecting the wider political and economic environment. Third, the consensus itself evolved: the faith of the creators of the NHS in rational planning, in giving free rein to the experts, became eroded. Fourth, while in the post-war era of economic growth governments were anxious to centralise credit – to claim responsibility for the improvements made possible by increasing prosperity – in the early 1980s the stress switched to diffusing blame for the inevitable shortcomings in an era of economic crisis: to decentralise responsibility is also to disclaim blame. Lastly, and perhaps most important, the combination of all these factors put new issues on the NHS policy agenda: the result was to set a question mark against assumptions which hitherto had seemingly been set in the concrete of a generally accepted conventional wisdom. If the consensus survived – changed, battered and moth-eaten – it could no longer to taken for granted.

References

1. Rudolf Klein, 'The Stalemate Society', *Commentary*, Nov. 1973, pp. 42–7.
2. The analysis here draws on Samuel Beer, 'In Search of a New Public Philosophy' in Anthony King (ed.), *The New American Political System*, American Enterprise Institute: Washington, DC 1978. Although Beer's analysis of the intellectual climate in the 1960s and 1970s is based on American experience, it is equally relevant to Britain.
3. Ministry of Housing and Local Government, *People and Planning*, HMSO: London 1969.
4. FWS Craig (ed.), *British General Election Manifestos, 1900–1974*, Macmillan: London 1975.
5. Anthony King, 'Overload: Problems of Governing in the 1970s', *Political Studies*, vol. XXIII, nos. 2–3, June–Sept. 1975, pp. 162–74.
6. Robert Bacon and Walter Eltis, *Britain's Economic Problem: Too Few Producers*, Macmillan: London 1976.
7. Chancellor of the Exchequer, *Public Expenditure to 1979–80*, HMSO: London 1976, Cmnd. 6393.
8. Social Services Committee Third Report, Session 1980–81, *Public Expenditure on the Social Services*, vol. 2, HMSO: London 1981, HC 324–11. Because of a change in the method of presenting figures in the Public Expenditure White Paper, the figure derived from this source is for England only.
9. Barbara Castle, *The Castle Diaries, 1974–76*, Weidenfeld & Nicolson: London 1980. See App. 1 for expenditure figures.
10. Expenditure Committee Ninth Report, Session 1976–77, *Spending on the Health and Personal Social Services*, HMSO: London 1977, HC 466; Social Services Committee Third Report, Session 1979–80, *The Government's White Paper on Public Expenditure: The Social Services*, HMSO: London 1980, HC 702.
11. Department of Health and Social Security, *The NHS Planning System*, HMSO: London 1976.
12. Department of Health and Social Security, *Priorities for Health and Personal Social Services in England*, HMSO: London 1976.
13. Rudolf Klein, 'Ideology, Class and the National Health Service', *Journal of Health Politics, Policy and Law*, vol. 4, no. 3, Fall 1979, pp. 464–91.
14. National Board for Prices and Incomes Report no. 166, *The Pay and Conditions of Service of Ancillary Workers in the National Health Service*, HMSO: London 1971, Cmnd. 4644.
15. Royal Commission on the National Health Service, *Report*, HMSO: London 1979, Cmnd. 7615.
16. Rudolf Klein, 'Incomes: Vive La Différence', *British Medical Journal*, 10 July 1976, pp. 126–7. Strictly, the figures given in the text refer to the median quartile of people in each group.
17. Review Body on Doctors' and Dentists' Remuneration, *Sixth Report, 1976*, HMSO: London 1976, Cmnd. 6473.
18. Review Body on Doctors' and Dentists' Remuneration, *Seventh Report, 1977*, HMSO: London 1977, Cmnd. 6800.
19. Review Body on Doctors' and Dentists' Remuneration, *Eighth Report, 1978*, HMSO: London 1978, Cmnd. 7176.
20. Review Body on Doctors' and Dentists' Remuneration, *Tenth Report, 1980*, HMSO: London 1980, Cmnd. 7903.
21. For a detailed narrative of this dispute see Susan Treloar, 'The Junior Hospital Doctors' Pay Dispute 1975–1976', *Journal of Social Policy*, vol. 10, no. 1, Jan. 1981, pp. 1–30.
22. *BMJ*, Report of Proceedings of the Central Committee for Hospital Medicine Services, *British Medical Journal*, 6 Dec. 1975, pp. 593–5.
23. Leading article, 'Industrial Action by Doctors', *British Medical Journal*, 6 Dec. 1975, p. 544.

24. Sir Theodore Fox, 'Industrial Action, The National Health Service, and the Medical Profession', *The Lancet*, 23 Oct. 1976, pp. 892–5.
25. *BMJ*, 'Discussion Document on Ethical Responsibilities of Doctors Practising in the National Health Service', *British Medical Journal*, 15 Jan. 1977, pp. 157–9.
26. *BMJ*, 'From the Council', *British Medical Journal*, 7 Oct. 1978, p. 1033.
27. *BMJ*, 'The Week', *British Medical Journal*, 3 June 1978, p. 1479.
28. Rudolf Klein and Janet Lewis, *The Politics of Consumer Representation*, Centre for Studies in Social Policy: London 1976.
29. Kathy Sayer (ed.), *The King's Fund Directory of Organisations for Patients and Disabled People*, King Edward's Hospital Fund: London 1979.
30. The analysis draws on Rudolf Klein, 'Ideology, Class and the National Health Service', op. cit. Where no sources are given in the text, they can be found in this paper.
31. Barbara Castle, *The Castle Diaries*, op. cit., p. 131.
32. DP Choyce, Letter in the *British Medical Journal*, 21 August 1976, p. 479.
33. Barbara Castle, *The Castle Diaries*, op. cit., p. 568.
34. Department of Health and Social Security, *The Separation of Private Practice from National Health Service Hospitals: A Consultative Document*, DHSS: London 1975.
35. Health Services Board, *Annual Report, 1979*, HMSO: London 1980, HC 354.
36. For details of the contract, see Review Body on Doctors' and Dentists' Remuneration, *Ninth Report, 1979*, op. cit.
37. Royal Commission on the National Health Service, *Report*, op. cit.
38. Royal Commission on the National Health Service, Research Paper no. 5, *Patients' Attitudes to the Hospital Service*, HMSO: London 1978; Research Paper no. 6, *Access to Primary Care*, HMSO: London 1978.
39. Royal Commission on the National Health Service, Research Paper no. 1, *The Working of the National Health Service* (Maurice Kogan *et al.*), HMSO: London 1978.
40. *Regional Chairmen's Enquiry into the Working of the DHSS in Relation to Regional Health Authorities*, DHSS: London 19 May 1976.
41. Committee of Public Accounts, *Ninth Report, Session 1976–77*, HMSO: London 1977, HC 532.
42. Expenditure Committee, Ninth Report, Session 1976–77, *Spending on the Health and Personal Social Services*, HMSO: London 1977, HC 466.
43. Social Services Committee, Third Report, Session 1979–80, *The Government's White Papers on Public Expenditure: The Social Services*, HMSO: London 1980, HC 702.
44. Social Services Committee, Third Report, Session 1980–81, *Public Expenditure on the Social Services*, HMSO: London 1981, HC 324.
45. Department of Health and Social Security, *The Way Forward*, HMSO: London 1977.
46. David J Hunter, *Coping With Uncertainty*, Research Studies Press: Chichester 1980; RGS Brown, *Reorganising the National Health Service*, Basil Blackwell/Martin Robertson: Oxford 1979; S Hayward and A Alaszewski, *Crisis in the Health Service*, Croom Helm: London 1980.
47. Social Services Committee, Third Report, Session 1980–81, op. cit., p. 104.
48. Peter D Fox, 'Managing Health Resources: English Style' in Gordon McLachlan (ed.), *By Guess or By What? Information Without Design in the NHS*, Oxford UP 1978; Michael Butts, Doreen Irving and Christopher Whitt, *From Principles to Practice*, Nuffield Provincial Hospitals Trust: London 1981.
49. Timothy Booth, 'Collaboration Between the Health and Social Services', pts 1 and 2, *Policy and Politics*, vol. 9, nos. 1 and 2, Jan. and April 1981, pp. 23–51 and 205–27.
50. Chancellor of the Exchequer, *The Government's Expenditure Plans, 1980–81 to 1983–84*, HMSO: London 1980, Cmnd. 7841.
51. Royal Commission on the National Health Service, *Research Paper no. 1*, op. cit.
52. Committee of Inquiry into Normansfield Hospital, *Report*, HMSO: London 1978, Cmnd.

7357. See also Rudolf Klein, 'Normansfield: Vacuum of Management in the NHS', *British Medical Journal*, 23 Dec. 1978, pp. 1802–4.

53. Jane Smith, 'Conflict Without Change: The Case of London's Health Services', *Political Quarterly*, vol. 52, no. 4, Oct. 1981.

54. N Korman and H Simons, 'Hospital Closures' in Royal Commission on the National Health Service, *Research Paper no. 1*, op. cit.

55. This analysis draws on Rudolf Klein, 'Health Services', Ch. 9 in PM Jackson (ed.), *Government Policy Initiatives 1979–80*, Royal Institute of Public Administration: London 1981. Where no sources are given in the text, they can be found in this paper.

56. Department of Health and Social Security, *Patients First*, HMSO: London 1979.

57. Department of Health and Social Security, *Health Service Development: Structure and Management*, Circular HC (80)8, July 1980.

58. *The Economist*, note on 'Health Services', 29 Aug. 1981, pp. 23–4.

59. Department of Health and Social Security, *Hospital Services: The Future Pattern of Provision in England*, DHSS: London May 1980.

60. Department of Health and Social Security, *Care in Action*, HMSO: London 1981. See also Rudolf Klein, 'The Strategy Behind the Jenkin Non-Strategy', *British Medical Journal*, 28 Mar. 1981, pp. 1089–91.

61. Department of Health and Social Security, *Democracy in the National Health Service*, HMSO: London 1974; Department of Health and Social Security, *Democracy in the National Health Service*, Circular HSC (IS)194, Sept. 1975.

Chapter 5

The politics of value for money

If the consensus about the NHS appeared to be giving cause for concern in the early 1980s, by the end of the decade it was dead. The date of its death can be fixed with some precision. The publication of the Conservative Government's White Paper, *Working for Patients*,[1] in January 1989 brought about the biggest explosion of political anger and professional fury in the history of the NHS. The subsequent insistence of the Government on driving the White Paper proposals through Parliament, with virtually no concessions to the critics, crystallised both the anger and the fury. By the time that the legislation was formally implemented – the changes took effect in 1991 – there was a widespread perception that the NHS, as conceived in 1948, had been transformed in ways that betrayed the principles on which it had been founded. For once the British Medical Association and the Labour Party were at one, defending the institutional values incarnate in the NHS against the subversive radicalism of Mrs Thatcher and her Ministers.

This chapter analyses the period leading up to Mrs Thatcher's decision, in January 1988, to set up the Review of the NHS which was to produce *Working for Patients*, leaving it to the next chapter to examine in detail the genesis and nature of those reforms. An appropriate starting point is 1983, when a clear shift in policy became apparent. This was symbolised by the publication of the Griffiths Report,[2] which marked the beginning of the NHS's managerial revolution. For whereas the main preoccupation previously had been with the organisational *structure* of the NHS, attention now switched to the organisational *dynamics* of the NHS.[3] In particular, policy came to be driven increasingly by the productivity imperative. Caught between rising demands on the NHS generated by technological change and the ageing of the population, on the one hand, and the financial constraints imposed by an ailing economy and the Government's commitment to restraining the growth of public expenditure, on the other, Ministers appeared to have only one option: to squeeze more out of existing resources by improving efficiency.[4] And if that meant reversing the previous drift to decentralisation – if it meant intervention by central government to force health authorities to be efficient – so be it. The search for ways of meeting rising demands while limiting the rise in public expenditure shaped policy.

This search is, of course, one of the themes that runs through the entire history of the NHS. It began, as we saw in Chapter 2, soon after its birth with Treasury pressure for measures to reduce demand and to eliminate waste.[5] And Treasury pressure on the NHS to contain spending and to cut costs is the one constant running through subsequent decades, seldom overtly evident but persistently and relentlessly exercised in the annual negotiations about the allocation of departmental budgets. What distinguished the 1980s was therefore not the concern about efficiency. It was that this concern increasingly dominated government policy: what had been a minor theme became the major one. If Ministers were to prevent the economic triumph in containing spending from turning into a political disaster – if their success in limiting the rise in the NHS's budget was not to be perceived as a failure to deliver an adequate health service to the people of Britain – they somehow had to demonstrate that outputs could be increased at a faster rate than inputs: to de-couple inputs and outputs. Only the philosopher's stone of efficiency – to be achieved by better management and by changing the system of incentives in the NHS – could do the trick by enabling the production of services to increase at a faster rate than the NHS's budget.

In pursuing this strategy Ministers were caught in a dilemma, however. To increase efficiency meant taking measures perceived as threatening by NHS providers – the medical profession, in particular. Providers reacted by advertising their discontent. And they did so, entirely predictably and in line with precedent, by proclaiming the imminent dissolution of the NHS. In turn, Ministers responded to the charge that they were starving the NHS of funds by introducing yet more changes designed to increase efficiency which, at the same time, threatened existing interests in the NHS. Thus was created the self-reinforcing and escalating cycle of suspicion, antagonism and confrontation between the Government and NHS providers that was to culminate in the grand finale of *Working for Patients*. A decade which had started in a low-key fashion, with changes designed to reduce the role of central government and to limit the responsibility of Ministers for what was happening at the periphery, ended in high drama with the NHS occupying the centre of the political stage as never before.

But, as always, the changes in the NHS mirrored wider political, social and economic changes. If this chapter takes 1983 as its starting point, it is not only because of events within the NHS. It was also the year which put the Thatcher imprint on the decade with her second General Election victory, to be repeated in 1987: the beginning of the process which saw Mrs Thatcher's transformation from being merely an assertive leader to becoming an authoritarian one, shaping a Cabinet in her own image.[6] The story of the NHS in the 1980s therefore provides an opportunity to tease out what (if anything) was distinctive about the contribution of 'Thatcherism'[7] to the evolution of health care policy, as against the role of those economic and social factors which helped to make 'Thatcherism' possible and which provided the environment in which both the Government and the NHS were operating. In what follows, therefore, the aim is to interpret the politics of the NHS not simply in terms of the ideological preferences or idiosyncrasies of Mrs Thatcher's administration but of seeing them also as the product of the changes in the environment which allowed her to win three General Elections in succession, albeit on a minority vote of the electorate, and to stay in office throughout the 1980s.

The changing environment

The NHS was born into a working class society only slowly emerging from war, where rationing and queueing were symbols not of inadequacy but of fairness in the distribution of scarce resources. It celebrated its 40th anniversary in 1988 in what had become an affluent consumer society where only access to work was rationed. Whereas in 1951 over 64 per cent of the occupied population were manual workers, by 1981 the proportion had fallen to less than 48 per cent.

Conversely, the same period saw the rise of the service class: the number of employers, people working on their own account, managers and professionals rose from just under 19 per cent of the labour force to over 31 per cent.[8] Again, whereas in 1947 only 27 per cent of the population owned their own homes, by 1981 the proportion had risen to 58 per cent.[9] Both trends were intensified during the 1980s. The decay of many of Britain's traditional industries, like coal and steel, meant also the disappearance of the manual jobs created by them; the Thatcher Government's policy of encouraging the sale of council houses further accelerated the growth of home ownership. The Beveridge report had assumed that the normal family economy would revolve around a male bread-winner but by the end of the 1980s almost as many women as men were in either full-time or part-time employment, while the number of households headed by women was soaring. Being a member of a two-earner family had, for many people, become the best protection against falling into poverty in a period when rising unemployment and rising poverty were going hand in hand.

The Britain of the Thatcher era differed from the Britain of the Attlee era in a number of other critical respects. It was a far more fractured society, with new cleavages cutting across or blurring traditional class divisions. It was a society exposed to a range of experiences and information – either direct or indirect – unimaginable in 1948, when mass-tourism did not exist and television ownership was an exotic rarity. It was a society in which scandal was less and less restrained by the self-censorship of the media and marked (whether as a cause or an effect) by the erosion of deference. All traditional institutions – whether the monarchy or the NHS – were exposed to the searchlight of publicity in a way which would not have been conceivable four decades earlier: élite, insider knowledge was being turned into public information for the masses far faster than ever before. If a 1980s doctor wished to protest about conditions in the NHS, he had an echo chamber of publicity denied to his predecessors in the 1940s. It was moreover a society whose members were far better educated than their predecessors, with expectations that had not been blunted by the experience of poverty and the depression of the 1930s, and where an increasing number could take it for granted that they would be able to control their own lives. It was a society experiencing rapid technological change – encapsulated, and perhaps over-simplified, in the notion of a switch from an economy based on manufacturing to an economy based on services – that was creating both new risks and new opportunities, encouraging the hopes of would-be entrepreneurs just as it was destroying traditions of lifetime employment in the same job.

Social change brought about political change. If there was a new consumerism in the economic market place – epitomised by the rise of the supermarket chains – so also was there a new consumerism in the political market place. Politics became marked by diminishing partisanship and an increasing willingness to shop around among the parties. It could no longer be taken for granted that those who identified themselves as working class – a diminishing proportion of the total population anyway – would vote Labour and even the proportion of voters identifying with the ruling Conservative Party fell.[10] Brand loyalty could no longer be taken for granted and support, increasingly, came to depend on perceptions of performance.

But it would be a mistake to assume that Mrs Thatcher's electoral successes meant that Britain had moved into the era of the politics of private consumption, dominated by self-seeking individualism and blind to poverty and collective needs. Mrs Thatcher herself certainly believed in the 'vigorous virtues' of energy, adventurousness and independence, rather than the 'softer virtues' of humility, gentleness and sympathy.[11] Moreover, she was voted into office in 1979 in part at least by an anti-Welfare State spending backlash and one of her consistent and persistent themes throughout the 1980s was to stress the import-ance of self-reliance and self-sufficiency as against dependency on the State. The aim was to create a country in which the 'vigorous virtues' could flourish and would be rewarded; the collective good would be promoted not by spending more on collective welfare provision but by unleashing the energies of individuals. Wealth creation – to be achieved by cutting taxes, by reducing the regulatory role of the State and by providing more scope for individual choice and initiative – was seen as the key to welfare. In all these, as in other respects, Thatcherism defined itself largely by reaction against the past: the collectivist, corporatist bias that had characterised Conservative and Labour administrations alike in the post-war era.

Surprisingly, however, there is little evidence that in all this Thatcherism either reflected or moulded public opinion. Indeed all the evidence suggests that the longer Mrs Thatcher remained in power, the greater became the gap between the values of her administration and those of the population as a whole. Take, for example, a survey conducted in 1988 in which people were asked which of two statements came closest to their ideal: 79 per cent chose 'a country in which caring for others is more highly rewarded', whereas only 16 per cent opted for 'a society in which the creation of wealth is more highly rewarded'. Again, when asked whether the government's most important job was to provide opportunities for everyone to get ahead or to guarantee everyone steady employment and a decent standard of living, 65 per cent opted for a government guarantee – a higher proportion than when the same question had been put in 1945.[12] If the Thatcher administration was the advocate of possessive individualism – as is often argued – it appears to have been singularly unsuccessful in winning over the people to its views. Similarly, support for the main institutions and programmes of the Welfare State – NHS, pensions and education – increased, if anything, during the Thatcher years, although views about benefits for the unemployed, single parents and children were rather more ambivalent.[13] Support for the NHS, as reflected in public opinion surveys throughout the 1980s, remained particu-larly strong.[14] On the one hand, any suggestion of moving towards a system of private insurance – while leaving the NHS to look after those with lower incomes – was overwhelmingly and consistently rejected: the proportion rejecting it rose from 64 per cent to 74 per cent between 1983 and 1989. On the other hand, the NHS invariably appeared as the leading candidate for extra spending when those interviewed were asked about their priorities: indeed a majority supported extra spending on the NHS even if this meant higher taxes.

The enthusiasm for extra Welfare State expenditure voiced by voters in response to public opinion polls was not altogether consistent with their behav-iour in the polling booths. So there must be some scepticism about the depth of the commitment. However, it is clear that one of the factors constraining the policy choices of the Thatcher Government was, throughout the 1980s, fear of antagonising voters by adopting measures that might appear as an overt attack on the Welfare State. Electoral pragmatism almost invariably tempered ideological impulses: Mrs Thatcher was quite clear that she owed it to future generations to stay in office as long as possible in order to complete the task that destiny had given her. The importance of this factor in shaping policy towards the NHS is explored further below: for most of her period in office, Mrs Thatcher treated the NHS like an unexploded bomb, liable to be set off by any imprudent move, which had to be handled with extreme care and caution. But much the same point can be made, if with less emphasis, about the other main institutions of the Welfare State. There were, indeed, important changes. The method of calculating the annual uprating of benefits became conspicuously less generous; there was increased emphasis on sharpening work incentives by reducing the scale and scope of entitlements; lavish tax incentives were handed out to promote private pensions; a mimic-market (*see* page 146) for schools was introduced. But the Welfare State was not dismantled: public expenditure on welfare programmes was considerably higher at the end of the Thatcher era than at the beginning, and not just because of the extra spending forced by high unemployment.[15] In short, the strategy – if a series of political compromises sharing a common bias can be called a strategy – was to maintain the institutions of the Welfare State intact, while seeking to change their dynamics: precisely the pattern of policy evolution evident in the NHS.

The preservation of the Welfare State's institutional structure owed, perhaps, more to political pragmatism than to any positive enthusiasm for maintaining the inherited structures. For Mrs Thatcher's Conservatism was of a peculiar kind; indeed some have questioned whether she was a Conservative at all.[16] While she conformed to type in her invocation of nation and family, she appeared more like a 19th century Liberal in her insistence that the market knew best and that government should be reduced in scope and scale. If the NHS was born in a period of nationalisation, it celebrated its 40th anniversary at a time when the industries which had been taken into State ownership in the 1940s were being sold off – with the pace quickening as the 1980s progressed. Moreover, Mrs Thatcher conspicuously lacked reverence for tradition as embodied in institutions: in this respect she was much nearer to Bentham than to Burke. Previous Conservative administrations had been characterised by the politics of the gentleman's club: insiders linked by a common background and ethos. But Mrs Thatcher was no gentleman; rather than seeking entry into the club, she was contemptuous of its rules and etiquette. So in the case of the NHS, as we shall see, her conduct of policy was distinguished by its repudiation of established rules of the game.

At the heart of Thatcherism there was a paradox. To reduce the role of government, she had to strengthen the power of the State. If the scope of government was reduced in some respects, as by the privatisation of the nationalised industries, its tread became heavier. If markets did not exist, they had to be created. Once created, furthermore, they had to be regulated. More fundamentally still, the Conservative Government can be seen as the equivalent of the Tudor Monarchy[17] asserting the power of the State in order to modernise a country previously dominated by feudal barons and corporate interests like the Church. As the Thatcherites saw it, the horrendous economic problem which swept them into office – rapid stagflation, soaring public expenditure, apparently irreversible economic decline – reflected the ability of corporate groups to subvert the public interest to their own: to perpetuate rigidities and to oppose change. The corporatist stalemate that had developed since 1945 – and which the NHS epitomised in many respects, as we have seen – had to be broken if Britain was not to be condemned to permanent economic sclerosis.[18] Similarly, if public services were to be run in the interests of consumers rather than in the interests of those working in them, provider power had to be smashed. But to achieve all this, the State needed more power, not less; the ability of central government to impose its own policies had to be strengthened even if this meant restricting the role of local authorities or crushing established interest groups. In the first Thatcher administration, a start was made on tackling and taming the trade unions. Next, the second Thatcher administration turned its attention to the soft underbelly of the professions and demonstrated the impotence of university and school teachers to resist government policies designed to reshape the educational system. Finally, the third Thatcher administration engaged in a head-on confrontation with the most ancient corporate interest groups: the professions of law and medicine.[19]

In short, the implicit vision of society was that of a strong, centralised State and strong, individualistic consumers but with the role of intermediary bodies – be they local authorities, trade unions or professional associations – sharply diminished. In this, consumers were both an end and a means. They were an end in so far as one of the aims of policy was to give them more choice. They were a means in so far as consumers were cast as the rank and file in the assault on provider power in the public services: the infantry who would follow up the ministerial artillery barrage. The strong State, in other words, would draw its power from mobilising the people, bypassing (and so undermining) the entrenched interests. The case of education, which was to provide Ministers with an exemplar when it came to the reform of the NHS, illustrates the strategy well.[20] By emancipating schools from the grip of local authorities, by extending the right to choose between schools and by providing more information to parents, it was hoped that parent power would act as a counterweight to teacher domination and so diminish the influence of what were perceived to be pernicious educational theories. However, as the case of education once again illustrates well, it was not an altogether coherent strategy. While the creation of a mimic-market implied a devolution and fragmentation of responsibility, the Government was at the same time introducing a national curriculum and a battery of national tests designed to ensure that the education system would make an appropriate contribution to economic growth. The result was not only to limit professional autonomy but also to restrict parental choice. Much the same kind of tension between the different policy aims of the Thatcher administration – with reality as often as not lagging a long way behind rhetoric – was to be evident, as we shall see, in the case of the NHS.

The Thatcher decade was also conspicuous for the rise of the good house-keeping State. If efficiency was seen as the key which would enable the Government to combine a tight budgetary constraint with expanding services in the NHS, the same formula appeared to provide the key to the more general problem of how to limit the growth of public expenditure while yet meeting the expectations of the voters to have their taxes but not their services cut. If the Welfare State could no longer live off the dividends of economic growth – the national income actually fell in the first two years of the 1980s and the average annual growth rate for the decade was, at 2.2 per cent, no better than in the dismal 1970s[21] – perhaps it could survive on the dividends of efficiency drives. But in order to achieve this policy aim, the Government once again had to forge new instruments of intervention. In pursuit of its value-for-money aims, it adopted and developed many of the techniques first introduced in the 1960s and early 1970s by the rationalist managers (*see* Chapter 3). If the new public management[22] heavily borrowed ideas from the private sector, it also built on concepts developed in the public sector in earlier decades. Consider, for example, the 1983 Financial Management Initiative.[23] This helped to transform adminis-trative style throughout Whitehall and beyond, with its insistence that each government programme should have explicitly stated objectives and measures of performance from which it would be possible to assess progress towards the goals that had been agreed. Measurement was the key to the control of performance, as if to emphasise the Benthamite streak in Thatcherism. The FMI prompted the mass production of performance indicators[24] throughout the public sector: in the case of the NHS this was achieved by the mass-baptism of all existing statistical series as performance indicators (PIs). And the FMI was, in 1988, followed by the *Next Steps* initiative[25] – the product of the Prime Minister's Efficiency Unit – designed to devolve as much of government activity as possible to independent agencies, although the full impact of this initiative was only to become evident in the post-Thatcher era.

The intellectual ancestry of these initiatives can, in fact, be traced back to the epoch of belief in central government planning which the Thatcher Government was so anxious to repudiate. Thus the notion of accountable units of management in the public sector was first put forward by the Fulton Committee on the Civil Service.[26] Similarly, the interest in such techniques as programme budgeting, which involved setting objectives and measuring progress towards their achieve-ment, dates back to the same period. The real difference was that, 20 years later, a very different kind of Government used these techniques to create a new Whitehall management culture. The result was to set a new agenda of questions about the purpose of government programmes: a ferret down the bureaucratic warren. Moreover, some of the new techniques could be, and were, used in the service of the Government's strategy of invoking public support against entrenched producer interests. Thus performance indicators could be used not only as instruments of accountability to Ministers, but also as tools of account-ability to the public: hence the innovation of producing PIs for local authorities and schools designed for public consumption – an approach subsequently adopted in the NHS as well. Whether the publication of such PIs made any impact on the public is, of course, another matter.

Many of these changes were made possible and reflected – to reiterate the central theme of this section – wider changes in society: in particular, the explosion in the availability of information technology. This not only made it possible – as it had not been in the 1960s – to collect and process the kind of information needed to devise systems of control based on performance data. But, more important and more generally, it also prompted new thinking about the management of complex organisations. For in pursuing a policy of centralising control over decision-making while decentralising activity, the Government was following some larger trends in society. The trend is well caught in the following quotation from an industrialist, Sir Adrian Cadbury:[27]

> We will want, in future, to break these organisations down into their
> separate business units and to give those units freedom to compete in

their particular markets. Large companies will become more like federations of small enterprises – not because 'small is beautiful' but because big is expensive and inflexible. . . . I would expect tomorrow's companies . . . to concentrate on the core activities of their business, relying for everything else on specialised suppliers who would compete for their custom.

In short, the trend – internationally – was from centralised institutions to networks, from hierarchic top-down models of organisation to looser constellations.[28] This fragmentation of traditional hierarchic models was not only facilitated by developments in information technology but was also accelerated by them: given a rapid diffusion of knowledge, and given also a rapid pace of change and uncertainty about the future, an adaptable peripheral learning model may in any case be more functional than a rigid central command model. And what goes for the private sector applies, if anything with greater force, to the public sector:[29] hence the transformation of the Welfare State into the Regulatory State, with increasing emphasis on the role of government not as a provider of services but as the regulator of services produced by others.[30] These developments were not driven or determined by changes in technology but they were certainly made possible by them. Already by 1982 it was possible to anticipate some of the main characteristics of *Working for Patients* by extrapolating technological trends:

> In the long run the development of microtechnology may permit the creation of information systems which permit the individual units within the NHS to operate as independent entrepreneurs in a kind of social market, buying services from each other (and perhaps the private sector as well).[31]

Such, then, were the main elements in the transformation of the NHS's environment in the 1980s. All were apparent at the beginning of the decade but their full logic was slow to work its way through. The puzzle addressed in the rest of this chapter is therefore not just how and why the NHS changed but also how far and why the NHS successfully survived pressures under which other institutions crumbled.

Political v. financial constraints

The Thatcher Government fought the General Election of 1983 – as it did the General Election of 1987 – firmly committed to the NHS. 'Let me make one thing absolutely clear', the Prime Minister proclaimed, 'The National Health Service is safe with us'.[32] The commitment was all the more emphatic because the Government felt itself to be vulnerable on this issue. In the autumn of 1982 the Central Policy Review Staff – the Government's internal think-tank – had produced a paper examining the options for cutting public expenditure. Among the options put forward was that of replacing the tax-financed National Health Service by a system of private insurance; further, the paper advocated increased charges. When presented to Ministers by the Chancellor of the Exchequer, it precipitated the 'nearest thing to a Cabinet riot in the history of the Thatcher Administration'.[33] The subsequent leak of the document to *The Economist* compounded private anger with public embarrassment. In particular, it infuriated

Norman Fowler, who in 1981 had succeeded Patrick Jenkin as Secretary of State for Social Services. Whereas Jenkin was described by one of his own officials as too good a bureaucrat to be an effective Minister, Fowler was a supple, entrepreneurial politician highly sensitive to public opinion. The CPRS's suggestions were, in his view, mischievously wrong-headed. His predecessor had sent a civil servant round Europe to examine different systems of funding health care; the resulting analysis confirmed the conclusion that 'in many ways our centrally financed system was the most effective in controlling costs'.[34] Moreover, any threat to the NHS would, given its popularity, be a political disaster. From this followed the need to be as emphatic as possible in shooting down the CPRS's kite[35] and reaffirming the Government's total devotion to the NHS.

Fowler's political instinct turned out to be correct. In the 1983 General Election, as in the 1987 one, the Opposition parties seized on the NHS as a battering ram for the assault on the Government.[36] In 1983, for example, the CPRS report featured largely in the Labour campaign as evidence that the Conservatives were planning to dismember the NHS. The spectre of privatisation rattled its chains in both elections. On both occasions, too, Labour charged that the NHS was about to collapse because of inadequate funding. The Conservative response on both occasions was to underline, hands on heart, their commitment to the NHS and to discharge a battery of statistics showing that funding had increased, that more doctors and nurses were being employed and that more people than ever before were being treated. The strategy did not carry conviction. In both elections voters gave Labour a strong lead when asked which of the parties they would prefer to deal with the NHS. This may have made no difference to the outcomes but it did underline the fact that the NHS was the issue where the Tories were at their weakest and Labour was at its strongest. In short, the election campaigns demonstrated the political vulnerability of the Conservative Party on the issue of health care and reinforced the Government's conviction that NHS policy-making was an exercise in walking on egg shells. If public opinion did not influence policy-making positively or directly,[37] it helped to shape ministerial perceptions of political feasibility.

Just as public opinion played a key role in defining the frontiers of the politically possible, so the Treasury largely determined the frontiers of the financially possible. The controversy about the adequacy or otherwise of NHS funding – the battle between the inputters and the outputters – is examined in detail in the next chapter. Here it is sufficient to note that the 1980s were indeed a period of relative deprivation for the NHS; Treasury policy reflected, albeit not always consistently, both the Government's determination to contain the growth of public spending and the fact that the performance of the national economy was poor during most of the years in question. The average increase in the NHS budget in the 10 years from 1978/9 to 1989/90 was just below 3 per cent a year in real terms and just over 1 per cent a year in volume terms.[38] The problem of knowing which is the most appropriate price index to use when calculating changes in the NHS budget – the GDP deflator, which measures all price changes (real terms) or the NHS-specific index, which measures changes in prices and pay specific to health care (volume terms) – is just one instance of the conceptual puzzles involved in evaluating the adequacy or otherwise of funding and of the opportunities for the selective use of statistics in political controversy. Crucially, however, the increase in the NHS's budget – whether measured in real or volume terms – represented a fall in the historical trend. It was thus a shock to the system, challenging the assumptions that had grown up over the decades of growth and optimism. In particular, it was a shock to the health service providers. Financial stringency thus reinforced the in-built incentives of doctors, nurses and other providers to denigrate the service – a tendency first noted by Enoch Powell 20 years earlier – and to advertise their own claims for extra resources by drawing attention to the NHS's shortcomings. The professional cries of pain and outrage, in turn, reinforced public apprehensions and increased the political price of successful financial cost containment.

Government policies can therefore best be understood, as argued at the start of this chapter, as a succession of attempts to resolve the dilemma of how best to limit both economic and political costs under the all-important constraint that radical reform had been ruled out of court. The policies can usefully be analysed under four headings. First, contrary to the trends of the early 1980s but in line with the general direction of government policy, there was a sharp turn to centralisation. Far from decentralising responsibility and thereby diffusing blame, the Department of Health and Social Security moved towards setting objectives and monitoring progress towards their achievement. Second, and linked to this, better and stronger management came to be seen as the key to greater efficiency, marking in many respects a revival of faith in bureaucratic rationality albeit in a new guise. Third, in line with the initiatives taken in the early 1980s, there was a continuing if unspectacular expansion in the private sector and in the contracting out of NHS services. Fourth, there was growing emphasis on the development of primary care and prevention as part of a wider strategy designed to reduce the rise in demands on the NHS. Alas for the Government, the timetable of change in the NHS and the political timetable did not coincide. Even the most optimistic protagonists of ministerial policies and the new managerialism had to concede that time was needed for results to become apparent. Meanwhile some of the policies themselves were feeding suspicions of the Government's intentions towards the NHS both among providers and the Opposition, so further reinforcing the resentment and antagonism created by financial stringency. The drive for efficiency, although designed to find a solution to the Government's political dilemma, in many ways compounded the problems faced by Ministers. In the sections that follow, which examine the four main strands of policy, it is therefore important to remember that the events and policies described have to be interpreted as much in terms of their symbolic significance as of their practical implications: the way in which they shaped the perceptions of the different actors in the health policy arena.

The return to centralisation

The rhetoric of delegation to the periphery and the retreat from prescription by central government that characterised the 1982 reorganisation were to have a short shelf-life. Even while the organisational changes were still in the process of being implemented so the new Secretary of State, Norman Fowler, and his new Permanent Secretary, Sir Kenneth Stowe, were in the process of introducing a series of measures designed to strengthen the grip of central government. From repudiating the language of norm setting, and insisting that health authorities must have freedom to make their own decisions within broad national guidelines, the DHSS moved towards a system of performance review designed to monitor progress towards the achievement of very specific targets: a tighter system of control and accountability than had ever existed in the previous history of the NHS.

The switch was, of course, very much in line with the general emphasis of government policy. If the DHSS was to have any credibility with the Treasury in the annual battle for funds, it had to demonstrate that it was taking the Financial Management Initiative seriously. Similarly, if Ministers wanted to squeeze more value for money out of the NHS's budget, they had to strengthen the capacity of the Department to ensure that its policies were being implemented by health authorities. But there was a more fundamental reason still, one endemic in the nature of the NHS as a tax-financed service. While Ministers might be tempted to diffuse blame in hard times, to flirt with the idea of decentralisation, Parliament would have none of it. From 1980 to 1982 the DHSS was the target of a series of reports from the Social Services and Public Accounts Committees of the House of Commons, which cruelly documented and scathingly criticised its failure to find out what was happening at the periphery.[39] In short, delegation of responsibility to the periphery proved incompatible – not for the first or the last time – with the Secretary of State's accountability to Parliament,[40] which is why the cycle of experiments with delegation quickly followed by reversion to centralisation provides, as we have seen, one of the themes running through the history of the NHS.

The centrepiece of the Department's new directive and interventionist strategy was the annual performance review, first launched in 1982.[41] The basic idea was simple. Each year Ministers and their officials would hold 'accountability meetings' with the regional chairmen and their officials. At these meetings targets were agreed and progress towards achieving them discussed. In turn, the regional authorities would have similar meetings with their constituent districts. Finally, district health authorities would be expected to do the same with all their own sub-units, so forging a hierarchy of review and accountability running from the individual hospital to the Secretary of State. These new arrangements were designed, the Secretary of State told the House of Commons,[42] to ensure that resources were used in accordance with the Government's priorities and 'that the Health Service obtains the maximum amount of direct patient care and the greatest value for money from the resources which the Government have made available to the NHS'.

Administrative innovation was supplemented by technical innovation: the introduction of a system of performance indicators.[43] Successive Ministers, almost from the birth of the NHS, had been frustrated by their inability to find out what was actually happening in the service. To the question of what was being delivered to whom, there were few and mainly unsatisfactory answers. To the further question of how to monitor, let alone assess, the changing performance of the NHS, there were even fewer, more unsatisfactory still, answers. In the 1970s there was a brief flicker of interest in developing more adequate instruments, but this quickly waned as the enthusiasm for the planning ideology of the 1974 reorganisation turned sour. As long as the aims of public policy were set in terms of desired inputs of resources (so many beds, so many doctors, so many nurses per 1,000 population), adequate controls could be exercised through the annual budget. But the growing preoccupation with value for money in the 1980s drew attention to the relationship between inputs and outputs. As Ministers faced hostile questioning from Parliamentary Committees about the adequacy (or otherwise) of NHS funding, so they increasingly switched to emphasising that improved productivity could yield more and better services even at a time of financial stringency.

The set of performance indicators (PIs), first issued in 1983 and subsequently revised, can be seen in part at least as a response to such pressures. They were, and long remained, an extremely crude set of instruments using the statistics routinely generated by the NHS: the innovation lay chiefly in bringing them together and using information technology to make them more accessible. They were extremely vulnerable to questions about their accuracy. The time lag between collecting the data and presenting it in the PI set invited the response that the information was of historical interest only, although this lag was to be slowly reduced over the next decade. Above all, the PIs excluded many dimensions of performance. They included much data about activity (the outputs of the NHS as measured by the number of patients treated and the number of operations carried out) but none about outcomes (the impact of the activities on the health of those concerned). Subsequent revisions to the PI set sought to introduce some indicators of outcomes – none very satisfactory – but did not change the overall bias. Similarly, the PIs were silent about the question of quality.[44] But, with all these reservations, the PIs allowed comparisons to be made – if only in a rough and ready way – between the performance of different hospitals and different health authorities on a number of criteria, such as the cost per case treated, staffing levels related to patient numbers, waiting lists, the availability of particular services to any given population, and so on. As such they provided the policy-makers and managers in the Department with tin-openers by allowing them to ask direct questions about what was happening at the periphery.

In all this, it is not just the role of technology in making this development possible or the revival of centralisation that is significant. It is the fact that the centralisation of the 1980s spoke a different language, with the accent on outputs. If in the 1970s priorities were expressed in terms of inputs, by the mid-1980s they were being expressed in terms of targets of activity. Both points can be illustrated by taking the example of the 1985–86 round of regional reviews and the output targets that emerged from them.[45] The Trent Region was set a target of 2,250 extra maternity patients, provoking somewhat ribald questions about who was to be responsible for increasing the birth rate; the West Midlands Region was set a target of 315 extra rheumatology patients, while the North Western Region was required to offer an additional 200 open heart operations and to provide an extra 315 patients with renal dialysis. Such targets were, of course, not arbitrarily imposed but were the product of negotiations between the Department and the regions: they represented figures which both sides believed to be attainable. But they were also part of a wider FMI strategy of setting objectives and monitoring progress towards their achievement. Thus the annual Public Expenditure White Paper set out targets for the NHS as a whole as well as for other services. For instance the 1988 White Paper included the following acute sector targets to be achieved by 1990: an increase in the annual number of coronary artery bypass grafts to 17,000 (from 10,500 in 1984), a rise in the number of hip replacement operations to 50,000 (from 38,000 in 1985) and an increase in the number of cataract operations to 70,000 (from 59,000 in 1985). Similarly, the DHSS set a target of 40 new renal patients per million population to be accepted annually for treatment.

As these examples indicate, the objectives were often set in response to political pressures or worries. They were, in effect, a reply to criticism about the lengths of waiting lists (in the case of hip replacement surgery) or excessively harsh rationing (in the case of end-stage renal treatment). In contrast to the 1974 reorganisation where the emphasis was on central planning by experts, the 1980s brand of central interventionism was much more directly political. The new review machinery was seen as an instrument for translating *ministerial* priorities into practice. Moreover, the review system was further reinforced as a transmission belt for the ministerial will by the gradual development, over the 1980s, of more direct contacts between politicians at the centre and district health authority chairmen at the periphery. Increasingly Ministers brought their influence to bear directly on those responsible for carrying out their policies. Perhaps this accounts for the fact that the new-style centralisation turned out to have more vigour and life about it than its predecessors.

This 'politicisation' of the NHS can be interpreted in a variety of ways. If Ministerial accountability to Parliament is to be more than a constitutional fiction, then Ministers must have the power to set objectives and the machinery required to ensure their implementation. Yet if Ministers do centralise decision-making, this is clearly at odds with the rhetoric of accountability to local populations. In short, there is a conflict between two different concepts of accountability which, as we have seen in previous chapters, have been at war with each other throughout the history of the NHS. And there is a further conflict. If the NHS is in any sense a 'democratic' institution (a dangerous because ambiguously fuzzy term) it is precisely because it is politically responsive. In turn, to make a service as large and complex as the NHS responsive to Ministers means creating a managerial machinery capable of carrying out ministerial aims. Yet the effectiveness of such a managerial machinery may depend, in part at least, on its ability to insulate itself from day-to-day political turbulence. In other words, there may be a trade-off between making the NHS so sensitive to immediate political objectives that it becomes incapable of pursuing even those longer-term aims which Ministers themselves want to pursue. In the next section, therefore, we turn to the managerial revolution in the NHS.

The new managerialism

In October 1983 there appeared a 25-page document which was to transform the management style of the NHS. This was the Report of the NHS Management Inquiry led by Sir Roy (as he subsequently became) Griffiths, managing director of one of the country's most successful supermarket chains, Sainsbury's.[46] The style of the inquiry set the tone for its recommendations. It involved only four people. It took a mere six months to complete its task. It worked quickly and informally, consulting a great many people but not taking any formal evidence. It thus marked a break with the tradition of setting up Committees and Royal Commissions, representative of all the interested parties, whose job it was to produce acceptable consensus reports: a break which was one of the hallmarks of the Thatcher administration. The new management style in the NHS was thus born of an equally new approach to decision-making in Government – brisk and decisive, if sometimes also peremptory – and mirrored many of those characteristics.

The Griffiths report's analysis was not new. In effect, it confirmed the diagnosis of institutional stalemate offered in Chapter 4. But it was expressed in blunt language. The NHS was suffering from 'institutional stagnation'; health authorities were being 'swamped with directives without being given direction'; the NHS was an organisation in which it was 'extremely difficult to achieve change'; consensus decision-making led to 'long delays in the management process'. In short, the report concluded in a phrase that was to reverberate through the media and across the years, 'if Florence Nightingale were carrying her lamp through the corridors of the NHS today she would almost certainly be searching for the people in charge'.

From this diagnosis followed a clear prescription: a general management structure from the top to the bottom of the NHS, i.e. individuals, at all levels, responsible for making things happen. At the top, within the DHSS, there was to be a Supervisory Board to be chaired by the Secretary of State, to set objectives, take strategic decisions and receive reports on performance. Below that, but still within the Department, there was to be a Chief Executive, to carry out the policy objectives, provide leadership and control performance. Lastly, and perhaps most importantly, there were to be general managers responsible for the operations of the NHS at all levels – regions, districts and units. The general managers, the report suggested, might well be recruited from outside the NHS or the civil service, while their pay should be linked to their performance.

The recommendations were to be carried out almost to the letter. Both a Supervisory and a Management Board were set up within the NHS. The arrangement proved unstable both in the short run and in the long term.[47] The division of responsibility between the two Boards was blurred; there was friction between the civil service hierarchy of the DHSS and the Management Board. The first Chief Executive of the NHS – Mr Victor Paige, who had been brought in from industry – resigned because it proved impossible to draw a clear line between management and politics. Subsequently the Minister of State for Health took over the Management Board – clear recognition that politicians were endogenous to the management process in the NHS – with a new import from the private sector, Mr Len Peach, as Chief Executive. The Supervisory Board effectively withered away.[48] But this new arrangement did not last. It was revised yet again following the NHS reforms (see Chapter 6). Nor is this surprising. There is little support in the academic literature for the idea that policy-making and implementation can be kept in separate compartments, instead of being seen as part of a continuing, dynamic process. And generalised scepticism is reinforced by the specific circumstances of the NHS. The instability of the central governance arrangements of the NHS – like the cycle of decentralisation leading to a reversion to centralism, and so da capo – reflected a basic tension embedded in the system of health care as revised in 1948. Given the financial basis of the NHS, management is inextricably political in the sense of involving Ministers who are accountable to Parliament.

Haunting the history of the NHS, therefore, is the dream that it might somehow be possible to de-politicise the management of the NHS by handing it over to an independent Commission. The 1979 Royal Commission considered the idea of an independent health commission to provide 'the permanent and easily identifiable leadership which the service at present lacks'[49] but rejected it as incompatible with parliamentary accountability. The Griffiths Inquiry would have liked to recommend such a solution but was persuaded that it was politically unaccep- table. At the end of his term as Secretary of State Norman Fowler came to the conclusion that a Commission was desirable but left office before he could do anything to bring his ideas about.[50] Even the implementation of the *Next Steps* Initiative – the wholesale transfer of government activities to freestanding agencies – left the NHS firmly embedded in the Department of Health.

Despite the problems at the top, the general management revolution swept through the NHS. Everywhere, at every level, new managers were appointed. The consensus teams born in 1974 effectively died 10 years later, and with them the attempt to institutionalise producer syndicalism: predictably so, given the Government's general suspicion of corporate interest groups. The mobilisation of consent for change, rather than consolidation of consensus, became the new style:[51] the 'vigorous virtues' came to be the sought-for qualities in the NHS as elsewhere. The medical and nursing representatives on the management committees lost their veto power; nurse managers, in particular, lost much of the ground they had gained after 1974. The new managers had, in contrast to their predecessors, a direct self-interest in the promotion of change. Their salaries and contracts were linked to performance. If they did not deliver the goods, they risked not having their contracts renewed – as happened to quite a few of them, in the outcome.

The impact of the new managerialism on the way the NHS conducted its business at district and hospital level was perhaps not quite as revolutionary as the rhetoric implied, and certainly not as immediate as Ministers might have hoped. The conversion of NHS administrators who had traditionally seen themselves as 'diplomats' – brokers between the conflicting provider interests – into active managers was slow.[52] Some of them, brought up to believe that the NHS's unique organisational characteristics automatically disqualified ideas imported from the outside, resentfully questioned the applicability of what they saw as a supermarket management style. For others, the Griffiths report was tainted by its association with Mrs Thatcher and her style of government. No understanding of any events in the 1980s, whether in the NHS or elsewhere, can be complete without taking into account the antipathy aroused by the Prime Minister: her very positive (not to say aggressive) style prompted, in turn, a very positive (not to say virulent) dislike in a significant section of the population. But for many managers the effects were liberating. As the following quotations from district general managers illustrate,[53] the implementation of the Griffiths recommendations brought about a new sense that change was actually possible, a readiness to challenge the professionals and a willingness to take risks:

> What made me want to get into general management was a porter I passed every day at the main hospital entrance. He always had a fag hanging out of his mouth, he was rude to everyone – he just grunted – and yet, as Chief Nursing Officer, I could do nothing about it – I tried but I failed. As general manager I can.

> A lot of Health Authorities spent most of their time talking about administrative and financial issues – and we were one of those. . . . One of the most significant changes in this Authority is the number of

items that relate to nursing specifically or to medicine specifically. . . .
Now, in fact, I ask the questions and demand the answers and dictate –
if need be – what the timetables are. So it's not the 'I'll do that when I
feel like it' sort of approach.

The new-style management is not about bringing clinicians to heel.
Instead it is about making them grow up. It's about making them take
responsibility for doing things which they know in their hearts are
right.

As these quotations suggest, the post-Griffiths era was marked by a more
assertive management style towards the NHS workforce. As far as relations
with trade unions are concerned, it is difficult to disentangle the effects of the
new managerialism from other developments in the 1980s. In this respect, as in
others, the NHS mirrored changes on the national stage. With a Government
determined to break the power of the trade unions, the days when they were
considered members of the policy club were clearly over. So while it would be
impossible to write a history of the NHS in the 1970s which did not take account
of the role of the trade unions – as Chapter 4 demonstrated – quite the reverse
was the case in the 1980s. The number of actors in the health care policy arena,
having expanded in the 1970s, shrank in the 1980s. The trade unions, despite an
explosion of militancy over wages in 1982, became predominantly passive
spectators of developments. They were often vociferous in their opposition to
the Government's policies but powerless to prevent their implementation. In
this respect, the corporate stalemate had been truly broken and the Griffiths
report should perhaps be seen more as the product than the cause of this new
situation.

   No such clear-cut conclusion is possible when it comes to examining the impact
of the Griffiths recommendations on the NHS's professional providers, i.e. doctors
and nurses. Griffiths himself was always anxious to assure them that the new
managerialism did not represent a threat to them but rather an opportunity to
participate more in the decision-making process. There was no reason, he argued,
why the new managers should not be recruited from the medical and nursing
professions. In the outcome, only 25 per cent of general managers were doctors or
nurses by 1987 – with the medical profession predominant – while 61 per cent
were former NHS administrators or finance people. A further 12 per cent had
been recruited from outside the NHS.[54] The hostility of doctors and nurses
towards the Griffiths report had, however, deeper roots. Nurses quite clearly
lost out: the effect of the Griffiths recommendations was that nurses lost both the
right to be managed exclusively by a member of their own profession and their
automatic representation on district management teams, both guaranteed by the
1974 corporatist arrangements. In the case of doctors, however, the antagonism
had rather different causes. Reflecting subsequently on his experience,[55] Sir Roy
acknowledged that 'The medical profession saw the report correctly as questioning whether their clinical autonomy extended to immunity from being questioned as to how resources were being used'. Furthermore, there was a
widespread sense – not limited to doctors – that ideas drawn from the private
sector were, by definition, inappropriate and injurious when applied to the NHS:
they represented, as it were, an invasion of the sacred by the profane. As Sir Roy
put it:

All the professions saw the report as the introduction of economics into the care of patients, believing that this was inimical to good care. There was a deep-seated feeling that what distinguished the Health Service from the private sector or business or commerce was the very immunity of the Health Service from the supposedly corrupting influence of profit making and that this very immunity guaranteed high quality. This denies the fact that the hallmarks of the truly great organisations in the private sector is that they have placed quality and customer satisfaction first and profit for a long time simply emerged as the by-product of effective services.

The Griffiths report thus marked not only the introduction of a new management style but also a challenge to some of the assumptions which had shaped the NHS ever since its birth. One of the report's central arguments was that the management task revolved around delivering a good product to the consumer: 'Businessmen have a keen sense of how well they are looking after their customers. Whether the NHS is meeting the needs of the patient and the community, and can prove that it is doing so, is open to question.' Thus Griffiths put two new questions on the NHS agenda, which became increasingly salient over the following decades. First, was the NHS producing the right kind of goods? Second, was the quality of the goods being produced adequate? Furthermore, the post-Griffiths reshuffle quite accidentally created a lobby for quality. Jobs had to be found for dispossessed nurse managers and quite a few of them re-emerged in charge of quality assurance. The concept was imported from the United States and enthusiastically adopted in the NHS, perhaps partly because its versatile ambiguity could cover a variety of activities.

But the NHS, throughout its history, had been characterised by the fact that its outputs were decided by the medical profession. Since the NHS existed to meet need, and since only professionals could define what need was, it followed that what doctors produced was *ipso facto* the right product. Moreover, even more self-evidently, only doctors could judge the standards of their peers. To ask whether the right goods were being produced and to question the adequacy of standards was, therefore, to threaten the secret garden of professional autonomy.[56] If supermarkets provide a good symbol for the 1980s it is because they can be seen as the embodiment of individual choice and the supremacy of the consumer. To import their values into the NHS – as, to some extent, the Griffiths report did – was therefore to introduce some extremely subversive notions. Specifically, they were potentially subversive of medical dominance. If management in the NHS was all about satisfying consumers instead of keeping doctors happy, then the implications were indeed profound.

The Griffiths report's importance thus lies as much in the philosophy which shaped its recommendations as in the recommendations themselves. It marked a shift from producer to consumer values. And precisely because the Griffiths report was articulating a more general social change, not specific to the NHS, its invocation of consumer values was to determine much of the health care policy agenda for the next decades. In particular, policy had to address a crucial question left unanswered by the report, a rather large hole in its chain of argument. If the NHS was to behave like a supermarket trying to satisfy its customers, and to deliver value for money, how best could managers and doctors be persuaded to behave appropriately? If a supermarket failed to satisfy its customers, or it ran its business inefficiently, it would eventually be taken over or go bankrupt. If an NHS hospital failed to satisfy its customers, or tolerated waste, there were no equivalent sanctions. There was much talk of changing the culture of the NHS. But where were the incentives and sanctions which would actually persuade managers and others to adopt the new ways? However elegant the Griffiths model may have appeared, it lacked an engine to drive it. Its weakness lay not so much in seeking to impose on the NHS an approach to management drawn from the private, for-profit sector of the economy – the view taken by most contemporary critics – as in assuming that it was possible to change the style without also re-engineering the dynamics of the system: precisely the defect which *Working for Patients* sought to remedy.

Not surprisingly, then, the impact of the Griffiths report turned out to be much less radical or dramatic than the ideas which had shaped its recommendations. Producer domination of the NHS did not end in the 1980s; indeed, as we shall see in the following chapters, a long struggle still lay ahead. But the search for efficiency – of which the Griffiths report was both the expression and a symbol – coincided with, and in part prompted, a series of evolutionary developments which fuelled the apprehensions of the medical profession. Consider, for example, the implications of the new system for setting objectives and targets and monitoring progress towards their achievement. The ultimate logic of such a system of review is to challenge the performance not just of particular health authorities or managerial units within them but also that of individual consultants. The point is well illustrated by the case of waiting lists, politically one of the most sensitive issues throughout the 1980s, as it had been for much of the NHS's history and as it was going to be again in the 1990s. The implications drawn for policy and practice from the existence of long waiting lists depends crucially on the diagnosis of the reasons for their length in the first place. If waiting lists in a particular district were long, it might be because the available resources were inadequate (for which the Government could be blamed, and where the solution was to inject more money into the NHS). Or the reason might be found in the way in which any given bundle of resources was managed by the district (for which the health authority could be blamed, and where the solution was to improve the quality of management). Or it might simply be because doctors were not treating as many patients as their counterparts elsewhere (for which individual consultants could be blamed, and where the solution was to change the pattern of clinical practice). In the 1980s all three diagnoses were offered and acted upon at various times: thus the Government provided some earmarked funds with the specific purpose of reducing the queues. But much of the evidence underlined the importance of clinical practice. For instance, one study[57] found that the number of cases treated by individual orthopaedic surgeons varied fivefold, from 200 to 1,000 a year. The same study suggested that long waiting lists reflected not so much a shortage of operating theatres but their under-use, an analysis subsequently confirmed by the National Audit Office.[58] And if it was the work practices of individual consultants which were responsible for long waiting lists – or for above average costs per case as revealed by the performance indicators – then, clearly, it was the responsibility of managers to challenge those practices: to subject clinical discretion, interpreted as the right of every doctor to decide how to treat his or her patients, to scrutiny.

The renegotiation of what was meant by clinical autonomy or freedom[59] – and how the demarcation line between managerial and professional responsibilities should be defined – was to continue into the 1990s and is still far from completed. However, the traditional right of consultants to determine which patients should be treated, and how, was being questioned from another perspective as well. Throughout the 1980s there was a rising interest in techniques designed to measure the relative impact of different procedures in terms of the cost of achieving specific outcomes. So, for example, one study compared the quality-adjusted life years (QALYs) yielded by heart transplants as against bypass surgery.[60] Rising interest did not lead to consensus about such techniques; there remained much doubt about their validity and usefulness. But, potentially at least, it seemed that the technicians – economists, epidemiologists and others – might be able to provide managers with tools for determining priorities: a threatening prospect for consultants. The ethical individualism of the medical profession (emphasising the doctor's responsibility to the individual patient) was increasingly being confronted by the utilitarianism of the economist and the epidemiologist (emphasising the impact of any individual decision on the population as a whole): a conflict endemic in the NHS from the start was beginning to come to the surface.[61]

In all this, the Griffiths report was perhaps more important in setting up signposts for the future rather than in making any immediate impact on the NHS's efficiency or productivity. And therein, of course, lies an irony. On the one hand, the changes produced by the new managerialism were not sufficient to acquit the Government of the charge that it was starving the NHS of funds. Quite possibly the new managerialism did lead to more value for money; almost certainly, it resulted in a more brisk approach to problem-solving in the NHS. But evidence to support such contentions was difficult to assemble. The politically most visible, if misleading, symbol of NHS inadequacy – long waiting lists – remained stubbornly impervious to managerial intervention. On the other hand, the changes were quite sufficient to provoke despondency among the NHS's providers and alarm among the Thatcher Government's political critics. As we have seen, they threatened provider dominance. And they appeared to herald the invasion of the NHS temple by the Thatcherite money-lenders, bringing with them a false set of values. As the Government saw it, the new managerialism was part of its strategy for saving the NHS: for ensuring its survival in hard times. As the Government's professional and political opponents saw it, the new managerialism was part of an insidious strategy for privatising the NHS without actually attacking it head-on.

A drift to privatisation?

So far the analysis has tended to identify change rather than continuity in the 1980s, or at least new strategies for trying to deal with familiar problems. But there was one issue where old political battles continued to be fought all over again, testimony perhaps to the longevity of symbols in politics. The word 'privatisation' still provoked the traditional reactions. In its 1983 manifesto the Labour Party pledged itself to 'remove private practice from the NHS and take into the NHS those parts of the profit-making private sector which can be put to good use'; in 1987, it took the view that 'privatisation means a Health Service run for profit rather than in the patients' interest'. Conversely, the 1983 Conservative manifesto welcomed the growth in private health insurance and promised to 'promote' close partnership between the State and the private sectors in the exchange of facilities and of ideas 'in the interests of all patients'. In 1987, however, Mrs Thatcher decided that 'The NHS was seen by many as a touchstone of our commitment to the welfare state and there were obvious dangers of coming forward with new proposals out of the blue'[62] and the manifesto accordingly took the safety-first line of stressing managerial and other improvements within the NHS.

The concept of 'privatisation' is, however, more complex than political stereotypes or rhetoric would suggest.[63] It has a number of different dimensions or meanings which it is important to distinguish in analysing developments in the 1980s. To start with, it is important to distinguish between the sources of funding and the ownership of the means of production. Both can be either public or private. The NHS is the paradigm case of public ownership accompanied by public finance. The private sector of acute health care is the paradigm case of private ownership and private finance: people (or their insurance policies) pay for the services they get in privately owned facilities. Then there are the mixed cases. On the one hand, there is the private funding of public services: people may be asked to pay charges, as in the NHS. Conversely, there is the public funding of people using private services: in the 1980s, social security played an increasingly important role in funding people in residential and nursing homes. Additionally, if inaccurately, the term 'privatisation' was increasingly used in the 1980s to describe, pejoratively, the public purchase of services from the private sector: for example, contracting out laundry or catering services. In what follows, we shall therefore distinguish sharply between these various definitions, since each raises a somewhat different set of issues.

Throughout the 1980s, both the provision of acute medical care in the private sector and the proportion of the population with insurance policies continued to grow.[64] In 1980, there were 154 private hospitals with 7,000 beds. By the end of the decade, there were 216 hospitals with almost 11,000 beds. The trend was not only upwards but also towards a different pattern of ownership. Whereas in 1980 the independent sector had been dominated by hospitals owned by charitable and religious organisations, by the end of the decade hospitals owned by for-profit groups predominated. However, the threatened take-over of the private sector by American companies – widely prophesied in the early 1980s and widely resented as the intrusion of rampant commercialism[65] – did not take place: the US companies, having first rushed in, soon sold up. The expansion in the size of the independent hospital sector reflected, in turn, the expansion in the insurance market. In 1980, only 6.4 per cent of the population were covered by private insurance schemes. By the end of the decade, the proportion had risen to 11.5 per cent and the figure was much higher still among professionals (27 per cent) and employers and managers (23 per cent). Significantly, however, both developments owed little to Government policies. Despite manifesto rhetoric, the Thatcher administration did nothing directly to encourage the growth of the private sector, apart from increasing marginally (to £8,500) the income limit below which tax concessions could be claimed for health insurance premiums.

To the extent that private sector activity can be interpreted as a commentary on the failure of the NHS to respond to consumer demands, then its continued expansion would suggest a widening gap between what the public sector supplied and what the customers wanted. This indeed was the interpretation put upon it by many of Mrs Thatcher's critics, who argued that the Government had starved the NHS in order to drive demand into the private sector: that there was a deliberate move, in other words, towards creating a two-tier health care system. And even those who did not embrace this conspiracy theory argued that the effect of the growth of the private sector, whether intended or not, was to weaken public support for the NHS and the principle of universalism. The most articulate and most exigent users of the NHS – the middle classes – would exit into the private sector rather than exercising voice to improve the NHS.[66]

These arguments need to be unpackaged, since they tend to conflate a number of different propositions. First, the 1980s saw little or no change in the nature of the demand for private health care. It remained, predominantly, for the treatment of those conditions requiring elective surgery where there were long queues in the NHS. The private sector, in short, continued to offer treatment to improve the quality of life for people of working age rather than dealing with life-threatening conditions in the population as a whole. In the mid-1980s, an estimated 16.7 per cent of all non-abortion elective surgery in England and Wales was carried out in the private sector, with the proportion rising to over 28 per cent in the case of hip replacement.[67] Second, the evidence suggests that the growth of the private sector reflected not just frustrated access but also a demand for consumer control over the non-medical aspects of treatment: personal privacy, the timing of an operation, and the right to insist on being treated by a consultant.[68] In all these respects, the private sector had the incentives – as well as the resources – to act out the Griffiths model for the NHS: to treat patients as customers. Third, and following on from this, an increase in such demands (and in the financial ability to satisfy them) might have been expected to follow from the social and economic changes in the population noted at the beginning of this chapter, i.e. the rising proportion of the population in middle-class occupations which either provided health care insurance as part of the pay package or paid salaries which made such insurance affordable.

The growth of private sector activity in the 1980s does not, therefore, necessarily mean that dissatisfaction with the NHS was rising. It may simply have reflected the spreading capacity to do what the wealthiest had always done, during the entire history of the NHS, which was to exit into the private sector when it suited them. There had always been a two-tier health care system in the UK; the difference in the 1980s lay in the fact that the private tier, rather like holidays abroad, became more widely accessible. Fourth, the fears that the increasing use of the exit option would erode support for the principle of a universal, tax-financed health care system were contradicted by the experience of the 1980s. As noted earlier, public support for the NHS, and for spending more tax-funded money on it, was stronger at the end of the decade than at the beginning. Even those with private insurance coverage continued to use the NHS for much of the time: more than half of their inpatient stays, and four-fifths of their outpatient attendances, were as NHS rather than as private patients.[69] In short, consumers did not exit into the private sector; they commuted between it and the NHS. As a result neither voice nor loyalty was weakened.

There is a further reason for scepticism about the assumption that use of the private sector can be directly equated with dissatisfaction with the NHS. Consumer demand in all health care systems is strongly influenced by medical decisions. If there is an increase in the number of doctors, and if they have an incentive to generate extra activity, one would predict an increase also in demand. And this is precisely what happened in the case of private practice. One of the first acts of the incoming 1979 Conservative Government, as we saw in the last chapter, was to relax the consultant contract so as to allow all contract holders to engage in private practice. So the supply of doctors available for private practice increased. At the same time, there were powerful incentives to increase activity: the fees that could be earned by so doing. If disputes over the pay of doctors were relatively muted during the 1980s, despite the fact that consultant salaries in the NHS were tending to lag behind earnings in many comparable occupations, it was no doubt because they were doing exceedingly well out of private practice.

Private hospitals did not prove a consistent Klondyke for their shareholders; many suffered from under-occupation, with occupancy often running at 60 per cent or less. The insurers were struggling to hold back the rise in premiums, as the market for insurance became more competitive and as claims multiplied. But the medical profession's earnings soared. In 1980 the insurers paid out just over £57 million in fees to doctors. By 1988 this figure was almost £245 million, a considerable rise even allowing for inflation. A study carried out in the early 1990s[70] showed that of all consultants with an income of more than £1,000 a year from private practice, 37.8 per cent earned less than £10,000, net of expenses; 33.4 per cent earned between £10,000 and £30,000; 24.6 per cent earned between £30,000 and £100,000 and 4.2 per cent earned more than £100,000. The distribution of earnings was, of course, skewed as between different specialties, as well as geographically. Surgeons had a good chance of doubling their NHS salaries, at the very least, while pathologists tended to be poor relations who were lucky if they earned some pocket money from private practice.

But consultant-induced demand can offer, at best, only a very partial explanation of the growth of private practice. The danger of looking for the causes of changes exclusively in the dynamics of the health care arena – or in the ideology of government – are illustrated when the focus of analysis is switched from the growth of the private acute sector to the expansion of the private sector of long-term care. The 1980s were marked by an explosion in the provision of residential and nursing home care far more dramatic than the rise in the acute sector. The number of places in these homes – owned by both for-profit and voluntary organisations – rose from 107,000 in 1980 to 318,000 in 1990.[71] But this had absolutely nothing to do with the medical profession, traditionally disinterested in long-term care. Nor does political ideology provide the explanation even though the growth of the private sector of long-stay care fitted snugly into the Government's preferences and was fuelled by a large injection of public funds through the social security system.

This injection of public funds was not the product of deliberate Government policy but the perverse and unintended effect of a series of decisions taken with quite different aims in mind:[72] the product of policy accident rather than policy intention. Under the 1948 National Assistance Act, social security offices had discretion to make allowances to those living in residential and nursing homes. From the 1970s onwards these payments slowly rose: by 1983 they had reached £39 million a year and were contributing to the cost of caring for 16,000 people. The Department decided to stop the creep. Each local social security office was asked to set a limit for the weekly payments, based on the highest reasonable charge for the area. The result was precisely the opposite of that intended. The maxima quickly became the minima. More important, what had previously been a low-visibility, discretionary payment overnight turned into a highly visible, as-of-right entitlement. Financial need, not medical or social need, was the only criterion. The result, not surprisingly, was a sharp rise both in the number of residents whose fees were being paid by social security and in the level of charges. In turn, new providers came into the market to meet the demand so generated: hence the expansion of private provision. The public spending creep turned into an avalanche. By 1990 expenditure was £1,270 million and still rising fast: it was to reach £2,530 million in 1992 before a change in the system put a lid on spending. And the social security system was paying for the care of 189,000 people, a figure which was to rise to 271,000 by 1992.

Contrary to its policy aim of containing public expenditure, the Government had stumbled into creating a demand-led, and therefore uncontrollable, spending explosion. Contrary to its declared policy of targeting spending on the most needy, the Government had created a new entitlement where there was no test of need for residential or nursing home care. Contrary to what might have been expected on the basis of its general ideological stance, the Government had furthermore stumbled into the most egalitarian policy commitment taken during its entire period in office. In effect the social security entitlement meant that the poorest had access to services which previously had only been available to the relatively well-to-do. In contrast to the expansion of the private acute sector, the growth of the private sector of long-stay care almost certainly diminished rather than accentuated inequalities: a warning against assuming that 'privatisation' must necessarily be equated with increased inequality and a reminder that the way in which access to the private sector is financed is crucial in determining its impact on equity.

Mrs Thatcher's Government might well have been able to exploit this policy accident by arguing that it represented a triumph for its vision of transferring power to the consumer in the market place. The social security payments could have been presented as the equivalent of vouchers, giving consumers the ability to choose between competing providers: the democratisation of choice. But nothing of the sort happened. When it came to choosing between economic and ideological imperatives, the former invariably triumphed. From a Treasury perspective, ideological opportunism would have come at too high a price. Additionally, the new system was strongly criticised as offering perverse incentives to both health and local authorities to encourage people to move into social security financed institutional care, instead of developing community care.[73] And indeed both seized the opportunity to run down their own long-stay facilities and to transfer the financial burden to social security. So the Government once again turned to Sir Roy Griffiths.[74] Somewhat at odds with the consumer thrust of his 1983 report, and the Government's distrust of local government, his formula turned out to be transferring responsibility for funding long-stay care to local authorities and ending the social security entitlement. It was a formula which was subsequently to be adopted, in large part, by the Government and implemented in the 1990s.

So the growth of private long-stay care for the elderly, and the decline of public sector provision, points to no simple ideological moral. It does, however, raise two general issues. First, it emphasises the importance of environmental factors in explaining what happens within the health care policy arena. Given the increase in the over-75 population, demand for institutional care might have been expected to rise irrespective of public policy. Given also that an increasing proportion of the elderly were becoming reasonably well-off,[75] often with capital in the shape of a house, demand for private institutional care might have been expected to rise even if the public sector had been more generously financed. As in the case of private acute hospitals, the geographical distribution of private institutional provision for the elderly reflected – among other factors – geographical variations in the social composition of the population:[76] the wealthier the population, the higher was private provision. Second, the story illustrates how developments in the private sector feed back into the public sector. In the case of institutional care for the elderly, the growth in the private sector provoked fears that vulnerable elderly people would be exploited by private proprietors anxious only to maximise profits. The result was legislation in 1984 tightening up the responsibilities of health and local authorities, i.e. for regulating the private sector.[77] This underlines one of the central paradoxes of the Thatcher years: that the expansion of the private sector led to increasing regulatory activity of the State. Additionally, however, the consequent debate about regulation raised questions about the extent to which the NHS was maintaining standards for the vulnerable elderly in its own care. The reports of the Health Advisory Service were far from reassuring;[78] neither were the reports of a succession of inquiries into conditions in individual hospitals.[79] If exploitation for profit was frequently perceived to be the original sin of the private sector, exploitation of patients by providers was often revealed to be the original sin of the public sector.

While the growth of the private sectors, both acute and long-stay, give little support to the notion that health care policy in the 1980s was driven by the Government's general style and ideological predisposition, the case of competitive tendering appears at first sight to provide more support for this thesis. In September 1983 the DHSS issued a circular instructing all health authorities to put out to competitive tender their cleaning, catering and laundry services, which between them accounted for about 12 per cent of the NHS's total expenditure.[80] It was very much a central government directive, specifying precisely the procedures to be followed, the criteria to be met and the timetable to be followed. Gone were the days when the DHSS merely offered guidance to health authorities, leaving them to interpret it in their own way and to proceed at their own pace; instead, the Department took a detailed and intensive interest in the process of implementation, frequently intervening directly and applying pressure to laggard authorities. In its execution the introduction of contracting out thus provides a neat case study of centralisation at work, with Ministers making it very clear that they were determined to push their policies through, whatever the resistance or scepticism among NHS staff or authority chairmen and members.

In the outcome, there was both resistance and scepticism. In particular, the principle of competitive tendering was seen as a direct threat by the NHS unions, NUPE and COHSE, which had been the leading actors in the battles of the 1970s (discussed in Chapter 4). Moreover, it was intended as such: competitive tendering challenged the monopoly of the in-house providers of services. The fact that the Government successfully pushed its policy through, despite a national campaign by the unions and local attempts to block the tendering process, provides further evidence of the shifting balance of power within the health care policy arena: a shift which reflected, in turn, the general decline in the influence of the trade union movement brought about by Government policy. Similarly, the Government's insistence on compliance with its policy directive on competitive tendering underlined its determination that national policy object-ives had to override local preferences. In the crusade for value for money, no deviations were to be allowed: health authorities which appeared to be biased towards in-house tenders from their own staff were sharply dealt with.

The direct financial yield of the new policy turned out to be modest. By 1986 annual savings had reached £86 million.[81] Furthermore, the policy did not 'privatise' the NHS's support services in the sense of transferring them to the private sector. Of all the contracts awarded by the end of the first cycle of the competitive tendering exercise, only 18 per cent went to private contractors. The rest were all awarded to bids coming from in-house teams which, by the end of the first round, were capturing over 90 per cent of all contracts. But if the direct effects were less than spectacular, the indirect effects were probably more significant – if difficult to pin down statistically. The exercise forced NHS managers to examine what they were doing. When it started most of them had never specified the standards of their services, let alone devised ways of defining quality of provision. For, although competitive tendering prompted many complaints about a consequent decline in quality, it was never clear on what these were based – since no previous benchmarks existed. In addition, apart from forcing improvements in the techniques of control, the contracting-out process gave confidence to managers by demonstrating that change could be introduced and resistance could be overcome. In this respect, it marked a clear break with the 1970s. The gains in efficiency may therefore have been larger if less visible than the figures of direct savings suggested. Conversely, the same may be true of the costs of the exercise. These tended to fall on the lowest-paid and most vulnerable workers in the NHS. The price of successfully defending in-house contracts tended to be lower earnings and redundancies.[82]

Overall, then, contracting out can be seen most accurately not so much as the product of an ideology of privatisation as the product of an ideology of managerial efficiency. After all, it was a Labour Prime Minister – Harold (subsequently Lord) Wilson – who pioneered the concept of contracting out when he decreed in 1968 that central government departments should find private contractors to take over their cleaning. The Conservative strategy appears to have been to introduce some of the disciplines of competition into the NHS – using the market as an instrument for so doing – but not necessarily to transfer the production of health care to the for-profit sector.

The Government's enthusiasm for privatisation also turns out to have been heavily qualified when one examines, finally, another sense in which the word has been used. This is the process of 'privatising' health care costs by charging patients: thus it has been argued that the increase in various charges to patients under the Conservative administration represented the 'backdoor privatisation' of services.[83] Leaving aside the question of whether or not this is an appropriate use of the term, some other qualifications need to be noted. The increases represented a policy of cautious incrementalism, gradually ratcheting up the level of charges, rather than a sudden rush of ideological blood to the head. Conspicuously, the increases fell most heavily on those services which – rightly or wrongly – have been perceived since the 1950s as most marginal to the purposes of the NHS: dental and optical charges.

In contrast, in the sensitive area of prescription charges, no attempt was made to increase the yield by narrowing the exempt categories: the old, the young, those on income support and some (but not all) of those suffering from chronic diseases who, between them, accounted for 80 per cent of the prescriptions issued by the end of the 1980s. Yet any Government determined to increase revenue – as distinct from avoiding political trouble – would surely have sought to restrict the scope of exemptions. Failing any such attempt, it is not surprising that this form of privatisation – if that is what it was – yielded only a modest income. In 1979–80 charges contributed 2.2 per cent of the NHS's total finance. By the end of the decade the figure had risen steeply to 4.5 per cent, but even so was less than it had been in the 1950s.[84] In the 1980s, as in the 1950s and succeeding decades, the level of charges was determined in the annual budget-setting tussle between the Department and the Treasury. A hike in the level of charges was the bone that Department civil servants could throw to the Treasury wolves in order to safeguard what they perceived to be the NHS's core interests. In the 1980s one of the Department's core interests was the development of primary care. This meant seeking extra funding to grease the engine of change – i.e. to buy the acquiescence of GPs – and increased charges was the price paid for Treasury agreement to this strategy. In the next section we examine this strategy in more detail.

Controlling the gatekeepers

One of the paradoxes of the NHS since its creation has been that it exercises least control over those who, in theory at least, exercise the greatest influence in determining the demands for health care: general practitioners.[85] One of the main reasons why Britain was able to spend less on health care than most comparable European countries, it was generally agreed, is that GPs have a unique role in filtering, shaping and controlling demands on the expensive hospital sector of care. GPs are, at one and the same time, the patient's agents in steering him or her to the appropriate specialists and the system's gatekeepers in that they determine who is referred where and for what. Yet at the same time, GPs are independent contractors and as such have a peculiar hands-off relation-ship with the NHS. In effect, they are small businessmen who – as noted in previous chapters – have fiercely and successfully defended this status ever since 1913. Despite changes in the small print of the GP's contract – especially those introduced by the Family Doctor Charter of the 1960s – general practice remained an autonomous enclave within the NHS: a fact recognised by the 1982 decision to make Family Practitioner Committees, the bodies responsible for the administra-tion of primary care, directly accountable to the DHSS. Tangling with general practitioners involved high political costs; ancestral memories of decades of bitter wrangling with the BMA were slow to die in the DHSS.

But as the 1980s progressed, it became increasingly clear that the financial costs of avoiding a confrontation with the medical profession over general practice might outweigh any political costs. The emphasis on strengthening management might allow the NHS to cope with more demand within any given budget by improving efficiency; the development of the private sector might provide a safety valve for excess demand. But none of these strategies could address the question of whether it was possible to limit the seemingly inexorable upward surge of demand itself. Was it inevitable that, given the rise in the over-75 population and given the new possibilities of treatment opened up by technological change, demand would go on rising? Or was it possible to devise other strategies which might at least limit the rate of expansion and, by so doing, curb the growth of public expenditure on health care?

As these questions became more urgent, so attention turned to primary health care and to prevention. The two were linked. Primary health care could itself be seen as a form of prevention, i.e. as a means of coping with conditions either before they became acute enough to call for more expensive hospital intervention or as a way of providing treatment more cheaply than in an institutional setting. In addition, primary care was a source of obvious concern for a Government anxious to control public spending. It represented an open-ended public expenditure commitment; there was no way of imposing cash limits on the amount spent by GPs on prescribing, just as there appeared to be no way to check the number of people they referred to hospitals. There were wide, seemingly inexplicable variations in the rate at which different GPs prescribed and referred – a range of 20 to 1, according to some studies – yet public policy appeared incapable of bringing discipline to the apparent chaos. The number of GPs in practice increased; average list sizes fell below the 2,000 mark; the number of, and salary bill for, supporting staff in surgeries shot up. Expenditure on the Family Practitioner Services (which included dentistry and ophthalmic services, though these are not considered here, as well as general practice) rose faster than spending on the rest of the NHS, with the result that their share of the total budget rose from 22 per cent in 1979–80 to 24 per cent in 1985–86. Yet, frustratingly, there was little evidence that the increased investment was yielding any returns. Neither prescribing nor referral patterns seemed to be linked systematically to such factors as list size.[86] Moreover, one by-product of the decision to make FPCs directly accountable to the DHSS – as part of the 1982 reorganisation – was to make the Department more aware than it had been before of the inadequacies in the management of primary care. At a meeting in April 1984, therefore, the Secretary of State, Norman Fowler, and his Minister for Health, Kenneth Clarke, decided that it was time to initiate a review of the family practitioner services.[87]

Prescribing provided the first demonstration of the Government's willingness to risk political costs in order to bring financial costs under control. Spending on prescribing accounted for almost half the total expenditure on primary health care; it was, furthermore, expanding at a rate of more than 5 per cent a year in real terms. The notion of restricting the established right of general practitioners to prescribe whatever they wished, regardless of the cost or efficacy of the drug and the availability of cheaper substitutes, had been floating around a long time. Successive Governments had, however, flinched from the prospect of a head-on conflict with the BMA on this issue. Hence the announcement of a 'limited list' in November 1984 caught everyone by surprise.[88] It created what Norman Fowler described as an 'eccentric alliance' in opposition to the proposal between the medical profession, the pharmaceutical industry and the Labour Party. The BMA, angered by the unprecedented failure of the Government to consult the medical profession before taking a policy decision, protested strongly at what its Secretary described as 'one of the biggest changes in the NHS since its introduction'. But Kenneth Clarke told them sharply that 'private formal consultation' in advance of publishing proposals was 'no way to run a system of parliamentary government'. The pharmaceutical industry campaigned vigorously against the proposal. It argued, imaginatively, that the proposal would introduce a two-tier system of medicine by discriminating against patients who could not afford to buy drugs excluded from the official list and, predictably, that the resulting cut in profits would restrict research and the development of new products. More surprisingly, the Labour front bench criticised the Government's scheme as a 'major threat to the NHS' and supported the drug industry's assertion that it would introduce the two-tier principle.

In the event, confrontation ended in compromise. Some of the Government's backbenchers were restive; the medical profession itself was divided, with some of the Royal Colleges supporting the idea of a limited list; the Opposition, too, was split. In February 1985 the Government announced that the limited list would be extended from 30 to 100 items and that the medical profession would be consulted about its precise composition; an Advisory Committee on NHS Drugs was set up to consider proposals for adding new drugs to the list; the estimate of likely savings was pared down from £100 to £75 million a year. But the Government had succeeded in imposing the principle of a limited list and thereby challenging the idea that clinical autonomy bestowed an automatic, unfettered right to use public resources without scrutiny or limits. It had, further, demon-strated that its willingness to take on corporate interest groups extended even to the medical profession. Although not intended to be a muscle-flexing exercise – it was an accidental rather than deliberate trial of strength with the medical profession – the limited list episode proved to Ministers that it was possible to take on the doctors without getting a bloody nose: a lesson Kenneth Clarke, in particular, was to remember when it came to implementing *Working for Patients*. Lastly, the Government had shown that, in its pursuit of efficiency, it was prepared to use any tools, whether or not consistent with its ideology of the market and minimum State interference: in this case, using the tools of bureau-cratic control to limit choice.

The tension between managerial and market strategies, between bureaucratic control and consumer choice, also marked the Government's proposals for the reform of primary health care first unveiled in 1986. The Government's Green Paper *Primary Health Care: an Agenda for Discussion*[89] set four main aims. The first two were consumer-orientated objectives. They were: 'to give patients the widest range of choice in obtaining high quality primary health care services' and 'to encourage the providers of services to aim for the highest standards and to be responsive to the needs of the public'. The second two were managerial object-ives. They were: 'to provide the taxpayer with the best value for money from NHS expenditure' and 'to enable clearer priorities to be set for the family practitioner services in relation to the rest of the NHS'.

The specific proposals reflected this mix of motives. On the one hand, there were the proposals designed to create more of a market situation for GP services. The incentives for GPs to be more sensitive to consumer preferences were to be sharpened by increasing the proportion of their income derived from capitation fees (which had sunk to 45 per cent by the mid-1980s) and by making it easier for patients to change their doctors. Similarly, there was much emphasis on improving the availability of information to prospective patients and thus strengthening their ability to shop around among competing GPs. On the other hand, there were the proposals designed to increase managerial control over the activities of GPs and other contractors. This was to be done largely by strengthening FPCs, hitherto viewed as managerial eunuchs whose chief responsibilities were to shuffle paper, to pay out money and to keep GPs happy. In future, it was proposed, they should be required to carry out a 'regular appraisal of the quality and quantity of services being provided' and 'to develop more systematic means of measuring quality and detecting shortfalls in the provision of services'. Passive administration was to be replaced by active management. Additionally, the 1986 Green Paper floated the idea that GPs themselves might be given a direct incentive to improve standards by being offered a 'good practice allowance'. Entitlement would be contingent both on objective measures like 'personal availability to patients' and a performance review which might include 'such things as prescribing patterns and hospital referral rates'.

The BMA reacted tetchily.[90] The Green Paper was criticised for showing 'signs of a faltering commitment to the NHS', no doubt because of its failure to give 'any hint that additional resources will be provided to fund the development of primary care'. Specifically, the BMA objected to giving FPCs a more active managerial role: 'As self-employed persons who have agreed to provide certain services, general practitioners are responsible for organising their practices to meet their patients' needs', it argued, 'FPCs assist and advise but do not direct or control.' Similarly, it rejected the idea of a good practice allowance and any move towards increasing the proportion of doctors' pay represented by capitation fees. If the BMA had had its way, little would have been left of the Government's proposals. However, this time the Government – in contrast to the limited list episode – adopted a conciliatory stance. There followed a highly visible exercise in consultation during which Ministers took evidence from 370 witnesses representing 73 organisations; the House of Commons Social Services Committee, too, weighed in with its own inquiry.[91] If the intention was to increase the Government's freedom of manoeuvre by promoting a babble of conflicting voices, the strategy succeeded. The White Paper published in 1987, *Promoting Better Health*,[92] remained faithful both to the objectives and to most of the proposals put forward in the discussion document. There were some clear concessions to the medical profession. The notion of a good practice allowance was dropped and, instead, the Department proposed to promote quality by introducing bonus payments linked to the achievement of specific targets and by paying special allowances to GPs working in deprived areas. But there was greater emphasis, if anything, on strengthening the role of FPCs and establishing managerial control over general practice:

> By ensuring that they receive more information about the services for which they are responsible and improving their means of control, the Government will require FPCs to exercise a stronger role in the management of those services. In this way the Government expects to secure continuing improvements in the level, quality and cost effectiveness of service provision and greater accountability.

Specifically, FPCs were to set disease prevention targets, to carry out surveys of consumer satisfaction and to monitor, with the help of professional advice, patterns of prescribing and hospital referrals.

Many of the Government's proposals proved to be unacceptable to the BMA's representatives in the negotiations that started in March 1988, following the translation of the White Paper into a draft contract for general practitioners. For example, the BMA rejected as 'totally unacceptable' the requirement that every GP should submit an annual report to the FPC on the grounds that 'this bureaucratic exercise could only serve to waste scarce resources and would stifle innovation'.[93] The negotiations wearily dragged on clause by clause, month by month. But just as it appeared that they might be inching their way towards agreement, the publication of *Working for Patients* created an entirely new situation. What had started out as a fairly familiar, if not particularly friendly, exercise in hammering out a settlement over pay and conditions between the profession and the Government turned into the fiercest confrontation between them in the history of the NHS.

One of the less controversial aspects of the 1987 White Paper was, however, the prominence it gave to a new but fast developing theme in the evolution of health policies. Its title, *Promoting Better Health*, provides the clue. By 1987 the Thatcher administration had become converted, with some enthusiasm, to the cause of health promotion. The White Paper added a new objective to those enunciated in the consultative paper. This was 'to promote health and prevent illness'. It gave much emphasis to the role of GPs, both in advising patients about lifestyle and in screening at-risk groups, particularly the elderly. Moreover, as we have seen, it reinforced rhetoric with financial incentives for GPs to achieve the targets for the rate of immunisation, vaccination and other preventive measures. 'The prevention of avoidable illness and the promotion of good health' even featured as the first of the six principles guiding Conservative policies on health care in the party's 1987 election manifesto. The point was further elaborated in a long catalogue of initiatives: for example a 'major campaign to tackle the problem of coronary heart disease'. It was a theme that was to be greatly amplified in the 1990s.

The new-found enthusiasm of the Conservatives for health promotion is, at first sight, somewhat puzzling. In previous decades, prevention had tended to be one of the enthusiasms of the Left and even in the first half of the 1980s the Government showed little enthusiasm. It quarrelled with the Health Education Council, and subsequently reformed it, in part at least because of the latter's obsession with the issues raised by the Black report on inequalities in health. There was a steady decline in the status and role of community physicians: the medical specialists who, in the 1974 reorganisation, had been cast in the role of the philosopher kings who would determine need and decide priorities according to their own, technical criteria.[94] Nor is this surprising: health promotion tends to be associated in the minds of many Conservatives with the Nanny State interfering with the way in which people run their lives, whether by trying to persuade them to take more exercise or to give up smoking. But then came the conversion. It appears to have had two causes: AIDS and money. By 1986 the Government had become intensely worried about AIDS,[95] responding perhaps less to the number of deaths (which were few) than to the number of column inches in the press (which were many). A Cabinet Committee was set up; a major House of Commons debate was held; the Prime Minister overcame her intense dislike of even discussing the subject. But what characterised this new epidemic – for such it seemed at the time – was that it was not amenable to laboratory science or medical treatment. The only policy instruments that appeared to be available were the traditional public health tools. Accordingly the Government committed itself to a major campaign of public health education, given that the only long-term protection against the spread of AIDS seemed to be a change in the population's sexual habits. Within the DHSS, the epidemic thus created a new constituency of support for preventive strategies and strengthened the influence of Sir Donald Acheson, the Chief Medical Officer, the main protagonist of the public health tradition as represented by community physicians.

The other reason which might explain the Government's new-found enthusiasm was, as always, money. If demand seems to be set on a collision course with supply, Governments will inevitably be drawn into a search for means of manipulating the former. The new emphasis on reducing demand by exercising more control over GPs was one such policy response; the new stress on preventing illness was another. Both, however, were long-term strategies. Neither could deliver results in the immediate future or ease the immediate pressures on the Government. Indeed in the case of general practice – as with the new managerialism – policy compounded those pressures: the efficiency dividend was a future promise while the medical profession's suspicions and resentment were a present threat. Almost unwillingly the Government was thus edged into addressing – as we shall see in the next chapter – the issue which it had sought to side-step so long: to examine the institutional foundations on which the NHS had been built in 1948.

References

1. Secretaries of State for Health, Wales, Northern Ireland and Scotland, *Working for Patients*, HMSO: London 1989, Cm. 555.
2. Roy Griffiths, *NHS Management Inquiry: Report to the Secretary of State for Social Services*, Department of Health and Social Security: London 1983, Mimeo.
3. Sir Patrick Nairne, 'Managing the DHSS Elephant: Reflections on a Giant Department', *Political Quarterly*, vol. 54, no. 3, July/September 1983, pp. 243–56.
4. Efficiency is here used colloquially rather than technically to mean the ratio between inputs and outputs, holding the quality and specifications of the products constant. In the NHS context efficiency is usually taken to be synonymous with productivity. If there is a rise in outputs for any given bundle of inputs, it is assumed that there has been a gain in efficiency.
5. For illuminating accounts of the role of the Treasury in the early days of the NHS, see Charles Webster, *The Health Services Since the War*, vol. 1, HMSO: London 1988 and Frank Honigsbaum, *Health, Happiness and Security*, Routledge: London 1989.
6. The best, if inevitably biased, description of Mrs Thatcher's evolving style as Prime Minister is provided by Nigel Lawson, *The View from No. 11*, Corgi Books: London 1993.
7. For a review of the literature on Mrs Thatcher's Government, see Jeremy Moon, 'Evaluating Thatcher: Sceptical versus Synthetic Approaches', *Politics*, vol. 14, no. 2, September 1994, pp. 43–9. Key texts are A Gamble, *The Free Economy and the Strong State: The Politics of Thatcherism*, 2nd edn, Macmillan: Basingstoke 1994, and D Kavanagh, *Thatcherism and British Politics: The End of Consensus*, Oxford UP: Oxford 1990.
8. Chris Hamnett, Linda McDowell and Philip Sarre (eds), *The Changing Social Structure*, Sage: London 1989.
9. AH Halsey, *British Social Trends Since 1900*, Macmillan: Basingstoke 1988.
10. Ivor Crewe, 'Voting Patterns Since 1959', *Contemporary Record*, vol. 2, no. 4, Winter 1988, pp. 2–6. The literature on voting patterns, and their significance, has grown

rapidly in size and discord. For a review see David Denver, *Elections and Voting Behaviour in Britain*, 2nd edn, Harvester: Hemel Hempstead 1994.

11. Shirley Robin Letwin, *The Anatomy of Thatcherism*, Fontana: London 1992. Written by someone sympathetic to Thatcherism – in contrast to most of the contributions to the literature – this provides some of the best insights into the phenomenon.

12. Ivor Crewe, 'The Thatcher Legacy' in Anthony King *et al.*, *Britain at the Polls 1992*, Chatham House: New Jersey 1992.

13. Peter Taylor-Gooby, 'Citizenship and Welfare' in R Jowell *et al.* (eds), *British Social Attitudes: the 1987 Report*, Social and Community Planning Research: London 1987.

14. Nick Bosanquet, 'Interim Report: The National Health' in R Jowell *et al.* (eds), *British Social Attitudes: the 9th Report*, Social and Community Planning Research: London 1992.

15. Chancellor of the Exchequer, *Public Expenditure Analyses to 1995–96: Statistical Supplement to the 1992 Autumn Statement*, HMSO: London 1993, Cm. 2219, Table 2.3. More specifically, on patterns of Welfare State spending, see John Hills (ed.), *The State of Welfare*, Clarendon Press: Oxford 1990.

16. For a persuasive attempt to assimilate the record of the Thatcher administration to the Conservative tradition, see David Willetts, *Modern Conservatism*, Penguin: Harmondsworth 1992. For the contrary argument, see John Gray, *The Undoing of Conservatism*, Social Market Foundation: London 1994.

17. Originality, it has been said, is a function of forgetfulness. In this case, alas, I have forgotten the source of this phrase.

18. For an influential analysis of the sources of sclerosis, see Mancur Olson, *The Rise and Decline of Nations: Economic Growth, Stagflation and Social Rigidities*, Yale UP: New Haven 1982.

19. For a comparative study of the Thatcher administration's policies towards the legal and medical professions, and their outcomes, see Margaret Brazier, Jill Lovecy, Michael Moran and Margaret Potton, 'Falling from a Tightrope: Doctors and Lawyers between the Market and the State', *Political Studies*, vol. XLI, no. 2, June 1993, pp. 197–213.

20. Jenny Brain and Rudolf Klein, *Parental Choice: Myth or Reality?*, Centre for the Analysis of Social Policy: Bath 1994, Bath Social Policy Paper no. 21.

21. Christopher Johnson, *The Economy under Mrs Thatcher*, Penguin: Harmondsworth 1991.

22. For the best overview of the impact of the Thatcher administration on the civil service culture, see Peter Hennessy's classic study, *Whitehall*, Fontana Press: London 1990. For a definition of the new public management, see Christopher Hood, 'A Public Management for all Seasons', *Public Administration*, vol. 69, no. 1, Spring 1991, pp. 3–19.

23. Prime Minister and Chancellor of the Exchequer, *Financial Management in Government Departments*, HMSO: London 1983, Cmnd. 9058. For an analysis of the implementation of these policies, see Andrew Gray and Bill Jenkins, with Andrew Flynn and Brian Rutherford, 'The Management of Change in Whitehall: the Experience of the FMI', *Public Administration*, vol. 69, no. 1, Spring 1991, pp. 41–59.

24. Neil Carter, Rudolf Klein and Patricia Day, *How Organisations Measure Success: The Use of Performance Indicators in Government*, Routledge: London 1992.

25. Patricia Greer, *Transforming Central Government: The Next Steps Initiative*, Open University Press: Buckingham 1994.

26. Lord Fulton (chairman), Committee on the Civil Service, *Report*, HMSO: London 1982.

27. Quoted in John Urry, 'Disorganised Capitalism', *Marxism Today*, October 1988, pp. 30–3. The whole issue of the journal is of great interest in its argument that what needs explanation is not Thatcherism as such but the social changes that made it possible. See, in particular, Charlie Leadbetter, 'Power to the Person', pp. 14–19.

28. The trend had, of course, been evident for some time: see Donald A Schon, *Beyond the Stable State*, Pelican Books: Harmondsworth 1973.

29. Geoff Mulgen, 'The Power of the Weak', *Marxism Today*, December 1988, pp. 24–31.

30. Patricia Day and Rudolf Klein, 'The Business of Welfare', *New Society*, 19 June 1987, pp. 11–13.
31. Rudolf Klein, 'Health Care in the Age of Disillusionment', *British Medical Journal*, vol. 285, 5 July 1982, pp. 2–4.
32. Norman Fowler, *Ministers Decide: A Memoir of the Thatcher Years*, Chapman's: London 1991.
33. Nigel Lawson, op. cit., pp. 303–4.
34. Norman Fowler, op. cit., p. 184. For an analysis of why the Conservatives were so committed to the NHS, see also Rudolf Klein, 'Why Britain's Conservatives Support a Socialist Health Care System', *Health Affairs*, vol. 4, no. 1, Spring 1985, pp. 41–58.
35. The episode is noted in Tessa Blackstone and William Plowden, *Inside the Think Tank*, Heinemann: London 1988 as marking the beginning of the end for the CPRS, which was subsequently abolished by Mrs Thatcher.
36. David Butler and Dennis Kavanagh, *The British General Election of 1983*, Macmillan: Basingstoke 1984; David Butler and Dennis Kavanagh, *The British General Election of 1987*, Macmillan: Basingstoke 1988.
37. For the role of public opinion in health policy making, see Lawrence R Jacobs, *The Health of Nations: Public Opinion and the Making of American and British Health Policy*, Cornell UP: Ithaca, NY 1993. This argues that public opinion was the engine of change in both the US and UK: a thesis which, however, is only tenuously supported by evidence in the 1940s and contradicted by events in the 1980s.
38. Karen Bloor and Alan Maynard, *Expenditure on the NHS During and After the Thatcher Years*, Centre for Health Economics: York 1993, Discussion Paper 113.
39. For example, see Social Services Committee Third Report Session 1980–81, *Public Expenditure on the Social Services*, HMSO: London 1981, HC 324 and Committee of Public Accounts Seventeenth Report Session 1980–81, *Financial Control and Accountability in the National Health Service*, HMSO: London 1981, HC 25.
40. The importance of parliamentary accountability in determining the introduction of new instruments of central control is stressed in the account of events by the then Permanent Secretary, Sir Kenneth Stowe, *On Caring for the National Health*, The Nuffield Provincial Hospitals Trust: London 1988.
41. David E Allen, 'Annual Reviews or no Annual Reviews: The Balance of Power between the DHSS and Health Authorities', *British Medical Journal*, vol. 285, 28 August 1982, pp. 665–7.
42. Quoted in Stowe, op. cit., p. 87.
43. Carter, Klein and Day, op. cit., Chapter 4. See also Rudolf Klein, 'Performance Evaluation and the NHS', *Public Administration*, vol. 60, no. 4, Winter 1982, pp. 385–409.
44. Christopher Pollitt, 'Measuring Performance: A New System for the National Health Service', *Policy and Politics*, vol. 13, no. 1, 1985, pp. 1–15.
45. Patricia Day and Rudolf Klein, 'Central Accountability and Local Decision-Making: Towards a New NHS', *British Medical Journal*, vol. 290, 1 June 1985, pp. 1676–8.
46. Sir Roy Griffiths, op. cit. See also Sir Kenneth Stowe, op. cit., p. 51, for his account of the genesis of the Griffiths Inquiry. Initially this appears to have been prompted by anxieties about the management of manpower – following a bitter pay dispute in 1982 – but subsequently changed its focus.
47. Rudolf Klein, 'What Future for the Department of Health?', *British Medical Journal*, vol. 301, 8 September 1990, pp. 481–4.
48. See the evidence given by Tony Newton, Minister of State for Health, to the Social Services Committee Session 1987–88, *Resourcing the National Health Service: Minutes of Evidence 8 June 1988*, HMSO: London, HC 264-XII.
49. Sir Alec Merrison (chairman), *Report of the Royal Commission on the National Health Service*, para 19.31, HMSO: London, Cmnd. 7615.

50. Norman Fowler, op. cit., p. 197.

51. Patricia Day and Rudolf Klein, 'The Mobilisation of Consent versus the Management of Conflict: Decoding the Griffiths Report', *British Medical Journal*, vol. 287, 10 December 1983, pp. 1813–16.

52. Christopher Pollitt, Stephen Harrison, David J Hunter and Gordon Marnoch, 'General Management in the NHS: The Initial Impact 1983–88', *Public Administration*, vol. 69, no. 1, Spring 1991, pp. 61–83.

53. All the quotations come from a valuable study of NHS managers: Philip Strong and Jane Robinson, *The NHS under New Management*, Open University Press: Milton Keynes 1990.

54. Stephen Harrison and Christopher Pollitt, *Controlling Health Professionals*, Open University Press: Buckingham 1994, p. 67.

55. Sir Roy Griffiths, *Seven Years of Progress – General Management in the NHS*, The Audit Commission: London, Management Lectures no. 3, 12 June 1991, Mimeo.

56. Patricia Day and Rudolf Klein, *Accountabilities*, Tavistock Publications: London 1987.

57. John Yates, *Why are we Waiting?*, Oxford UP: Oxford 1987. For a more recent study, see Stephen Frankel and Robert West (eds), *Rationing and Rationality in the National Health Service: The Persistence of Waiting Lists*, Macmillan: Basingstoke 1993.

58. National Audit Office, *Use of Operating Theatres in the National Health Service*, HMSO: London 1987, HC 143. See also Chris Ham (ed.), *Health Care Variations*, King's Fund Institute: London 1988.

59. Sir Raymond Hoffenberg, *Clinical Freedom*, The Nuffield Provincial Hospitals Trust: London 1987.

60. Martin Buxton, *et al.*, *Costs and Benefits of Heart Transplant Programmes*, HMSO: London 1985.

61. Rudolf Klein, 'The Conflict between Professionals, Consumers and Bureaucrats', *Journal of the Irish Colleges of Physicians and Surgeons*, vol. 6, no. 3, January 1977, pp. 88–91.

62. Margaret Thatcher, *The Downing Street Years*, Harper Collins: London 1993, p. 571.

63. Rudolf Klein, 'Privatization and the Welfare State' in Christopher Johnson (ed.), *Privatization and Ownership*, Pinter Publishers: London 1988, pp. 30–46.

64. All the statistics about the private sector are drawn from that invaluable compendium, *Laing's Review of Private Healthcare, 1994*, Laing & Buisson Publications: London 1994.

65. Joan Higgins, *The Business of Medicine*, Macmillan: Basingstoke 1988.

66. Rudolf Klein, 'Models of Man and Models of Policy: Reflections on Exit, Voice and Loyalty Ten Years Later', *Milbank Memorial Fund Quarterly: Health and Society*, vol. 58, no. 3, 1980, pp. 416–29.

67. JP Nicholl, NR Beeby and BT Williams, 'The Role of the Private Sector in Elective Surgery in England and Wales, 1986', *British Medical Journal*, vol. 298, 28 January 1989, pp. 243–7; ibid. 'Comparison of the Activity of Short-stay Independent Hospitals in England and Wales, 1981 and 1986', *British Medical Journal*, vol. 298, 28 January 1989, pp. 239–43.

68. David Horne, *Public Policy Making and Private Medical Care in the UK since 1948*, PhD thesis, University of Bath 1986. The findings reported in this have been confirmed by Michael Calnan, Sarah Cant and Jonathan Gabe, *Going Private: Why People Pay for their Health Care*, Open University Press: Buckingham 1993.

69. Office of Population Censuses and Surveys, *General Household Survey, 1982*, HMSO: London 1984.

70. Monopolies and Mergers Commission, *Private Medical Services*, HMSO: London 1994, Cmnd. 2452.

71. The source for the data on the private long-stay sector is, once again, Laing, op. cit.

72. Patricia Day and Rudolf Klein, 'Residential Care for the Elderly: A Billion Pound Experiment in Policy-making', *Public Money*, March 1987, pp. 19–24.

73. Audit Commission, *Making a Reality of Community Care*, HMSO: London 1986.
74. Sir Roy Griffiths, *Community Care: An Agenda for Action*, HMSO: London 1988.
75. GC Fiegehan, 'Income after Retirement', *Social Trends*, no. 16, HMSO: London 1986, pp. 13–18. For a critical view of this interpretation, see Paul Johnson and Jane Falkingham, *Intergenerational Transfers and Public Expenditure on the Elderly in Modern Britain*, Centre for Economic Policy Research, Discussion Paper no. 254: London 1988.
76. Duncan Larder, Patricia Day and Rudolf Klein, *Institutional Care for the Elderly: The Geographical Distribution of the Public/Private Mix*, Centre for the Analysis of Social Policy, Bath Social Policy Paper no. 10: Bath 1986.
77. Patricia Day and Rudolf Klein, 'Maintaining Standards in the Independent Sector of Health Care', *British Medical Journal*, vol. 290, 30 March 1985, pp. 1020–2.
78. Patricia Day, Rudolf Klein and Gillian Tipping, *Inspecting for Quality: Services for the Elderly*, Centre for the Analysis of Social Policy, Bath Social Policy Paper no. 12: Bath 1988.
79. JP Martin, *Hospitals in Trouble*, Basil Blackwell: Oxford 1984.
80. For this analysis, I have relied on the excellent account in Kate Ascher, *The Politics of Privatisation*, Macmillan: Basingstoke 1987.
81. National Audit Office, *Competitive Tendering for Support Services in the National Health Service*, HMSO: London 1987, HC 318.
82. Robin G Milne, 'Competitive Tendering in the NHS', *Public Administration*, vol. 65, no. 2, Summer 1987, pp. 145–60.
83. Stephen Birch, 'Increasing Patient Charges in the National Health Service: A Method of Privatizing Primary Care', *Journal of Social Policy*, vol. 15, part 2, April 1986, pp. 163–85.
84. Successive Public Expenditure White Papers provide data about the proportion of the NHS's income derived from charges in the 1970s and 1980s; for earlier data, see Merrison, op. cit., Table E11.
85. Patricia Day and Rudolf Klein, 'Controlling the Gatekeepers: The Accountability of General Practitioners', *Journal of the Royal College of General Practitioners*, vol. 36, March 1986, pp. 129–30.
86. For an analysis of general practice at this period, see David Wilkin, Lesley Hallow, Ralph Leavey and David Metcalfe, *Anatomy of Urban General Practice*, Tavistock: London 1987.
87. The best account of primary health care policy is that given by the civil servant responsible for it, Bryan Rayner, 'The Development of Primary Health Care Policy in the 1980s: A View from the Centre' in Patricia Day (ed.), *Managing Change: Implementing Primary Health Care Policy*, Centre for the Analysis of Social Policy: Bath 1992.
88. John Wheatley, *Prescribing and the NHS: The Politics of the Limited List*, MSc thesis, University of Hull 1985. In what follows I have drawn on this excellent study for both analysis and quotations.
89. Secretaries of State for Social Services, Wales, Northern Ireland and Scotland, *Primary Health Care: An Agenda for Discussion*, HMSO: London 1986, Cmnd. 9771.
90. General Medical Services Committee, *Report to Special Conference of Representatives of Local Medical Committees on 13 November 1986*, BMA: London August 1986.
91. Social Services Committee First Report 1986–87 Session, *Primary Health Care*, HMSO: London 1987, HC 30.
92. Secretaries of State for Social Services, Wales, Northern Ireland and Scotland, *Promoting Better Health*, HMSO: London 1987, Cm. 249.
93. General Medical Services Committee, *Report to a Special Conference of Representatives of Local Medical Committees on 27 April 1989*, BMA: London February 1989.
94. Jane Lewis, *What Price Community Medicine?*, Wheatsheaf Books: Brighton 1986; Sarah Harvey and Ken Judge, *Community Physicians and Community Medicine*, King's Fund Institute: London 1988.
95. Patricia Day and Rudolf Klein, 'Interpreting the Unexpected: The Case of AIDS Policy Making in Britain', *Journal of Public Policy*, vol. 9, part 3, July/September 1989, pp. 337–53.

Chapter 6

The politics of the big bang

There are a number of different ways of telling the story of how, in January 1989, the Government came to precipitate the most serious conflict in the history of the NHS by publishing its manifesto for change, *Working for Patients*.[1] First, there is the Cleopatra's nose version.[2] If Mrs Thatcher's temper had been on a longer leash, and if it had not been tried so severely by a sustained barrage of criticism about her Government's management of the NHS, she might not suddenly have surprised television viewers of *Panorama* (and some of her Cabinet colleagues) by announcing her Review while appearing on that programme in January 1988. Second, there is the economic determinism version. Caught between the imperative of containing public expenditure and the pressure to expand the NHS's activities, the Government had no option but to consider ever more radical ideas for the financing and organisation of health care. Third, there is the ideological 'outing' version. The Government, its confidence boosted by a third election victory, finally felt strong enough openly to pursue its ideological commitment to the market, having previously only been able to do so by stealth. Fourth, there is the policy-learning version.[3] From its own experience both in the health policy arena and in other policy fields like education, the Government could draw the lesson that it was possible to overcome obstacles to change previously considered to be insurmountable: the horizons of the possible had widened out. Fifth, there is the policy soup version.[4] By the end of the 1980s, the Government was able to draw on a rich mix of ideas, home grown and imported, which allowed it to choose from a wider policy menu than when it had first come into office: the clear (if thin) consommé of ideas that had shaped the NHS in 1948 had become a thick (if confusing) minestrone. Lastly, there is the organisational predestination version. Nothing that the Government did should have surprised anyone aware of the changes in theory and practice, largely made possible by information technology, that were transforming large organisations everywhere.

All these interpretations contribute to an understanding of the circumstances that led to the Review and to the publication of *Working for Patients*, if with varying degrees of plausibility. They are complementary rather than competitive, in that they help us to understand different aspects of the policy-making process. Some help to identify the factors that precipitated action and led to the decision to set up the Review; some help to identify the factors that predisposed Ministers to adopt particular policy options during the course of the Review; others help to identify the factors that enabled the Government to implement particular policy solutions. None can claim any exclusive explanatory monopoly. In what follows, therefore, this chapter will draw on the different modes of explanation, as appropriate, in tracing the evolution of policy from the decision to set up the Review to the implementation of the proposals set out in *Working for Patients*.

Consider, first, the circumstances that precipitated Mrs Thatcher's decision to overcome her own reluctance to address the reform of the NHS head-on. The 1987 General Election had been 'a bruising experience so far as the NHS was concerned' for the Conservatives.[5] Subsequently every Tuesday and Thursday, at Prime Minister's Question Time in the House of Commons, Mrs Thatcher 'had thrown at her case after case of ward closures, interminably postponed operations and allegedly avoidable infant deaths, all of them attributed to Government parsimony'.[6] The newspapers and television programmes, too, served up 'horror stories about the NHS on an almost daily basis' and Mrs Thatcher's irritation was further compounded by the failure of the DHSS (as she saw it) to come up with effective replies to criticisms.[7] Finally, bringing her exasperation to boiling point, she felt outraged when the Presidents of the Royal Colleges publicly denounced the Government's policies. This represented, in her view, a repudiation of the implicit concordat between the State and the medical profession forged by the creation of the NHS, whereby the former accepted the autonomy of the medical profession in decisions about the use of resources while the latter accepted the right of the State to set the budgetary constraints within which it worked.[8] The basis of the accommodation between the State and the medical profession had been betrayed.

But if the media pressures and the *pronunciamento* of the Presidents of the Royal Colleges all helped to push Mrs Thatcher over the precipice, she had already been moving towards the edge for other reasons. Her Chancellor of the Exchequer, Nigel Lawson, took the view that 'we had reached the point where the pressures to spend more money on the Health Service were almost impossible to resist'. But the Treasury was reluctant to agree to more money for the NHS without an assurance that this would yield 'real value for money in terms of improved patient care'. Hence, Lawson argued over dinner with the Prime Minister, the case for a review of the NHS.[9] However, according to Mrs Thatcher's own account, she did not need prompting from her Chancellor. She had started discussions about how to ensure better value for money from the existing system with her new Secretary of State for the Social Services, John Moore, soon after the General Election: while 'Norman Fowler was much better at publicly defending the NHS than he would have been at reforming it', his successor was anxious to have a fundamental review.[10] It seemed to her that 'the NHS had become a bottomless financial pit', where the providers blamed the Government for all that went wrong. It was thus a political liability and, with her thoughts turning to a fourth General Election victory, she saw advantages in quick action that would put any reforms in place before the time came to face the voters again.

The proximate cause for the decision to set up the Review can therefore be seen as the Prime Minister's resolve to escape from what was becoming an ever more embarrassing political situation. But what created that situation was the failure of the Government's policies, analysed in the previous chapter, to resolve the tension between constrained budgets and expanding demands. Despite the Government's value-for-money crusade, despite the statistics about the increasing number of doctors and nurses employed and the rising number of patients treated which the Prime Minister reeled out whenever challenged about the NHS, the public obstinately continued to see the Health Service as a casualty of the Thatcher administration's parsimony. Given the crucial importance of the issue, the next section therefore examines in more detail the debate about NHS funding.

A dialogue of the deaf

The increasingly fierce political debate about NHS funding that characterised the 1980s was revealing not so much for any conclusions reached about the adequacy or otherwise of its budget but for its demonstration that it was impossible to come to anything like an agreed verdict. It was a reminder – if a reminder was needed – of the view taken by the 1979 Royal Commission that 'There is no objective or universally acceptable method of establishing what the "right" level of expenditure on the NHS should be'.[11] But failing such a formula for resolving argument, or any set of agreed criteria or benchmarks against which the level of funding could be assessed, the political dispute inevitably turned into a dialogue of the deaf. In these circumstances, the medical profession – as so often before in the history of the NHS – was able to impose its interpretation on the situation. If there was no agreed way of using statistics to give an accurate picture of the adequacy or otherwise of funding, if there was no authoritative evidence that would command general assent, doctors (and, to a lesser extent, nurses) were the obvious witnesses. Who, after all, was better placed than they to provide testimony based on their own day-to-day experience? If they declared the NHS to be on the point of collapse – as they did with increasing stridency as the decade went on – who could question their authority? In short, the ambiguity of the evidence available – and the lack of consensus about how to assess it – reinforced the power of those able to impose their interpretation of reality: unsurprisingly the proportion of the public declaring themselves to be dissatisfied with the NHS rose from 25 per cent in 1983 to 46 per cent in 1989.[12]

But why was it so difficult to assess the evidence? The simplest way of answering this question is to examine further the debate between the 'inputters' and the 'outputters', between the Government's critics and successive Secretaries of State, already briefly referred to in the previous chapter. The criticism of the Government's expenditure plans, as articulated by the all-party Social Services Committee of the House of Commons in a succession of reports, drew attention to a widening gulf between the inputs of resources and what was deemed to be required. To define what was required the Committee used a formula first devised in the 1970s in order to extract money from the Treasury: an exercise in ingenuity by civil servants which came to haunt their departmental colleagues in the 1980s. The formula suggested an annual growth in the NHS budget of about 2 per cent in real terms. As one much quoted Ministerial statement[13] put it:

> One per cent is needed to keep pace with the increasing number of elderly people; medical advance takes an additional 0.5 per cent and a further 0.5 per cent is needed to make progress towards meeting the Government's policy objectives (for example to improve renal services and to develop community care).

Comparing actual spending levels with the expenditure needed to produce an annual growth of 2 per cent, it was then a simple arithmetical exercise to calculate the deficit. Using this method, the Social Services Committee in 1986 produced a figure of £1.325 billion as the cumulative under-funding of the hospital and community services. It was a figure which was to reverberate throughout the entire debate, feeding alike the sense of grievance within the NHS and the indignation of Opposition politicians. And when the Social Services Committee repeated its exercise in 1988, it came up with the still more dramatic figure of £1.896 billion as the accumulated deficit.

The Government, in contrast, put the emphasis on outputs, i.e. on what the NHS was actually producing. This, of course, was the logic of a value-for-money approach, hinged on the *relationship* between inputs and outputs, which defined performance in terms of activity rather than the level of resources. Already in 1983 the Government's preparation for the General Election included the publication of a document setting out the increase in activity.[14] And this remained the Government's response to criticisms of inadequacy throughout the 1980s and into the 1990s. In its evidence to the 1988 Social Services Committee inquiry,[15] the DHSS provided figures showing the increase in the number of patients treated and specific operations carried out, arguing that rising productivity – the efficiency savings produced by the new managerialism, the resources freed by competitive tendering and other initiatives – had allowed the NHS to provide more and better services despite tight budget constraints.

The arguments proved impossible to resolve. The Government's logic in directing attention to the outputs of the NHS was impeccable. The level of inputs tells us nothing of itself; the adequacy or otherwise of any given bundle of resources depends on how they are used. However, the Government's line of reasoning was vulnerable on two counts. First, its story about increasing activity and improved productivity could say nothing about the adequacy of what was being produced. Given the lack of any measure of demand – let alone need – increasing activity could still be compatible with a shortfall in what was required. Moreover, the persistence of waiting lists – and the growth of the private sector – seemed eloquent evidence of the NHS's failure to meet demand. Second, the Government was vulnerable to the criticism that quantity was being achieved at the expense of quality, as lengths of stay in hospitals fell and as the proportion of operations carried out on a day care basis rose. It was an argument which could neither be proved nor refuted: the required benchmarks of quality simply did not exist.

The case for the prosecution was also flawed. The demonstration of under-funding by the Social Services Committee depended crucially on the baseline chosen.[16] Yet there was no particular logic about choosing 1980 as the starting point for the exercise; there was no conceivable way of telling whether the NHS was over- or under-funded in that year. So the deficit could just as easily have been twice as large as claimed or non-existent: given the Social Services Committee's methodology, there was no way of telling. Moreover, the method extrapolated into the future costs based on past practices at a time when it was public policy to change those patterns of service delivery. Lastly, the calculations ignored some significant inputs into health care. They did not include either the growing primary health care budget or the billions flowing into the long-stay sector via the social security system. And no one even raised the question of whether or not the extra spending on private health care should be brought into the reckoning.

Nor could appeal to comparisons with other countries settle the matter. By international standards Britain was indeed a low spender on health care.[17] Expenditure on health care in the mid-1980s was, at 6 per cent of the Gross Domestic Product, significantly lower than in France (9 per cent) or Germany (8 per cent) – let alone the United States (10 per cent). Such comparisons were indeed much invoked by the Government's critics, political and professional. But, again, the figures did not speak for themselves. It was quite possible to mount a counter-attack. Britain's apparent parsimony could be seen as a tribute to the ability of the NHS to keep down costs and to stretch the available resources to better effect than other health care systems. By successfully containing salary and wage increases, by avoiding the excesses of American medicine, the NHS was able to deliver more care for each unit of input than other systems. There was no way of resolving this clash of views on the basis of the available evidence. As the study by the Organisation for Economic Co-operation and Development, the source of most of the data used by both parties, concluded, somewhat lamely:

> The difficulties in measuring health outcomes, appropriateness of medical care, efficiency and distributional objectives . . . mean that there is an insufficiently solid basis for making strong policy recommendations – other than to improve the quality of data and studies concerning the measurement of the key aspects of health care.[18]

If the 1980s debate was a dialogue of the deaf it was therefore because there was no agreement about the currency of argument and no consensus about how to define key terms like adequacy, need or quality. Lacking such an agreed vocabulary and generally accepted measuring rods, no resolution was possible. There was little that the technicians – whether statisticians or epidemiologists, economists or social policy experts – could do to resolve the dispute. It was inevitably politicised. And therein precisely lay the real significance of the debate. Its nature was defined less by the issues involved than by the characteristics of the policy arena.

The characteristic of the health care policy arena that determined the nature of the debate about NHS funding in the 1980s – as in previous decades – was the central role of the providers. It was they who largely orchestrated and shaped the perception of crisis. There was nothing new in this. What needs explaining about the 1980s – and, in particular, the climactic confrontation between the medical and nursing professions and the Government that precipitated Mrs Thatcher's decision to set up the Review of the NHS – is the scale and ferocity of that conflict.[19] It was marked by a concerted and determined attempt by the providers to demonstrate that the NHS was (yet again) on the point of collapse and thus to mobilise public opinion in a campaign for extra funding. It was, moreover, an extremely successful campaign: as previously noted, the evidence of public opinion surveys during this period shows an increase in the proportion of people declaring themselves to be dissatisfied with the NHS *and* supporting an increase in spending on the service.

It was, in retrospect, a battle that the Government was bound to lose. While Ministers depended on abstract statistics, the critics could translate their concerns into human terms and concrete images. In so doing, they could furthermore exploit the bias of the media towards the dramatic. The extent and intensity of the media coverage were, indeed, unprecedented in the history of the NHS. There was a succession of reports about hospital wards which had to be closed because of cash crises. There was a procession of consultants complaining about being unable to carry out life-saving operations because of inadequate resources. The BMA's Central Committee for Hospital Medical Services commissioned a survey to document the impact of financial stringency and came up with statistics of bed closures, cancelled operating sessions and staff shortages.[20] The picture that emerged forcibly and vividly from all these accounts was that of a Health Service where the staff felt themselves unable to deliver care of adequate quality, where patients were being turned away and where morale and standards were both plunging.

Never mind that the NHS had been closing beds throughout its entire history: for example, as many beds were closed in 1977 and 1978 as in 1987 and 1988.[21] Never mind that temporarily closing wards, or cancelling operating sessions, was a routine phenomenon towards the end of the financial year. Never mind that Ministers could point out, quite correctly, that the budget of the NHS had not been cut: that, in real terms, it had gone up every year during their period in office – and that it was running at the historically respectable figure of 4 per cent a year in 1987–88. There always appeared to be an argument or evidence that contradicted the case for the defence. So the Ministerial claim that the NHS's budget had gone up in real terms – using the GDP deflator to iron out the effects of inflation – was countered by the argument that the Government was using the wrong index. Applying the NHS's own price index, instead of the GDP deflator, sharply reduced the claimed increase – from 4 to 1.3 per cent in 1987–88.[22] Again, it always was possible to find some health authorities which were indeed being squeezed financially. One of the perverse outcomes of the 1970s RAWP formula for equalising resource distribution (*see* Chapter 4) was that the process of moving towards this objective inevitably meant reducing allocations to those health authorities which were deemed to be over-provided in order to increase the budgets of those who were judged to be relatively under-funded. A formula devised in a period of optimism about the upward trajectory of public expenditure, and so designed to achieve a politically painless redistribution of resources through differential growth rates, thus came to mean budget cuts for some districts in a period of financial austerity.[23]

But, of course, the NHS balance sheet offers – at best – only a partial explanation of the conflict between the Government and the providers. The pressures on the NHS in the 1980s were not different in kind – though perhaps more intense and certainly more sustained – from those in previous decades. It was the willingness of the medical and nursing profession to accept those pressures which appears to have diminished drastically. Similarly, the 1980s were marked by disputes about pay: for example, the Government modified or delayed the implementation of the recommendations of the Review Body on Doctors' and Dentists' Remuneration for six consecutive years between 1981 and 1986.[24] This certainly was not calculated to improve the temper of the medical profession. But, again, it does not convince as an explanation of the profession's increasingly violent criticisms of the Government: pay disputes had, after all, been a chronic condition in the NHS ever since its creation. If doctors and nurses perceived the NHS to be in a state of crisis, it was predominantly if not exclusively because they saw themselves threatened by the Government's policies for solving that crisis. In 1979 Mrs Thatcher's administration had quite deliberately decided to avoid any kind of radical reform of the health care system – as we have seen – because of the political risks involved. Instead, it had adopted a series of strategies which had succeeded only in antagonising the NHS's providers and so increasing the political costs. By 1988, therefore, the Government appeared to have little to lose – and perhaps much to gain – from taking the step it had so long tried to avoid: the stage was set for Mrs Thatcher's announcement of her Review of the NHS. Far from marking the triumphalist fulfilment of a long-standing ideological ambition, the announcement was in effect a confession of failure: the Government had been driven to adopt a posture of radicalism which it had strenuously sought to avoid. And reluctant radicalism was to characterise – as we shall see in the next section – the Review itself.

Reviewing the options

The central paradox of the Review of the NHS was that, although prompted by the widespread perception of financial crisis, no proposals for change in the method of funding emerged from it. The 1948 model was preserved: the NHS remained a universal, tax-financed health care system. Instead, the aim of *Working for Patients* – very much in line with the policies that had preceded it in the 1980s – was to change the dynamics of the 1948 model. Specifically, it introduced two major – and highly contentious – reforms. First, there was the separation of the purchaser and the provider roles: health authorities would in future be responsible only for buying health care from the providers. The providers, both hospitals and community services, would be transformed into autonomous trusts, whose budgets would depend on their competitive efficiency in getting contracts from purchasers. Second, general practitioners were given the option of becoming fundholders, i.e. of getting a budget from which to purchase the services required by their patients, excluding only the most expensive or long-term treatment. Thus was created the notion of the internal or mimic market: the NHS was to mimic those characteristics of the market that would promote greater efficiency within the framework of a public service committed to the non-market value of distributing access to resources according to need. Financial incentives would be used not to generate profits, as in the market place, but to sharpen the incentives of everyone working in the NHS to make more efficient use of public funds. *Working for Patients* introduced a number of other changes as well – discussed below – but it was precisely this central thrust of its proposals, the attempt to introduce financial incentives into the NHS, that coloured perceptions of the reform package as a whole and led to it being denounced both by the medical profession and the political opposition as a betrayal of the principles of 1948.

There is a real puzzle, therefore. Why were reforms that preserved the basic constitution and commitments of the NHS widely seen as destructive of its ethos and a threat to its principles? The best way to start answering this question – before moving on to consider the options on offer – is to look at the form that Mrs Thatcher's Review took, since this largely determined the reactions to its outcome. In its style, though not in its outcome, the Review marked a brutal break with the past. Whereas the history of the NHS up to 1979 can be largely written – as previous chapters have argued – as an attempt to maintain a consensus, however fragile at times, about the main elements of health care policy, Mrs Thatcher explicitly repudiated the notion that consensus-seeking was a desirable form of political activity. In doing so, she also repudiated the traditional instruments of consensus-engineering: Royal Commissions. None were appointed during her tenure in office. The Review of the NHS was carried out by a Cabinet Committee of five: the Prime Minister, Nigel Lawson and John Major from the

Treasury, John Moore and Tony Newton from the DHSS (the latter two being replaced by Kenneth Clarke and David Mellor half way through the review, following John Moore's resignation and the decision to hive off Social Security from the Department of Health, as it then became). Sir Roy Griffiths and John O'Sullivan, a member of the Prime Minister's Policy Unit, were also regular attenders.[25]

The very notion of setting up a Cabinet Committee was, of course, an affront to the tradition embodied in the Royal Commission approach. The membership of Royal Commissions invariably incorporated representatives of the main interests. In contrast, a Cabinet Committee excluded precisely those – notably the medical profession – who had come to think of themselves as participating in the policy-making process as of right. It was this sense of exclusion, the feeling of being denied their proper place at the top policy-making table, that shaped the medical profession's perceptions of the whole process. In this respect, there is a close parallel with the bitter confrontation between the Government and the medical profession that led up to the creation of the NHS (*see* Chapter 1): much of the hostility to Bevan reflected as much resentment of his style as disagreement over substance. In short, the way in which Mrs Thatcher set up her Review was a direct challenge to the medical profession's view of its own position in the constellation of power.[26] Nor was the style of conducting the Review likely to smooth down resentment. As part of the exercise, there were two meetings at Chequers with NHS doctors and managers respectively. However, those invited to these meetings were selected not because they were representative of the professional interests involved (the Royal Commission model) but precisely because they were unrepresentative in their sympathy for ideas of radical reform.

Everyone could, of course, contribute to the policy soup of ideas from which the Cabinet Committee itself was drawing. And many did so: the announcement of the Review precipitated a variety of policy cooks into action, each ready with his or her own recipe for what needed doing about the NHS.[27] Analysing the various contributions does not necessarily establish the paternity of the proposals in *Working for Patients*: ideas often become politically acceptable only when they have become part of the common intellectual currency, their precise origins long since forgotten. But it does illustrate the extent to which the debate about the NHS widened out in the course of the 1980s to embrace ideas not even considered by the 1979 Royal Commission. And it thus allows the reforms that finally emerged from the Review to be placed in the spectrum of options – from the conservative to the radical – available to Ministers.

The medical profession, speaking through the voice of the BMA, stood firmly at the conservative end. Having raised the spectre of radical reform, it took fright. In its evidence to the Government Review, the BMA argued that only 'a relatively small percentage increase in funding' was needed and that it would be 'a serious mistake to embark on any major restructuring of the funding and delivery of health care in order to resolve the present difficulties',[28] though some form of hypothecated taxation might be desirable. In making the case against radical reform, the BMA provided an eloquent testimonial to the NHS, 40 years after having fought its introduction:

> While many of the alternative systems have shown superficially attractive features, we have always been led to the inescapable

conclusion that the principles on which the NHS is based represent the most efficient way of providing a truly comprehensive health service, while at the same time ensuring the best value for money in terms of the quality of health care. They also enable the cost of health care to be controlled to a much greater extent than has been achieved with other systems, as has been shown by the experience of other countries.

At the radical extreme were a number of proposals for privatising the finance of health care, and giving the consumer the ability to choose between competing schemes, by increasing the role of private insurance. The role of the State should be limited, it was argued, to ensuring that everyone had the resources required to buy health care. Decisions about the appropriate level of spending on health care would be largely de-politicised because diffused among consumers, the NHS's budget would depend on its ability to attract customers in the face of competition from other providers.[29] It was a model which had first been put forward 25 years previously by the Institute of Economic Affairs, an independent research organisation set up to propagate libertarian market doctrines, and generally dismissed as one more example of the IEA's eccentricity in trying to revive nineteenth-century ideas. By the 1980s, however, the IEA's championship of market liberalism seemed to have triumphed.[30] Its ideology appeared to be the Prime Minister's. In practice, Mrs Thatcher was a somewhat wayward disciple – all too ready to listen to the seductive voices of Think Tanks more prepared to bend their notions to political expediency. But the IEA remained the voice of ideological conscience: the home of the Old Believers in the doctrines of market liberalism. Its ideas therefore provided a touchstone for testing the Government's policies for ideological purity: a test which (as in the case of health care reform) the Government frequently failed. Its influence was, moreover, also apparent in other variations on the theme of giving more power to the market and the consumer. These included the notion, put forward by a former Conservative Cabinet Minister,[31] of funding the NHS through a National Health Insurance Scheme while giving everyone the right to opt for equivalent or greater private insurance cover: a model very similar to that already adopted by the Government for pensions.

If some of the policy recipes were primarily designed to change the method of financing health care, others were more concerned with changing the dynamics of the existing health care system drawing largely on American ideas. This import of American ideas was, in many ways, surprising: it was very much a case of experts on obesity advising a patient suffering from anorexia. American experience in trying to contain (unsuccessfully) a health care cost explosion was not self-evidently relevant to the British debate about under-funding. Perhaps, however, it was the frustrating failure of American policy which prompted the development of a highly sophisticated body of theory that proved to be highly contagious, as transmitted by globe-trotting economists, and influenced opinion in Britain and elsewhere. Two different types of policy approach, derived from this body of theory, must be distinguished. There were those who saw change as being driven by consumers while others saw it as being driven by managers. In the former (arguably more radical) category were proposals for allowing citizens to choose their own health care providers, who would then be reimbursed on a capitation basis by a central funding agency. The appropriate health care providers might be either GPs or specially formed Health Maintenance Organisations (HMOs) on the American model. In the latter category came the proposal for giving district health authorities a budget with which to buy the health services required by their populations from independent providers, thus leaving health authority managers (rather than consumers) to make the choices. Again, the American inspiration was evident: the notion of such an internal market had been first put forward by a visiting American academic, Alain Enthoven, in 1985.[32] It was a quite deliberate compromise between what Enthoven himself perceived as the greater advantages of the more radical, consumer-driven HMO approach – known, in the American context, as managed competition – and what he considered to be politically feasible in Britain. But it did address the central weakness of the NHS, as perceived by most policy cooks and by Ministers, which was that money did not follow patients.

It was a diagnosis with which the all-party House of Commons Social Services Committee – which in 1988 conducted its own review of the various options in parallel with the Cabinet Committee – largely agreed. The Committee rejected the more radical proposals for change in the funding or organisation of health care. But it gave a qualified welcome to the notion of an internal market as an idea which deserved further exploration and development. Specifically, it proposed 'limited experiments' to test its practicability, urging that 'it should not be introduced nationally before a thorough piloting had been done'.[33] Given the need to maintain consensus on the all-party Committee, in order to produce a unanimous report on a politically explosive topic, even such a degree of cautious interest was perhaps somewhat surprising. Certainly it would have been difficult to predict, on the basis of this Parliamentary report, the denunciations of the Government that followed its decision to adopt the internal market option in *Working for Patients* six months later.

The decision came only after the Cabinet Committee had wasted some months, in the view of some of those involved, exploring a series of policy dead-ends. For contrary to the view that the contents of *Working for Patients* were predetermined by the Government's ideological agenda, the Review of the NHS appears to have been a singularly rudderless operation. Far from steering a pre-set course, the Review tacked rather erratically between different options, only settling down to developing something approaching a coherent package towards the end of its existence. There certainly was an ideological *bias* among many of those taking part, in that they tended to share a belief in the merits of markets and competition. But there was nothing like an ideological *programme*. One of the most striking characteristics of the Review was that no one – not even the Prime Minister – appears to have had a clear agenda, apart from wishing to find some formula that would bring peace and prosperity to the NHS. There were lots of problems in the NHS; there was a long list of possible solutions. But matching problems and solutions turned out to be a fumbling process.

There were a variety of reasons for the Review's uncertain start. The Department of Health, which might have been expected to take the lead in shaping the agenda of any Review of the NHS, turned out to be ineffective in this role. Although John Moore, the Secretary of State, was anxious to demonstrate his credentials as an aspiring Dauphin by demonstrating his ideological radicalism, his health broke down; it was not until the much more pragmatic Kenneth Clarke replaced him that there was an effective Department of Health voice and that the Review moved towards developing a more coherent approach. Furthermore, the memoranda submitted by the DHSS civil servants were felt, by most of the Review's members, to be inadequate in their analysis and timid in their pre-scriptions. Instead, they tended to rely on the advice pouring in from other sources: the Treasury, Mrs Thatcher's No. 10 Policy Unit and various Conservative Think Tanks.

But perhaps the most important reason for the meandering start of the inquiry had nothing to do with the characteristics of the Review or of the actors involved. This is that there is no magic formula for health care reform[34] and that any attempt to devise one inevitably turns into a conflict between competing claims and interests. This became clear early in the life of the Review when, in a somewhat half-hearted way, it examined alternative ways of funding health care, looking at the experience of other countries. It quickly became apparent that the weakness of the funding system for the NHS in the eyes of its critics (the fact that it kept health care on short rations) was precisely its strength in the eyes of the Treasury (the fact that it could not be bettered as an instrument of public expenditure control). 'It did not take long to conclude that there was surprisingly little that we could learn from any of the other systems', Nigel Lawson noted,[35] 'To try to change to any of the sorts of systems in use overseas would simply be out of the frying pan into the fire.' In turn, when the DHSS sought to argue the case for funding health care by means of a hypothecated tax – which would have guaranteed the NHS a stable and increasing income – this was strenuously resisted, after an initial show of flirtatious interest, by the Treasury, whose control would have been threatened by any such move. Accordingly, the Prime Minister soon decided that the Review should concentrate 'on changing the structure of the NHS rather than its finance'.[36] This did not stop her from grinding her own favourite axe – tax reliefs for those taking out private insurance – throughout the rest of the Review. Nor did it stop the Treasury from resurrecting the case for increasing and extending charges throughout the NHS, as it had done regularly for the previous 40 years: a proposal on which the Prime Minister firmly stamped, as she records, as threatening to discredit any reforms. But it did mean that the most radical options – i.e. those designed to transform the way in which the health care system in Britain was funded and organised – had been ruled out of court.

The rejection of changes in the methods for funding health care – and the veto on further discussion of moving towards either the European social insurance model or a voucher-based market model – did not lead to the instant adoption of the internal market notion. The internal market emerged as the *by-product* of policies designed to change the NHS's dynamics, by giving more autonomy to the providers and introducing more incentives to efficiency. In this respect, the White Paper that emerged from the Review – *Working for Patients* – accurately mirrored its proceedings. All the emphasis is on specific measures, like splitting the purchaser and provider functions and giving hospitals independence, not on the abstract notion of creating a market. Specifically, the measures followed from the Review's diagnosis of the NHS's central weakness: that money did not follow the patient, thereby penalising rather than encouraging productivity. Increasing activity sent up costs in a hospital, operating under a budget fixed by the health authority, without increasing its income. There were no incentives to be sensitive to demands, particularly those coming from outside the authority's administrative boundaries. The logic of the analysis suggested devising a system of internal NHS finance that would relate hospital incomes more directly to their activities and giving hospitals more freedom to behave entrepreneurially in responding to new opportunities.

The idea of giving more independence to hospitals, and allowing them to emancipate themselves from bureaucratic control, was in itself calculated to appeal to a Conservative administration.[37] The model had already begun to be tested in the case of education where the Government had earlier given schools the right to opt out of control by the local education authorities and to become self-managing institutions whose budgets would depend on the number of pupils they managed to attract. So here there was a ready-made example, and there is no doubt that it influenced Kenneth Clarke and other Review members. There were significant differences between health and education, not least that in the case of schools the rationale behind the changes was that they would transfer power to parents by giving them the ability to choose between schools. But education was, in a sense, the laboratory in which Conservative Ministers first invented internal or mimic markets, subsequently drawing what they perceived to be the appropriate lessons for health.

It was not at all self-evident how the general principle of giving hospitals more independence or autonomy should be translated into practice. Who would own them? Who should run them? A Treasury paper, which caught the Prime Minister's fancy, suggested that hospitals should be contracted out: staff consortia, private companies and charities would all be able to bid. Again, as so often with the Review, a more cautious option prevailed. There was to be no competition for the right to manage hospitals; the final solution adopted was that of self-governing Trusts, with the Secretary of State nominating the board and retaining the ultimate power of control. Similarly, there were various ways in which the principle of money following patients could be translated into practice. One was the solution finally adopted: the purchaser–provider split, with hospitals dependent on the contracts obtained in a competitive market in which private providers could also compete. For once the Review chose the bolder option. The Treasury had argued for a less radical solution. Under its scheme hospitals would have continued to receive their basic budget from health authorities, but there would additionally have been a central funding pool from which they would have been paid for meeting, or exceeding, performance targets set by central government. This, the Treasury argued, would give them an incentive to greater activity while yet retaining the capacity to plan the NHS's strategic direction and maintaining expenditure control. Rejected by the Review team, a very similar formula was subsequently to be adopted by the Labour Party.[38]

Overall, however, Mrs Thatcher worried that 'we were losing our way' and 'moving away from, rather than towards, radical reform'.[39] Accordingly she seized upon the idea of GP budgets[40] with some enthusiasm, when this surfaced halfway through the life of the Review. The idea had been urged upon her by the No. 10 Policy Unit; Kenneth Clarke independently had also come to embrace this option, which he came to see as very much his own contribution to the reform cocktail. The primary health care policy stream had been going its own way, as we saw in the previous chapter, long before the Review had been set up. A complete reform agenda was already on the table. Many of the Review members, the Treasury Minister in particular, thought that their inquiry should concentrate on the hospital sector. But the notion of GP budget holding appeared to offer something which none of the other contemplated reforms could do: it brought the choice of what was to be purchased nearer to the consumer. The general practitioner would be the consumer's voice and consumers would be free to change their GP if they did not approve of his or her use of resources on their behalf. GP budget holding was thus much nearer the education model than any of the other reforms introduced by the Review. There were objections. The Treasury questioned whether GPs would be able to manage large budgets and worried about the creation of a powerful new lobby for extra health spending. However, the objections were over-ruled and GP fundholding became one of the most contentious parts of *Working for Patients*, not least because the BMA felt betrayed by the injection of this new element into the negotiations over the future of primary health care that had preceded the Review.

A number of other matters were settled as well, before the Cabinet Committee completed its labours after 24 meetings. The White Paper, as we shall see in the next section, which analyses its proposals in more detail, put forward managerial and organisational changes that were to prove almost as contentious as its introduction of the internal market and GP budgets. But there was also a private, internal battle to be settled. Pressed hard by the Prime Minister to introduce tax relief for private health care, the Chancellor of the Exchequer overcame his objections of principle to any such concession and offered a compromise: no change in the tax treatment of the benefit of company health insurance schemes but tax relief for policies taken out by the over-60s. It was a concession that Nigel Lawson subsequently came to regret, even though its financial implications were insignificant. Nevertheless the Treasury felt satisfied enough with the outcome of the Review to announce, as an overture to the publication of the White Paper, a 4.5 per cent increase in real terms in spending on the NHS, the first in a series of similar announcements over the next three years. The Review may have done nothing to change the system of financing health care that had provoked the 'under-funding' crisis but, ironically, the Government's determination to ensure the success of its reforms brought about a rare period of rapid growth in the NHS's budget.[41] But, as if to underline that the 'under-funding' crisis had been as much about the changing balance of power within the NHS as about the money, the generous financial settlement did nothing to ease the acceptability of the Government's plans. The antagonisms aroused by those plans ran too deep, as the reception of *Working for Patients* and the subsequent months were to show, to be assuaged by money alone.

An explosion of opposition

When launching their White Paper – an exercise carried out with a fanfare of publicity, at considerable cost to the public purse – Ministers faced a dilemma. Should they stress the radicalism of their proposals and thus claim credit for their boldness in changing the health care system? Or should they emphasise the strong element of continuity and thus claim credit for their determination to preserve the NHS? In the event, the strategy adopted in *Working for Patients* was to present the specific policy proposals as building on the achievements of the past: as a way of releasing the full potential of the NHS. There was a re-affirmation of the 1948 settlement and a celebration of the success of the NHS: 'The principles which have guided it for the last 40 years will continue to guide it into the twenty-first century. The NHS is, and will continue to be, open to all, regardless of income, and financed mainly out of general taxation.' Echoing Bevan, the White Paper further proclaimed: 'The Government wants to raise the performance of all hospitals and GP practices to that of the best.' The twin aims of the proposals were to give patients 'greater choice of the services available' and to secure 'greater satisfaction and rewards for those working in the NHS who successfully respond to local needs and preferences'. Who could possibly disagree with such general, benevolent aims?

The answer came quickly: almost everyone. The Labour Party position as enunciated by Robin Cook, its front-bench spokesman, was simple. The Government's strategy, he argued, was 'to destabilise the National Health Service and replace it with a commercial one'. The logic of the changes would lead inexorably to the ultimate horror: 'market medicine as it is practised across the Atlantic'. The conclusion was clear: 'We are in danger of losing a Health Service that is motivated by dedication and replacing it with one that is driven by financial targets'.[42] Much the same charges were made by the BMA – which throughout worked in a curious, unspoken alliance with the Labour Party – in an advertisement campaign that more than matched the Government's own expenditure on publicity. On the hoardings a poster picturing a giant steamroller carried the legend: 'Mrs Thatcher's Plans for the NHS.' In the newspapers, full-page advertisements carried the message: 'The NHS. Underfunded, Undermined, Under Threat.' In GP surgeries, a BMA pamphlet – designed to be handed out to those waiting – asked, among other questions, 'Do you want the cheapest treatment or what is best for you?' The BMA's indictment of the Government's proposals was comprehensive.[43] The proposals, argued the BMA, ignored the issue of under-funding. They would 'lead to a fragmented service', 'destroy the comprehensive nature of the existing NHS' and 'cause serious damage to patient care'. Instead of increasing patient choice, the changes would limit it. Political and professional voices spoke with a rare unanimity and with the same intent: to induce terror and apprehension at the thought that the Government was planning to replace the primacy of the patient with the primacy of the pound, forcing doctors to subordinate the search for health to the search for solvency.

Nothing like it had been seen in the NHS policy arena since the opposition provoked by Nye Bevan 40-odd years before. Nor was the intensity of the conflict the only similarity. In both cases, the degree of hostility appears – in retrospect, at least – disproportionate to the causes. In both cases, too, the ostensible pretexts for the conflict concealed other motives. Disentangling the reasons for the extreme reaction to the White Paper reforms is therefore complex. Some were not specific to the NHS. A generalised hostility to Mrs Thatcher – who by 1989 was widely seen as a domineering autocrat intent on imposing her own vision on the world – spilled over into the health care arena. Any proposal which carried her stamp of approval was therefore automatically tainted in the eyes of many. More directly, the circumstances in which the Review had been set up and carried out tended to condition the response to it. If the Royal Commission procedure was a device for creating consensus, the Review method was designed to provoke schism. The British style of adversarial politics was further calculated to amplify disagreement. So, too, was the combative style of the two leading political protagonists – Kenneth Clarke and Robin Cook – whose verbal violence seemed to escalate with each encounter. The Government's insistence that it would drive through its reforms, whatever the criticisms, strengthened in turn the root-and-branch opposition to the principles that shaped the plans. Thus was created a cycle of mutual and mounting antagonism. Ministers were strengthened in their conviction that engaging in discussion was futile. The Government's critics, conversely, were confirmed in their belief in a conspiracy to undermine the NHS. It was not a situation calculated to encourage discussion of how the reforms might best be introduced, even though it was clear that the impact of the Government's somewhat sketchy outline proposals would largely depend on the way in which they were implemented.

Opposition to the Government's plans cannot, however, be dismissed as an artefact of the political situation. The fact that the Opposition saw an opportunity for further exploiting public reservations about the Thatcher administration's record on the NHS and the medical profession's sense of outrage at its exclusion from the policy process both explain much. But the reasons for the hostility go deeper. Some were specific to particular policy areas: the special case of the reform of primary health care is examined separately in the next section. Others revolved around fundamental questions about the nature of the NHS. Was it possible to maintain the historic facade while gutting the building behind it without also destroying those characteristics of the NHS which made it special? Would not the reforms destroy the web of assumptions, loyalties and relationships, built up over the decades, which had sustained the NHS and allowed it to perform better than might have been expected from the size of its budget?

There is an irony in the evocation, by the Government's critics, of the traditions of the NHS: a Burkean defence of an existing institution on the grounds that the introduction of changes based on a priori ideas would threaten to unravel the delicate fabric woven by history. For this appeal to history as embodied in an existing institution was very much at odds with the origins of the NHS. The NHS, as we saw in Chapter 1, was the product of faith in scientific rationalism. It was designed as a machine for making generally available the benefits of scientific medicine,[44] using the tools of planning as an instrument for doing so. Services were to be free at the point of delivery precisely in order to ensure that treatment would be determined by scientific judgements about need, not by the financial resources of the patient. But by the 1980s, most of the assumptions built into this design were under challenge. There was increasing scepticism about the scientific basis of much of medicine and increasing resistance to accepting the judgement of doctors about need. Planning, as an instrument of public policy, was discredited. Feminism joined consumerism to question the medical determination of how patients should be treated. Conversely, a new form of rationalism was in the ascendant: that of the econocrats.[45] The rise of the economists in the policy arena in the 1970s has already been noted. By the 1980s they had become the Savonarolas of public policy, denouncing inefficiency and ignorance as the ultimate sins. Efficiency in health care, it was argued,[46] was not just desirable: it was an ethical imperative, since wasting resources meant losing the opportunity to provide beneficial treatment to someone. It was this new-style rationalism – the Benthamite streak in Thatcherism – that helped to shape the Government's proposals.[47] And the proposals were seen as threatening – rightly – to many of the assumptions on which the NHS rested. The real threat came not from ideology conceived in the narrow and limited sense of the Conservative Party's belief in markets and privatisation but from ideology seen as a way of defining problems and devising solutions.

Perhaps the most important founding myth of the NHS was that it divorced the practice of medicine from money. It did no such thing, of course. The NHS's great achievement was rather different: it largely cut the links between the practice of medicine and the income of doctors, thus removing any perverse incentives for either the selection or treatment of patients. Money remained, as the whole history of the NHS demonstrated, the great constraint on medical practice: hence the events leading up to the Review. However, the Government's internal market proposals rested on the assumption that doctors (like everyone else) would be responsive to financial incentives, even if these did not touch their personal incomes. The internal market thus raised the spectre that medical practice would be corrupted by a competitive drive to attract custom, setting doctor against doctor, with treatment being determined by financial considerations rather than need. The criticism betrayed a certain lack of faith in the moral fibre of doctors and their dedication to the code of medical ethics. Equally, it ignored the fact that competition between consultants for funds, beds and merit awards had characterised the NHS throughout its entire history and that one of the aims of the reforms was precisely to change the currency of that competition. In future (if the reforms worked out as intended) the currency would be the ability of consultants to attract patients rather than to attract research grants or to wave shrouds. But suspicions of a deep-laid plot to subvert the values of medicine, as embodied in the NHS, were further fuelled by GP fundholding. For here undeniably there appeared to be perverse financial incentives. If GPs were to stick within their budgets – or to make a surplus, which they could then plough back into improving their surgeries – they might be tempted either to deny their patients expensive treatment or to recruit only the healthiest patients to their list.[48]

So, for anyone with ideological hackles to raise, there was plenty of provocation in the White Paper. There might well be ways of dealing with the potential threats to the NHS's values posed by the reforms. Everything, it could be argued, would depend on their implementation: in the event, as we shall see, few – if any – of the prophesied disasters happened. But in 1989 one of the casualties of the political situation was precisely any willingness to discuss the nuts and bolts of implementation; the Government's insistence on driving through its proposals, without much attention to the mechanics of change, meant that all debate tended to be framed in apocalyptic terms. Discussion revolved around a mythologised past (an NHS in which money did not matter) and a demonised future (an NHS in which medical practice was driven by money).

The 1989 reform package could also be seen as a challenge to the traditions of the NHS in another respect. It marked the transformation of an organisation based on trust into an organisation based on contract.[49] Symbolic of this transformation were the changes proposed by the White Paper in contracts for consultants. Previously, such contracts had been held at the regional level, so in effect insulating consultants from the managers of their institutions. Now, however, the Government took the view that 'it is unacceptable for local management to have little authority or influence over those who are in practice responsible for committing most of the hospital service's resources'. In future, therefore, local management (which soon came to mean the management of the provider Trusts) would negotiate and monitor contracts. These would include 'a fuller job description than is commonly the case at present' and specify the responsibilities of consultants 'for the quality of their work, their use of resources, the extent of the service they provide for NHS patients and the time they devote to the NHS'. It was a more stringent form of control than anything that the Labour Government had dared to suggest when it was trying to limit the private practice activities of consultants in the 1970s (*see* Chapter 4). And Trusts, in particular, were to have discretion to depart from national agreements in negotiating contracts with staff, including consultants. Moreover, managerial influence was to be strengthened in other ways as well. The criteria for distinction awards were to be changed so that, to put their feet on the first rung of the ladder, consultants would have to demonstrate 'not only their clinical skills but also a commitment to the management and development of the service'. And, further, managers would – for the first time in the history of the NHS – be included in the membership of the committees making these awards. Finally, the quality of professional practice would in future have to be demonstrated, rather than being taken for granted: all consultants would be expected to take part in medical audit, reviewing their own practices, the use of resources and the outcome for patients.

Medical audit turned out to be an example of the profession's ability to modify – if not to subvert – the Government's intentions during the process of implementation. Consultants displayed only a fitful and erratic interest in audit, despite generous financial subsidies.[50] But there were plenty of other reasons for the apprehensions of doctors and others about the shift from trust to contract, from professional to managerial values, implied by the White Paper. The logic of market competition reinforced the logic of many of the managerial changes introduced before the Review. If there was to be market competition, there would have to be more and better information about activities and costs. It would therefore mean giving visibility to, and putting a price on, what the professionals were doing. Moving from a culture based on trust to one based on contract was therefore inevitably threatening to those working in the NHS in so far as it represented a switch of emphasis from autonomy to accountability: the books of the NHS were to be opened, literally as well as metaphorically, with the activities of both purchasers and providers being made subject to the scrutiny of the Audit Commission. It was an opportunity which the Audit Commission was to exploit with enthusiasm, issuing a series of reports that questioned medical practices.[51] Looking at the way in which resources were used turned out to be a singularly effective tool for challenging the way in which doctors went about their business.

The sense that the 1989 White Paper represented a turning point in the history of the NHS, a deliberate repudiation of the past, was further strengthened by changes in the composition of health authorities. Reviving a debate about the role of health authority members that went back to the 1974 reorganisation of the NHS, the White Paper argued (correctly) that 'at present they are neither truly representative nor management bodies'. So out went the representatives of the professions working in the NHS and the members nominated by local authorities. The new authorities were to be modelled on company boards. Their membership would be split between non-executive members chosen for 'the strength of the skills and experience they can bring to an authority's work', and paid on a part-time basis, and the authority's own executives. The new vocabulary of the NHS – as epitomised in the linguistic transformation of the one-time administrators into, first, general managers and subsequently into chief executives – seemed to represent not only a change of style but also the triumph of an alien set of values. It confirmed the fears of those who saw the reforms as threatening to turn the NHS into a business corporation and saw the new composition of health authorities as heralding an influx of hard-faced men (and women) concerned only about money and lacking in sensitivity towards the wider interests of the community.

Much of the criticism of the Government's proposals on this score rested, yet again, on an invented past. The notion that previously health authorities had derived democratic legitimacy from the presence of a few members nominated by local authorities – as though the fact of election to one body turned them into all-purpose representatives of the public – was never convincing. Nor did the record suggest that health authorities had been particularly effective in either making policy or monitoring management: membership tended to be a frustrating experience.[52] But the Government's new-style boards did mark a significant break with the past in that none of their non-executive members had an independent base or constituency. Both in the case of health authorities and of the new Hospital Trusts, there could no longer be any doubt about their exclusive accountability to the Secretary of State: the reforms represented the ultimate logic of Nye Bevan's principle that health authority members were the 'creatures' of the Minister. What is more, they underlined the collective accountability of the new boards, via the regions, to Head Office, i.e. the NHS Management Executive, the new incarnation of the NHS Management Board. It was the NHS Management Executive – headed by Sir (as he subsequently became) Duncan Nichol, a former regional general manager – which was to have the responsibility for implementing the *Working for Patients* programme.

The question of how and at what pace the White Paper proposals should be implemented was almost as contentious as its substance. The Government presented its reforms as a remedy for the NHS's ills which had to be swallowed whole and at a gulp. Ministers made few concessions of substance during the passage of the National Health Service and Community Care Act, which gave effect to *Working for Patients*, and the new legislation came into effect on 1 April 1991. The time between conception and birth was short. Yet the White Paper's proposals were little more than outline sketches, even when supplemented by a series of Working Papers put out by the Department of Health that sought to put some administrative flesh on the skeleton of ministerial ideas.[53] No one really knew how an internal market would work; almost everyone (including the Prime Minister) agreed that the NHS's existing information system was incapable of meeting the new demands that would be made on it. It was a timetable which, the Government's critics argued, was driven more by political expediency – a desire to get the NHS reforms in place before the next General Election – than by any regard for the good of the service: a brutal assault on the fragile fabric of the NHS, calculated to lower morale even further. The Government, argued the Social Services Committee in its report on the White Paper,[54] was trying to do too much, too fast: 'we have serious fears that the stability of the services and continuity of patient care may suffer during the years of transition to a new, untested system.' Instead of gambling with the future of the NHS by introducing untested ideas wholesale, it was argued, the Government should have first experimented with pilot projects. The refusal of Ministers to do so was widely seen as the victory of political brute force over rationality in policy-making.

The Government's strategy did indeed raise questions about rationality in policy-making, but the arguments could cut two ways. Ministers could, and did, point out that introducing change would be a gradual, incremental process. Only a minority of hospitals would initially opt to become Trusts; only a minority of general practitioners would choose to become fundholders. In practice, however – as we shall see when we look in more detail at the implementation process – this did not prevent considerable confusion and some chaos. Some of this confusion and chaos might indeed have been avoided if the changes had first been evaluated on a pilot basis. But such pilot experiments would have been able to test only the *components* of the new system: so, for example, they might have ensured the availability of adequate information. They would not, however, have been able to evaluate the new system as a whole: it would have been like putting a car on the market on the basis of having tested every component, without ever having made sure that it would actually run on the road. Even had there been a pilot of the whole system in one region, there would still have been a problem: the length of time needed before coming to any conclusions about the viability or otherwise of the experimental design. Given that even four years after the introduction of the internal market nationally, it was still extraordinarily difficult to evaluate its effects,[55] it seems implausible to assume that any firm conclusions could have been drawn from pilot schemes restricted to a politically realistic time-table. The rational model of policy-making – first experiment, then evaluate, finally decide – may thus be based, the case of the NHS suggests, on a series of irrational assumptions about the feasibility of applying it. In contrast, ministerial strategy seems to have been based – no doubt unconsciously – on a very different model of rationality in policy-making.[56] This sees policy-making itself as an experiment – the testing of theory by putting it into practice. From this perspective, no apology was needed for using the NHS as a laboratory for testing the Government's ideas, since there was no other way of finding out what would or would not work – and what adaptations were required to improve the design. If the 1948 NHS reflected the period's certain confidence in its ability to design institutions that would mould the future, the 1989 model reflected the loss of this confidence and decreasing certainty about what the future would bring. The Government had created – whether by intention or by inadvertence – an institution which would invent its own future in a process of trial and error.[57]

General practitioners on the rampage

The case of general practice provides a sub-plot in the drama of confrontation between the Government and the medical profession that followed the publication of the White Paper. The separate policy stream that had been meandering along for the previous three years now joined the main river and helped to turn it into a raging torrent. The medical profession's general suspicions of the reforms were reinforced and fuelled by specific grievances about the proposals for primary health care. Most disturbingly for the medical profession, the battle over general practice demonstrated with particular clarity – indeed brutality – that they had lost their ability to veto change in the NHS. In April 1990 the Secretary of State for Health, Kenneth Clarke, imposed a new contract on GPs, while the following year the rest of the White Paper reforms were introduced. Apart from winning some minor and marginal concessions on points of detail, general practitioners, as represented by the BMA, suffered a humiliating defeat. It was, in many ways, a repetition of the story of the events leading up to the introduction of the NHS 40 years earlier: the leaders of the profession could summon their troops to battle but could not make them fight.

The Review proposals for general practice were, in the main, variations on themes already developed in the previous policy documents and thoroughly explored in the negotiations that had followed (*see* Chapter 5). They were the product largely of evolutionary, departmental thinking rather than of Conservative ideology. If there was any ideology shaping the general practitioner proposals, it was largely that of the public health profession, with its emphasis on encouraging preventative medicine and on improving the quality of practice in inner cities. The draft contract for GPs, prepared by the Department following the publication of the White Paper, contained few surprises, though the profession was irritated by what it considered to be modifications of previously agreed positions. Throughout the country, local meetings of GPs voiced their hostility to the new contract; in April a special conference of representatives of Local Medical Committees 'overwhelmingly confirmed the profession's widespread opposition', though the meeting 'rejected by a large majority a proposal for doctors to resign from the NHS' if the Government insisted on going ahead.[58] Negotiations with the General Medical Services Committee of the BMA continued, although from the start the Government made it clear that it would impose the new contract unilaterally if no agreement was reached with the profession. The Department of Health made some concessions to the GMSC. For example, it modified the proposal that the proportion of GPs' incomes derived from capitation payments should be increased from 47 per cent to 60 per cent, in order to increase sensitivity to patient requirements, by widening its definition of what was to be included under this heading. Similarly, it abandoned the attempt to abolish seniority allowances for GPs, though reducing their value. At a 10-hour meeting between Kenneth Clarke and the GMSC negotiators on 4 May 1989, agreement about the new GP contract was reached, to the surprise of the participants.[59]

The agreement, however, was repudiated by the rank and file of GPs. Another special conference of Local Medical Committees voted by 166 to 150 votes to reject the compromise deal and called for a referendum of all GPs. The result was an overwhelming vote – by 76 per cent to 24 per cent – against the revised contract.[60] Once more the cycle was repeated. A further round of talks followed. Some minor concessions on the fine print of the contract were offered by the Government: for example, the methods of calculating the incentive payments for immunising children were revised. The GMSC leaders once again recommended acceptance of the terms, albeit with little enthusiasm; the special conference of Local Medical Committees, called to consider the deal in March 1990, once again rejected them 'without a dissenting vote . . . as being ill considered and harmful to patients'.[61] However, the conference also rejected – if only by 153 to 148 votes – a call for a ballot on sanctions against the imposition of the new contract. If the GP leadership could not deliver their troops to the Government – if their recommendations were consistently repudiated – neither could they make them fight. In advertising its opposition to the Government – by taking, literally, to the hoardings – the doctors had succeeded only in advertising their collective impotence. Unperturbed by the rejection of the GP contract by the profession, the Government simply went ahead. The new GP contract duly came into effect in April 1990.

GP hostility to the new contract both reflected, and reinforced, the profession's antagonism to the Review as a whole. The various issues involved boiled up in the same cauldron of discontent and it would be futile to try to disentangle the reasons for GP opposition from those which led the medical profession as a whole to battle against the NHS reforms. All sections of the profession resented their exclusion from the policy process, a resentment that was compounded in the case of GPs by the Government's imposition of the new contract without the agreement of the profession. All sections of the profession shared in the suspicion that the Government was corrupting the principles of the NHS by introducing the notion of buying and selling services, a suspicion strengthened in the case of GPs by the introduction of fundholding – even though they themselves had always seen themselves as small shopkeepers, running their own businesses with a keen sense of how to wring the most money out of the Government. Most important perhaps, all sections of the profession feared that their autonomy was being eroded by the new managerialism, a fear further fuelled in the case of GPs by some of the provisions in the new contract and in the White Paper.

The last point can be simply illustrated. In the regulations laid before Parliament in the autumn of 1989 – and which came into effect at the same time as the new contract – the responsibilities of GPs were spelled out as never before.[62] Family Practitioner Committees (FPCs) simply had the duty to ensure that GPs provided 'all the necessary and appropriate personal medical services of the type usually provided by general medical services'. In other words, the responsibilities of GPs were defined in terms of what they did, i.e. their own professional customs. But the Family Health Service Authorities (FHSAs) – which replaced FPCs in 1991 – had the duty of policing a contract which laid down in great detail what general practitioners were expected to do. So, for example, the contract not only required GPs to carry out an annual health check on all patients over 75 but also spelled out how that assessment should be carried out. FHSAs could call individual practitioners to account and indeed had a statutory duty to do so. It was quite clear that FHSAs, in contrast to their predecessors, would be expected actively to manage primary health care.

Nor was this all. In pursuit of its policy aim of making GPs more responsive to their patients the Government, in addition to strengthening the incentives in the remuneration system, introduced a series of changes calculated to induce alarm. GP practices would in future have to submit an annual report; changing one's doctor, and complaining against him or her, would be made easier. The spectre of consumer power appeared to be stalking through the country. Further, much alarm was caused by the Government's decision to introduce indicative prescribing budgets. All GPs were to be allocated shadow budgets to cover their prescribing costs; exceeding the budget would not stop the flow of medicines but would trigger off an inquiry into the GP's prescribing practices. The proposal revived the BMA's fears that the Government's hidden agenda – in line with the Treasury's long-standing and ill-concealed ambition – was to cap primary health care spending in the same way that expenditure in the hospital and community services had long been controlled. The result would be, the BMA argued, that doctors would not be able to afford to prescribe appropriate but expensive drugs and that expensive patients would be turned away: an argument designed to cause much unnecessary, as it turned out, anxiety among Britain's elderly population, in particular.

To compound the profession's apprehensions, all the changes would be implemented by FHSAs which – like all the other authorities in the NHS – were to be managerial, not representative, bodies. The old FPCs had been true children of the 1974 reorganisation, embodying the corporatist principle of representation for the professions. Of their 30 members, eight were appointed by the Local Medical Committee representing GPs while a further seven were nominated by the other primary health care professionals, dentists, opticians and pharmacists. In this respect, they were true successors of Lloyd George's Insurance Committees and a monument to the medical profession's success in 1911 (and subsequently) in gaining a strong voice in the administration of general practice.[63] FHSAs, in contrast, were to be small, managerial bodies with a total membership of 11. Only one of these 11 would be a general practitioner and even that solitary figure would be appointed by the regional health authority, serving in a personal, not representative, capacity.

Working for Patients, as subsequently translated into legislation, thus marked a double defeat for the medical profession. Not only did it signal the end of the medical veto in the national policy process. But it also weakened the doctor's voice in the local administration of health care. If the medical profession had shown itself strong in the distributional conflicts that had followed the creation of the NHS in 1948, it had proved powerless to prevent the introduction of a new constitutional settlement.[64] Its power, it turned out, was contingent on the arena in which it was exercised and the issues involved. When the health care policy arena was widened out – when reform of the NHS was put in the wider context of modernising Britain's institutions – the medical profession lost its central place on the stage: it simply became an actor, and not necessarily the most influential, among many. To the extent, however, that the Government needed the medical profession's co-operation to implement its policies – *within* the health care policy arena – so the balance of power might be expected to shift yet again to reflect the mutual dependence between the two parties. Indeed even while engaged in the battle over the GP contract, Kenneth Clarke – like Bevan before him – made an agreement with the Royal Colleges. The legislation going through Parliament was to be amended to include provision for the creation of a multi-professional clinical standards advisory group to monitor the impact of change.[65] It was a move rich in symbolism, if nothing else. It marked the acceptance by the Government, on the one hand, that the professions were the guardians of clinical standards in the NHS and by the Royal Colleges, on the other hand, that the reforms did not mean the end of the world. Despite the furore over the Government's policies, despite the apocalyptic prophecies of impending doom, the way was being prepared for a return to business as usual. Once the new GP contract came into force, the Department and the BMA resumed the routine of haggling, year after year, over the small print, modifying its application if not its principles. And GPs could find consolation in the fact that their defeat had been highly profitable: in the first year of the new contract their income exceeded the intended target by £6,000 a head.[66] Militancy was doused by prosperity.

Implementation as learning

Launching the new-style NHS proved to be a fraught exercise. The Government had provided a bold, outline sketch. The civil servants of the Department of Health had translated the sketch into legislation: the 1990 NHS and Community Care Act. But long after the official launch in April 1991, the managerial engineers were still hard at work plugging the leaks and adapting the design even while the ship was lurching through heavy seas. Of necessity, the NHS became a learning system, inventing itself as it went along. The process of adaptation began before the launch. As evidence grew about the unpreparedness of most health authorities and the risk of a market crash if the pace of change was forced too fast,[67] so the timetable was relaxed. With a new Secretary of State, William Waldegrave, taking charge of the Department of Health – under a new Prime Minister, John Major – the emphasis was on avoiding turbulence. On 1 April 1991, 57 NHS Trusts and 306 GP fundholders came into operation.[68] But the internal market did not. The NHS was not to be plunged suddenly into competition between providers. The instructions from the centre were that purchasers should stick to their existing providers, rather than switching around in search of the best buy. The emphasis was on achieving a 'soft landing' by maintaining a 'steady state'. There was to be no sudden leap into a market but incremental progress towards it.

In effect, the Department of Health (through the NHS Management Executive) was conceding that lack of knowledge and lack of expertise dictated caution. The concrete of the managerial foundations laid by the Griffiths report had hardly had time to dry; the introduction of new management techniques – notably the Resource Management Initiative, designed to involve clinicians in decisions – had proved to be more difficult than expected.[69] The transformation of a system based on control through a managerial hierarchy to one based on negotiating contracts between purchasers and providers would clearly take time. So, too, would the development of an information system capable of generating quick and accurate data about which patients were being treated, where and at what cost. It was a situation that compelled evolutionary adaptation. Set adrift without a compass, and with only the most rudimentary instructions to guide them, NHS managers faced a tough survival course. Their salaries rose dramatically. But their occupational life expectancy fell. Working on short-term, performance-linked contracts, their prospects depended – more directly than ever before – on carrying out government policies. In its managerial style the new NHS was a more merciless organisation than it had been before 1991. Both the opportunities offered to managers, and the demands made on them, increased sharply as the tempo of life in the NHS accelerated in the 1990s.

Nevertheless, by 1994 the separation between purchasers and providers – the cornerstone of the NHS's new architecture – was to be complete, despite the initial caution. By then more than 400 providers accounting for about 95 per cent of the NHS's activities had become self-governing Trusts. Two separate lines of accountability ran to the Secretary of State: one from the district health authorities (via the regions) and the other directly from the Trusts. By that time, too, over a third of the population belonged to fundholding GP practices. Both developments took place in the face of fierce initial resistance from the medical profession and despite some early disasters in the first year of the reforms. In a succession of ballots, consultants overwhelmingly voted – by two to one – against their hospitals becoming self-governing Trusts.[70] General practitioners who opted to become budget holders were seen as professional deviants who had betrayed their colleagues. Nor was the Government's cause helped by the initial experience of Trusts. Two of them – Guy's, a leading teaching hospital in London, and Bradford – announced that they would have to retrench by cutting 900 posts.[71] Dramatic stories of Trusts facing bankruptcy, and the Government being forced to rescue them with an infusion of funds, filled the media. But, as one wave of Trusts succeeded another, both the resistance and the disasters diminished. In the case of GP fundholding, the experience of the pioneer first generation[72] – and succeeding waves – tended to encourage others to follow their example. Both successes, as we shall see, were expensively achieved: management costs in the NHS rose sharply and fundholding GPs were treated with great generosity. However, the twin pillars of the institutional framework of the new NHS – Trusts and fundholders – had been firmly established.

But changing the labels on institutions proved easier than changing the dynamics of the service. Early critics of the Government's proposals had been quick to point out that the NHS – like other health care systems – had a number of features that made the notion of an internal market problematic. The theory of the internal market was that it would be driven by purchasers, thus reversing the dominance of providers that had characterised the NHS in the previous four decades. It was the purchasers who would determine what their populations required in the way of services, and then shop around accordingly. No longer would service developments be driven by the interests and ambitions of consultants. In practice, however, it was the providers who had the expertise and the information about services. In the words of one district health authority manager: 'in the early days, it was like going blindfold into a supermarket with a trolley and asking the staff to fill it up.' There was, in short, a problem of information asymmetry,[73] compounded by an asymmetry of managerial resources: the most able and ambitious staff tended to opt for managing provider units rather than purchasing authorities. Further, talk of an internal market over-simplified a complex situation. In 1991 the NHS was a collection of different types of markets,[74] making generalisation a high-risk activity. In some services, providers tended to have a monopoly: ambulance and accident and emergency services fell into this category. In others, an oligopoly of providers dominated local markets: most conventional acute services and regional specialties fell into this category. Lastly, there were the services where there was genuine competition: elective surgery, pathology and some community services fell into this category.[75] And cutting across this classification, there was the geographical factor. In London and other conurbations with a high concentration of NHS providers, there was clearly much competition. Conversely, in more rural areas providers may have had what were in effect geographical monopolies. Lastly, there was the biggest monopoly of all: the medical profession, which strictly regulates competition among its members.[76]

The vocabulary of official rhetoric soon came to adapt, with some subtle modulations, to the complex reality. Purchasers became transformed into commissioners: a recognition that monogamy rather than polygamy characterised the internal market, with most purchasers and providers locked into permanent relationships in which both partners sought to modify the other. The internal market became the managed market: a recognition that purchasing was all about shaping the nature of the services available to the local population over the long term, rather than buying off-the-shelf to satisfy immediate wants. Competition became replaced, as the key word, by contestability: acknowledging that the NHS internal market appeared to be creating regulated local monopolies rather than a free-for-all, it was argued that this did not matter as long as new providers could move into the market and purchasers could threaten to switch their custom. Competition, it was increasingly stressed, was a means, not an end to be pursued for its own sake. In turn, the linguistic shifts marked a significant switch of emphasis in public policy. The adoption of a market model for the NHS represented, in a sense, the apotheosis of a blame diffusion strategy. The logic of the model was clear if brutal: political decisions about the future configuration of the NHS would be replaced by market decisions. It would be impersonal market forces, not politicised planning decisions, that would decide which hospitals would survive and which went under. But in the event, public policy repudiated the logic of the model. The managed market, in which commissioning and contestability replaced purchasing and competition as the hurrah words, turned out to be one in which politicians were active actors rather than passive spectators of events. Although the introduction of the internal market had appeared to be a death certificate for the whole notion of planning, planners soon re-emerged in a new incarnation as commissioners. The NHS market, it had become clear, was not about driving the best bargain on offer, or going round the supermarket shelves, but about shaping the future.

The point can best be illustrated by the story of health services in London. If the logic of the internal market could be expected to work anywhere, it was in inner London. Here there was a plethora of providers and long-standing evidence of considerable over-capacity in the provision of acute care. Yet over the decades, successive governments had shirked the challenge of getting rid of redundant beds and institutions: Ministers of all parties had regarded the task of taking on the prestigious teaching hospitals in central London as an invitation to political suicide. But market competition promised to do what Ministers had failed to do: by taking away custom from the inner-city hospitals, it threatened their viability. If the logic of the market had been allowed to work its way through, therefore, the problem of over-supply would have been solved as hospitals went bankrupt. But, in the event, the Government intervened. Far from being left to the market, the re-structuring of London's health service was to become one of the most ambitious planning exercises in the history of the NHS.

Historically, the capital's over-supply of acute beds reflected the concentration of teaching hospitals in inner London, as already noted in Chapter 4.[77] There was much debate about the scale of the 'over-bedding' and about the extent to which the over-provision of expensive acute beds, compared with the rest of the country, was compensating for the inadequacies of primary care and long-stay facilities in London. But there was little doubt that London was relatively over-funded: it received 20 per cent of the NHS budget for hospital and community services, although Londoners made up only 15 per cent of the English population. The excess could not, moreover, be justified in terms of London's social problems or the population's health status. Before the 1991 reforms, however, London was to an extent sheltered from the pressures to cut back because the RAWP formula used for allocating funds to the regions (which in turn allocated funds to the districts) made allowances for cross-boundary flows.[78] This meant that the London regions and their districts benefited from the fact that they provided services for a wider population than that contained within their boundaries. However, the logic of the 1991 reforms required the budgets of purchasing authorities to be based exclusively on the needs of their own populations: if patients used providers in other districts, money would have to follow them. Accordingly, the 1991 reforms introduced capitation funding, i.e. a formula for allocating funds to district health authorities, via the region, based on their population characteristics and disregarding cross-boundary flows. This meant a re-distribution of resources from the historically over-provided districts which had been importers of patients (mainly in London and other big cities) to the historically under-provided districts which had been exporters of patients (mainly in the shires). Even though the new funding formula was to be phased in over five years, the impact on London was drastic: many districts, particularly those in the inner city, faced severe cuts in their budgets. The impact of this re-distribution of resources was reinforced by the fact that purchasers now had to pay the full costs of any services they bought. There was therefore a strong incentive for purchasers, particularly those on the periphery of London, to repatriate services: to stop buying from expensive inner London teaching hospitals and to contract with less expensive, and more accessible local providers. Purchasers were, in effect, voting with their money against the existing configuration of services in the London conurbation. The existing pattern of provision in London, it became clear, could not survive the introduction of the internal market.

The issues involved were first identified, and analysed, in a series of research reports produced for the King's Fund Commission: an inquiry set up in 1990 by an independent foundation with special interests in the capital's hospitals.[79] The ground was thus prepared when the Secretary of State for Health, William Waldegrave, announced in October 1991 an inquiry into London's health services: an inquiry prompted by Waldegrave's realisation that with London's teaching hospitals competing for capital funding for new developments, it was essential to have a framework within which decisions about the rival claims could be taken. The Tomlinson Inquiry[80] reported a year later to Waldegrave's successor, Virginia Bottomley. Its conclusions, building on and echoing those of the King's Fund Commission, were radical. By the end of the 1990s, it concluded, between 2,500 and 7,000 beds in inner London hospitals could become surplus. There would, therefore, have to be a rationalisation of hospitals, involving the closure or merger of several prestigious teaching institutions. Conversely, there would have to be some compensatory investment in developing primary and community care in London. Finally, the Tomlinson report recommended that the process of change should be supervised by a specially created implementation group.

Most of the Tomlinson recommendations were accepted, within five months, by the new Secretary of State, Virginia Bottomley.[81] A Review of six specialties was carried out; a London Implementation Group was set up with a former regional manager, Bob Nicholls, as chief executive; a London Initiative Zone was created to promote the development of primary health care. Special funding was allocated: some £100 million for redundancy payments to staff and £170 million for the development of primary care. Despite vigorous campaigns by some of the teaching hospitals faced with extinction, despite continuing debate about the pace of change and the scale of London's need for beds,[82] the scene was set for a radical transformation in the capital's health care provision: a transformation prompted by the changes introduced in 1991, and the dynamics of the market, but carried out as the result of a central government initiative. To manage the market – to avoid disruption to existing services, to ensure that London's population had appropriate services and to prevent competition from having perverse side effects on teaching and research – planning, it seemed, was essential.

The case of London illustrates another facet of the reforms: the process of introducing them was expensive. In London, as noted above, greasing the wheels of change involved considerable expenditure. More generally, creating the managerial infrastructure of the new model NHS meant a considerable invest-ment, partly in information technology and partly in manpower. Extra spending directly attributable to the implementation of the Review, according to the Department of Health's own calculations,[83] was some £600 million in the two years starting April 1991. Additionally, the new model NHS required more people to manage it, both centrally and locally. Staff numbers at the Department of Health – including the NHS Management Executive – rose from 3,680 in 1988–89 to 4,570 in 1993–94, an increase of almost a quarter; the number of adminis-trative and clerical staff in the NHS rose from 116,800 in 1989 (14.7 per cent of the total labour force) to 135,000 in 1992 (17 per cent of the total labour force).[84] Further, the NHS of the early 1990s was the setting for a gold rush by manage-ment consultants exploiting the service's needs for IT expertise, managerial training and reassurance. The consultants panning for gold were rarely disap-pointed, though those who employed them frequently were. The expenditure was diffused through the NHS, and is difficult to calculate even roughly, but it certainly helped to swell the total managerial budget. Whereas before 1991 the NHS could boast of being extraordinarily lean managerially – spending a lower proportion of its budget on administration than almost any other health care system – by the mid-1990s the Government was trying to trim off some of the accumulated fat. The under-managed NHS of the decades preceding the reforms (as the Government saw it) had become the over-bureaucratised NHS of the 1990s (as the Government's critics perceived it). The investment in management, Ministers argued, would pay for itself in increased efficiency: better management meant better patient care. Spending on management, the critics replied, was money diverted from patient care: only by spending more on employing doctors and nurses would patient care improve.

It was, yet again, a dialogue of the deaf, incapable of resolution by an appeal to evidence. For while it was quite clear that the cost of introducing the 1991 reforms had been high, there was no agreement about what the currency of evaluation should be: how, for example, could the impact on services of the new management structure, as distinct from that of all the other changes introduced in 1991, be measured? If reckoning up the total investment in the management of change was difficult, calculating the dividends turned out to be impossible.

New themes in the health policy arena

If the years following 1991 can in part be characterised as a period of adaptive policy learning, they were also marked by the emergence of two new themes in the language of health policy debate. First, there was the adoption of a new health policy paradigm which – like the new economic policy paradigm that had been so influential in the early 1980s – had its roots in the nineteenth century. Second, there was the transformation of NHS patients into consumers. Both these themes were, of course, 'new' only in the limited sense that ideas that had previously floated on the margins of debate became increasingly central as the 1990s went on. Both, however, were important in setting the agenda for the 1991 model NHS and shaping expectations about its performance. Both, furthermore, demonstrated the impact of the modulation of policy style that followed the fall of Margaret Thatcher and John Major's succession to the premiership.

The publication of *The Health of the Nation* White Paper[85] in 1992 – following a Green Paper of the same title a year before – marked a significant shift in public policy. Starting from the premise that the population's health was the product of a variety of factors – ranging from lifestyle to the environment – the White Paper embraced a strategy of social mobilisation. Within Government, a Cabinet Committee was to co-ordinate departmental policies that might have an impact on health. Outside Government, local authorities, voluntary organisations, employers and the media were all to play their parts in a campaign to create healthy cities, healthy schools, healthy workplaces, healthy homes and healthy environments. The roots of this strategy went back to the nineteenth century public health movement and the resurrection of this tradition internationally reflected the growing awareness that the role of medicine in producing health (as distinct from making the consequences of decay and disease more tolerable) was limited.[86] In short, the Government acknowledged that it had responsibilities for the health of the population that went beyond the provision of a health care system. Moreover, the White Paper translated this general responsibility into 25 specific policy targets. For example, by the year 2000 the death rate for coronary heart disease and stroke in people under 65 was to be reduced by at least 40 per cent, while the suicide rate was to be reduced by 15 per cent. Other targets included reductions in the proportion of smokers, heavy drinkers and overweight men and women in the population.

The White Paper provoked some cynicism. Conspicuously absent from its catalogue of factors associated with ill-health or premature mortality was any mention of income distribution or unemployment. The targets appeared to be largely based on extrapolations of past trends, designed to make sure that the Government would be able to congratulate itself on good progress in moving towards them: as, indeed, it did.[87] Any improvements in health might, in any case, be more attributable to changes in the social and economic structure of the country – such as the virtual disappearance of heavy industries like mining and steel – than to government policies. Still, a puzzle remains. Advocacy of the new health care paradigm, with its emphasis on State intervention, fitted neatly into the ideology of the Labour Party. So, for example, it was under Barbara Castle's auspices in 1976 that the Department of Health published a consultative document on prevention.[88] And it was the Labour Government which set up the Black Working Group on Inequalities in Health,[89] whose 1980 report argued that improving social conditions was a necessary pre-condition for improving health. But now a Conservative administration was committing itself to a programme of social engineering. The frontiers of Thatcherism, not of the State, were being rolled back. There could be no clearer signal that the temper of the times in the 1990s, as reflected in the health care policy arena, was significantly different from what it had been in the 1980s. If both Mrs Thatcher's economic paradigm and Mr Major's health paradigm had their roots in the nineteenth century, they grew from opposing traditions: those of individualism and collectivism.

The conversion to the new health care paradigm – like the conversion to the new economic policy paradigm a decade earlier – no doubt reflected, in part, a sense of frustration. The NHS, like Keynesian economics, had not delivered the goods. Contrary to early expectations (*see* Chapter 1), the NHS had become an institution for generating more demands: every leap forward in medical technology extended the scope for more expenditure. No wonder that a strategy which appeared to promise turning off the tap of demand at source – by tackling the causes of morbidity and mortality – appealed to Ministers. Whatever the reasons, and however tentatively the strategy was pursued, there were some significant implications for the NHS. First, it marked a shift of focus from the specialist exercising his or her magic in the hospital to the general practitioner and others involved in health promotion and prevention in the community. Second, it put further pressure on purchasers to test the demands of providers for extra resources against the White Paper's criteria that any services bought should make a demonstrable contribution to the population's health. If only at the level of symbolic rhetoric, the adoption of a new health policy paradigm therefore marked a further shift in the balance of power within the NHS.

If the *Health of the Nation* strategy seemed to be based on a collectivist view of the world, the other new theme to emerge in the 1990s was based on a more individualist model. The mimic market produced, in turn, a mimic consumerism. This reflected a national policy initiative involving the public sector as a whole as well as development within, and specific to, the NHS. With the publication of the *The Citizen's Charter*[90] in 1991, carrying the imprimatur of the new Prime Minister, the Government committed itself to defining the standards of service delivery of public services. The overall policy still remained to promote choice and responsiveness by privatisation, competition and contracting out. But where this was not possible, the citizen must be told what he or she could expect in terms of service standards. Although the Charter delicately skirted around using the word 'rights', it implicitly endorsed the notion of a menu of entitlements. Performance targets would be published; aggrieved citizens would have 'well-posted avenues for complaint'. In turn, the Citizen's Charter spawned a series of others specific to particular services. There were Charters for parents, tenants, jobseekers, railway travellers and a host of others. For the NHS, there was the *Patient's Charter*[91] which, more boldly than the parent document, explicitly set out a decalogue of rights. These ranged from the right 'to receive health care on the basis of clinical needs, regardless of ability to pay' to the right 'to be guaranteed admission for treatment by a specific date no later than two years from the day when your consultant places you on a waiting list'. In addition, there were nine national charter standards, setting out service specifications to be striven towards rather than establishing any entitlements. One such standard, for example, was that in emergencies ambulances should arrive within 24 minutes in urban areas or 19 minutes in rural districts. Another was that outpatients should be 'given a specific appointment and be seen within 30 minutes of that time'. District health authorities were to set local standards and publish an annual report on progress towards achieving them.

The rights and standards published in the *Patient's Charter* were not particularly exigent. Like the *Health of the Nation* targets, they appear to have been chosen largely because they were achievable. In any case, the standards themselves were revised and extended in subsequent years. But, again like the *Health of the Nation*, the symbolic importance of the charter outweighed its immediate impact. It introduced a new rhetoric and a new set of expectations in the NHS, marking precisely the kind of shift of power from providers to consumers envisaged in the Griffiths report. The point is well illustrated by the standard for individual outpatient appointments. The fact that it was even necessary to make this a standard demonstrated the extent to which the NHS had been dominated by providers for the previous 40-odd years: the persistence of the custom of booking a batch of patients for the same appointment (usually the start of the clinic session) reflected the assumption that not a second of the consultant's time must be wasted but that the time spent by the patient waiting was of no account.

The Department of Health followed up the *Patient's Charter* in 1994 by publishing a comparative performance guide, showing the extent to which individual hospitals (and departments within them) had achieved its standards as well as various performance targets set by the NHS Management Executives, such as those for increasing the proportion of people treated as day patients. By consulting the guide,[92] which was widely distributed and available free of charge, anyone could establish how his or her local provider had performed in 1993–94 relative to other NHS Trusts: the guide helpfully adopted a starring system, awarding five stars to the best performers. So, to take the example of a generally above-average hospital, at Bath's Royal United Hospital 78 per cent of the patients were seen within 30 minutes of their outpatient appointment (one star), 42 per cent of the patients coming in for hernia repairs were treated as day patients (four stars), while only one per cent of those getting their cataracts extracted were treated as day cases (one star). Similarly, the guide set out the waiting times for different types of surgery. Thus at Bath's Royal United Hospital, only 24 per cent of the patients were admitted for orthopaedic surgery within three months of being put on the waiting list (one star), whereas 61 per cent of those coming in for urological procedures were admitted within three months (three stars).

In effect, then, the performance indicators first introduced in the 1980s had gone populist by the 1990s: what had started as a tool of managerial control had become a way of giving the public information about the activities of the NHS. The information provided was designed, as the guide told its readers, to 'help you and your family doctor make informed decisions about your health care'. The invocation of the well-informed consumer, able to choose among the competing supermarkets, was unfortunately somewhat misleading. The family doctor – particularly if he or she was a fundholder buying services on behalf of his of her patients – might well be able to use the information about the performance of NHS Trusts to exert pressure for improvement. But there was nothing that the consumer could do directly: there were no decisions, informed or otherwise, to take – except, possibly, to opt out of the NHS and go private. In short, both the *Patient's Charter* and the guide underlined that the consumerism of the internal market was of a very peculiar kind: it was top-down consumerism. Just as district health authorities were exhorted by the NHS Management Executive to become the voices of their local populations[93] in making their purchasing decisions, so in turn the Executive was mobilising popular opinion to apply pressure on providers. But it was local, regional and central managers – not consumers – who had the power to impose sanctions when calling inadequate performers to account.

A new hierarchy of command

One of the paradoxes of the new model NHS, as of the Thatcher enterprise as a whole, was that only an assertive government could carry out the policy of reducing the role of the State. If the logic of the mimic market appeared to be to devolve decision-making in the NHS – to allow the Government to defuse blame by claiming that the allocation of and use of resources were matters for local purchasers to determine in the light of the needs of their populations – the administrative logic of working this transformation was ever-more intervention by the centre.[94] If the rhetoric of devolving decision-making persisted throughout the first half of the 1990s, the reality was hyperactivity by the NHS Management Executive driving, directing and dominating the agenda of the service as it implemented the policies of Ministers. It was the Executive which was responsible for launching successive waves of NHS Trusts. It was the Executive which was responsible for pushing through the unfinished business of the 1980s, such as the introduction of resource management and the reduction of waiting lists. It was the Executive which took the lead in pushing through the new agenda of the 1990s, such as various initiatives designed to make the NHS more quality conscious. It was the Executive which sent out the annual priorities and planning guidance for the purchasing authorities: an exercise notable for the proliferation of priorities, which increased year by year.[95] It was the Executive which was responsible for the flood of hortatory instructions – on matters ranging from land sales to staff motivation – that engulfed the NHS. As Duncan Nichol, the Chief Executive, put it in 1989: 'We want to give clear and decisive leadership to the health service to achieve more effective management.'[96] And no one, in the years that followed, could be left in any doubt about where leadership in the NHS was coming from: the centre.

If the first half of the 1990s were therefore years of expanding managerial activities, they were also the years that tested the energies of managers to the point of exhaustion. For no sooner had the new model NHS been put on the road – itself a daunting task – than the process of modifying it started. Again, the NHS proved to be a self-inventing institution, constantly adapting and modifying its own structure. Hardly had the new district health authorities started working than they began to merge; hardly had the mergers started, than the new combined authorities began to incorporate the family health service authorities. And what started as an exercise in cohabitation – the new commissioning authorities were living in sin, since there was no legal sanction for the new arrangements – soon became incorporated in government policy. In November 1993, following a review of functions and manpower, Virginia Bottomley announced a series of constitutional changes.[97] Legislation was to be introduced not only to allow all DHAs and FSHAs to merge but also to abolish the statutory regional health authorities. Instead of 14 RHAs, there were to be eight regional offices of the NHS Management Executive, thereby providing an opportunity to cut down staff members. The regional directors were, in turn, to be members of the Executive.

The changes were presented as part of 'the continued drive towards decentralisation in the NHS, with responsibility and decision-making devolved as far as possible to local level'. As local purchasers became stronger so, it was argued, the need for a regional tier diminished. But they can also be interpreted rather differently as the apotheosis of a process of centralisation that had gradually, almost stealthily, been creeping up. Almost 50 years after the NHS was first created, in the second half of the 1990s it became a *national* service. Instead of a loose conglomeration of different services – with no integration of primary and secondary care – there was to be one unified managerial structure. It was a structure, moreover, where the lines of accountability ran firmly and unambiguously to the centre: where in the last resort authority chairmen and non-executives owed their position exclusively to Ministerial favour. A complex baroque building, incorporating the architecture of many previous generations, had been transformed into a neat brutalist structure. The process of architectural simplification was completed in 1994 with the publication of the Banks report on the Department of Health.[98] This addressed one of the remaining sources of confusion and tension: that between the Department itself and the NHS Management Executive. In theory, the division of labour between them was simple. The Department was responsible for helping Ministers to develop policy, while the Executive was responsible for its implementation. In practice, and entirely predictably, the line between policy and implementation turned out to be blurred. Accordingly, the Banks report recommended that in future the Executive should be responsible for both policy formulation and implementation, leaving the Department with a miscellany of other responsibilities. It was a development which, to an extent, marked the victory of the NHS over the civil service. It was former NHS managers – not civil servants or outsiders imported from management consultancy firms and business – who dominated the new Executive. It was also a development which marked the rejection, yet again, of the more radical option of hiving off the NHS and the Executive as an independent *Next Steps* agency. Once more this was rejected on the familiar grounds that given the scale of public spending on the NHS, any such quasi-independent status would mean a reduction in parliamentary and public accountability.

So was completed another cycle in the NHS's oscillating progress between devolution and centralisation, and back again, which had characterised the service ever since 1948. But, as we shall see, it was not the last. For it reflects, as we have seen in previous chapters, the tensions built into the constitution of the NHS. On the one hand, its dependence on public funds inevitably centralises accountability. On the other hand, the public perceptions of the shortcomings of the service equally inevitably persuade Ministers that it would be best to devolve responsibility for how the money is spent at the periphery. Even while the Secretary of State for Health was completing her new design for the management of the NHS, she was also trying to decentralise pay bargaining.[99] Similarly, she was vigorously repudiating the notion that the centre should define the menu of NHS services, i.e. what should or should not be offered, in the name of purchaser autonomy.

The Conservative legacy

In 1996 Stephen Dorrell, who had succeed Virginia Bottomley as Secretary of State for Health the previous year, published a White Paper setting out the Conservative Government's vision for the future of the NHS.[100] For the Government, the NHS was an electoral liability: survey after survey showed that voters put their trust in Labour, rather than the Conservatives, to run the NHS successfully. With a General Election looming up, the Government was therefore anxious to demonstrate its credentials as the guardian of the NHS. The White Paper, *A Service with Ambitions*, was born of this anxiety: it was an exercise in political persuasion and reassurance. But it was more than that. It also demonstrated the extent to which Conservative attitudes and policies had shifted since the publication of *Working for Patients* and the subsequent introduction of the 1991 reforms. The change in attitudes in part reflected the different, more emollient tone set by John Major as Prime Minister: compared to Mrs Thatcher, he was less ideological and aggressive in style. Similarly, his Secretary of State for Health, Dorrell, was a pragmatic, middle-of-the-road politician. But the change in policies also reflected policy learning: the lessons drawn from the process of implementing the 1991 reforms. From this perspective, the 1991 reforms can be seen as a policy experiment that disappointed some of the hopes of their sponsors (as well as the dire prophecies of their critics) but also created new opportunities. The agenda set out in *A Service with Ambitions* largely built on the experience gained as a result and, in so doing, anticipated many of the themes that New Labour was to claim as its own.

The main political goal of *A Service with Ambitions* was, as already noted, to provide reassurance. It represented in effect an attempt to recreate (and reclaim for the Conservatives) the consensus about the NHS that had seemingly been shattered by the introduction of the 1991 reforms, stressing the Government's commitment 'to build on the founding principles' of the NHS. These were defined as being to provide a universal service, available to anyone who wishes to use it; delivering high quality; applying the latest knowledge and the highest professional standards; and being available on the basis of clinical need without regard for the patient's ability to pay. Decisions were to be guided by three 'clearly defined values': equity, efficiency and responsiveness. 'No better model than the NHS has been found', it argued, 'for adapting to change and development and making the best use of available resources to meet demand for health care'. And it stressed that its intentions could be achieved without 'further radical change' by building on 'the best of current practice'.

The overriding aim was to create 'a high-quality, integrated health service which is organised and run around the health needs of individual patients, rather than the convenience of the system or the institution'. It was to be a 'seamless service' based on 'partnership' between the primary and secondary care sectors of the NHS. It was to work across 'the boundaries of health, social care and voluntary organisations'. It was to promote a 'well-informed public' since 'having more information not only helps people have a greater say in the way health care is provided, it also helps them to make more appropriate and responsible use of services and take greater responsibility for their own health' and 'knowledge-based decision-making', as well as being 'sensitive to the needs and wishes of patients'. Further, the White Paper put great emphasis on 'managing for quality', improving the NHS's information system and investing in professional development. All these phrases were to find an echo in the policy statements of the Labour Government when it took office in 1997: both parties were drawing on a common stock of 'hurrah words'. And most significant of all – in terms both of substantive policy change and of what was to come – the White Paper stressed the trend 'towards a primary care-led NHS': the top priority in the planning guidelines sent out the same year by the NHS Executive to health service managers.[101]

But as significant as the words used in the White Paper were the words that did not feature. There was no invocation of the market, of competition or choice. Instead there was an invocation of the softer virtues. The new vocabulary of partnership, seamlessness and sensitivity could offend no one. The language of *Working for Patients* had softened; the aims of policy had subtly shifted. Why this should be so, political expediency apart, is explained by the evolution of policy in the light of experience in implementing the 1991 reforms.

From the start of the 1991 experiment, as we have seen, the emphasis of Department of Health policy was on controlling the pace and direction of change, rather than allowing the market to disrupt or dictate the pattern of service provision. Moreover, stability was not the only policy goal in conflict with promoting competition between providers. So, too, was the continuing priority given to slimming down the NHS: mergers between trusts were likely to be sanctioned if they promised to reduce capacity even though the result was to limit competition[102] – ignoring the fact that competition in the US had succeeded most in bringing down prices and improving efficiency in precisely those states which, like California, had massive surplus capacity. NHS parsimony and competition turned out to be incompatible bed-fellows. Moreover, although health authorities were powerful purchasers in theory, in practice they were greatly constrained in using their financial clout to switch their contracts or threatening to do so.[103] They were inhibited precisely because local provider trusts were financially dependent on them, just as they themselves were dependent on those trusts to provide services to their populations. Even a small shift of resources to another provider might, however, endanger the viability of their 'home' trust because of the interdependence of services, reinforced by the requirements of professional training and accreditation. And a threat to viability would almost inevitably bring political intervention. The logic of market competition and the logic of NHS politics were pulling in different directions. The former required decisions to be devolved to the market; the latter forced decisions to the centre in the name of accountability.[104]

The result was that health authorities tended to use their fiscal muscle with great caution. They tended to rely heavily on block contracts, i.e. buying specified levels of activity, rather than shopping around.[105] Contrary to the intentions of *Working for Patients* money did not necessarily follow patients: once the specified level of activity had been achieved, providers had no incentive to treat more patients. The pre-1991 pattern of hospitals stopping operations near the end of the financial year persisted. Increasingly health authorities became more concerned to shape provision to fit into their long-term plans rather than reacting to what the market had to offer. To do so, they worked to establish long-term, stable relationships with trusts, even if this meant contracting with fewer providers – and thus less competition and less choice for consumers.[106]

No wonder, then, that when Alain Enthoven returned to Britain to see what had come of the ideas he had helped to seed, his verdict was that the reforms had failed to deliver the hoped-for transformation of the NHS.[107] In this he echoed the conclusions of other American observers.[108] There had indeed been some important gains, Enthoven maintained – a point further explored below, when drawing up an overall balance sheet of the costs and benefits of the 1991 reforms. But the essential conditions for a market to operate, he argued, were not fulfilled. The necessary foundations had not been laid; in particular, information systems continued to be woefully inadequate. Incentives for purchasers and providers alike were too weak and the constraints imposed by central government too strong. 'Purchaser decisions were mostly about balancing the books and preserving institutions', he concluded, 'not about health gains or quality improvements'. The internal market, as he saw it, was the work of politicians in a hurry – more concerned with the election cycle and avoiding blame than with building the foundations for the kind of long-term evolutionary changes needed to make the notion work.

In one largely unanticipated respect, however, the 1991 reforms did transform ways of thinking about the NHS, if not its structure. The introduction of GP fundholding turned out to be the joker in the pack of reform. It was fundholding, rather than the much contested new GP contract, which proved to be the catalyst for a series of changes that were to nudge the NHS towards being 'primary care led' – the theme of the outgoing Conservative Government which was to be taken up *fortissimo* by the incoming Labour administration. GP fundholding, as already noted, had been denounced by both the BMA and the Labour Party (which in 1989 could still be classified as Old Labour, although the process of reinvention had begun). It was seen as introducing the cloven hoof of financial self-interest into general practice: GPs would have an incentive, it was argued, to scrimp on treatment and to weed out expensive patients in order to maximise their budget surpluses. While these surpluses could not be used to swell the income of GPs, but had to be ploughed back into the practice, they nevertheless could be used to increase the value of the premises (to the ultimate profit of the practitioners). Further, it was maintained, the scheme would lead to a 'two-tier' NHS, inasmuch as fundholders would be able to buy accelerated access for their patients: the result, in effect, would be to promote queue jumping.

Despite the virulent opposition, fundholding turned out to be a success story for the Government. Step by step the conditions for GPs to become fundholders, in particular the minimum number of patients required for eligibility, were relaxed. Their budgets were set generously, initially at least, on the basis of the past costs incurred by the practices concerned. The process of setting up as fundholders was lubricated by grants for management and information technology: a total of £232 million had been paid out in this way by the middle of the 1990s.[109] The profession's collective hostility to the project waned and even the BMA was forced to modify its position of uncompromising opposition as GPs voted with their feet in favour of the scheme. By the time the Conservatives left office about half the GPs in the country were members of fundholding practices, covering, in turn, something like 50% of the population.

GPs became fundholders for a variety of reasons. Some signed up because they were eager to exploit the opportunities offered by this new status. Others signed up as a defensive strategy because they did not want to be left out. Their attitudes towards fundholding, and the ways in which they responded, varied accordingly.[110] Like GPs in general, fundholders were a very heterogeneous lot. And it was this very heterogeneity that made evaluation of the experiment especially problematic.

Fundholding covered a wide range of practice strategies, ranging from that of the innovative entrepreneurs to that of the cautious traditionalists. Nor was any comprehensive evaluation commissioned by the Government; indeed any such evaluation might have been difficult given that the conditions of fundholding kept on changing in the light of experience. However, from a prolixity of one-off studies,[111] some tentative conclusions can be drawn. Most of the initial fears prompted by the introduction of fundholding proved unfounded. There was little evidence of 'cream skimming', i.e. selecting out expensive patients. Nor did fundholders as a whole appear to be short-changing their patients in search of surpluses: there was little, if any, difference in the increase in referrals to hospitals or prescribing costs between fundholders and other GPs. There was, however, some evidence that fundholders were able to buy preferential – i.e. fast track – access for their patients. Whether this should be considered as creating a 'two-tier NHS' is another matter. Individual GPs have always differed in their ability to negotiate access on behalf of their patients and, in this sense, the phenomenon of a 'multi-tier NHS' long predates fundholding.

If the fears prompted by fundholding proved to be largely unfounded, so did some of the more optimistic expectations. Some fundholders turned out to be more critical purchasers than health authorities: the very fact that their budgets represented only a small proportion of the income of any trust made it easier for them to switch providers without destabilising them. For the most part, though, they tended to be cautious purchasers, loyal to their local institutions. What is more, they appear to have been more sensitive to quality – defined in terms of process, such as speedy treatment for their patients and prompt discharge notes – than to prices. It is therefore difficult to know to what extent fundholding prompted efficiency gains among providers to set against the expense of introducing and running the scheme: to the setting-up costs of the scheme must be added the administrative costs to providers of dealing with a multiplicity of small contracts. Only an agnostic verdict is therefore possible on the economic impact of fundholding.

The main impact of fundholding must, however, be measured in a different currency of appraisal. First, it gave GPs an opportunity to enlarge the scope of primary care. Fundholders used their resources to buy extra services, ranging from physiotherapy to consultant sessions in their surgeries, for their patients. Second, it changed the balance of power between GPs and hospital consultants. The financial leverage enjoyed by fundholders meant that consultants had to respond to the wishes of GPs under threat of losing income. Third, it gave health authorities a strong incentive to involve GPs in their own purchasing decisions. Since fundholding allocations came out of the budgets of health authorities, the ability of the latter to devise a coherent purchasing strategy became increasingly dependent on the participation of GPs in the decision-making process – a dependency reinforced as the NHS Executive set itself the goal of moving towards a 'primary care-led' service[112] and transferred ever more purchasing power to fundholders. Specifically the scope of fundholding was gradually extended. Initially fundholding budgets covered only a limited range of services. But over time GPs were given the opportunity to opt for an ever-widening range. In 1995 Total Purchasing Pilots were introduced. Under this experimental scheme groups of fundholders could purchase virtually the entire package of NHS services on behalf of their health authorities.

The result of all these developments was to encourage a multiplicity of purchasing patterns and a devolution of fiscal power from health authorities.[113] Many health authorities embraced the notion of 'locality commissioning' or 'GP commissioning'. This took a variety of forms, as well as having a variety of labels. In some cases purchasing power was devolved to GPs in a particular geographical area; in other cases GPs' views were sought out and fed into the health authority's purchasing strategy. Significantly, it was a trend that embraced all GPs and not just fundholders. At the same time, fundholders and other GPs were forming themselves into larger consortia or groups in order to strengthen either their purchasing power or their collective voice. Already by the middle of the decade it was being predicted that a movement that had started with health authorities purchasing with the assistance of GPs would end with GPs purchasing with the assistance of health authorities and that the latter's role would centre around strategy and regulation.[114] When the Labour Government unveiled Primary Care Groups as its answer to fundholding – and the centre-piece of its strategy for the NHS (*see* next chapter) – it was therefore as much a christening as a birth: building on and institutionalising what in effect was an unplanned by-product of the 1991 reforms.

There was also an unexpected footnote to the Conservative Government's policies for primary care. The Government legislated to introduce salaried GPs. More surprisingly still, it did so at the suggestion of the medical profession. Fifty years after Bevan's plans for the NHS had almost been shipwrecked by the BMA's hostility to the very idea of salaried GPs (*see* Chapter 1), only five years after the medical profession had bitterly fought a contract which seemed to derogate from their status as independent small shopkeepers, the profession had not only accepted but instigated what it would once have denounced. True, the Government launched its legislative plans only after an elaborately staged consultation exercise about the future of primary care.[115] True, too, the introduction of salaried GPs was initially to be only on a small-scale experimental basis and formed part of a larger package designed to make more flexible contractual arrangements possible.[116] But even so the fact that the BMA effectively co-sponsored such a symbolically charged change – which in a few cases could and did lead to GPs being employed by nurses[117] in a reversal of accepted hierarchy – suggests that there had been a shift in the profession's perception of its own interests and role. It was a shift from which the successor Labour Government was to benefit, as we shall see.

Generally, though, the Government did not try to test the limits of the medical profession's acceptance of change. Stephen Dorrell's period in office was an era of conciliation rather than confrontation. Some of the 1991 policy commitments were quietly abandoned or diluted. So, for example, the provision for trusts to set their own conditions of pay and service was implemented so half-heartedly as to become virtually a dead letter: in effect, the medical profession successfully defended its much cherished system of nationally negotiated contracts. Similarly, the medical profession was in effect left in control of clinical audit. This, despite a large injection of funds by the Government, remained a somewhat undirected activity reflecting the interests of individual clinicians taking part rather than providing a systematic review of performance.[118] The result was to ensure that it would not become a tool of management for controlling the activities of doctors, thereby largely subverting the original policy goal. So in 1996 the Department of Health made an attempt to breathe new life into audit. Health authorities were made responsible for audit and their performance was to be monitored by the NHS Executive. This was part of a wider departmental initiative, reflecting its conversion to 'evidence-based medicine', a worldwide enthusiasm. The aim was to provide 'an evidence-based service which provides the best quality health care for the population'.[119] In pursuit of this objective the Department invested heavily in research, in promoting the production of guidelines and in developing outcome indicators, as well as trying to revive the audit process. Research would produce the evidence needed to identify clinically effective practices, the evidence would be incorporated in guidelines and audit would monitor medical performance (with better information about outcomes feeding into the process).

The design was neat but was to be overtaken by Labour's more directive strategy for quality before it could be tested. Two features, however, should be noted. First, the emphasis was strongly on making services 'more cost-effective'. In short, the enthusiasm for 'evidence-based medicine' was driven, in part at least, by the hope that it would drive out waste: science in the service of economy (not surprisingly, economists were among the strongest supporters of the new movement). Second, it crucially depended on the co-operation of the medical profession.[120] The participation of the medical profession's élite was required in the production of guidelines: without such participation, the guidelines would not carry authority. Equally, the adoption of guideline recommendations would depend on whether they were accepted by rank-and-file doctors. There was a tension between these two features of the strategy. To the extent that the new initiatives were seen (rightly or wrongly) by doctors as a tool of management and cost-cutting – as well as a threat to their autonomy – so they could be expected to react with scepticism at best and hostility at worst. Government and management had to tread cautiously.

The continued dependence of Ministers and managers on the co-operation of the medical profession was, in one important respect, reinforced by the 1991 reforms.[121] Rationing emerged as a headline issue. There was nothing new about the fact of rationing, defined as decision-making about the allocation of scarce resources.[122] It was built into the very design of the NHS: rather than demands (professional and public) driving the budget, a fixed budget made it necessary to choose among the competing demands for treatment. The case of renal dialysis (*see* p. 63) illustrates the point. Here a deliberate decision was taken to limit the availability of the service: to ration access. But such rationing attracted little debate. It was accepted as one of the facts of life in the NHS. And it was accepted as such largely because political decisions about the allocation of resources were translated into clinical decisions about which patients should get treated and how. Ministers and managers were able to shelter behind the doctrine of clinical judgement. The care that patients received (or did not receive) was presented to them as reflecting their doctor's assessment of the appropriateness of particular interventions rather than the scarcity of resources. Doctors, in turn, internalised scarcity in their judgements about appropriateness.[123] Only waiting lists gave visibility to the fact of scarcity in the NHS: rationing by delay.

The 1991 reforms, however, brought rationing into the public domain. Health authorities were required to publish their purchasing plans, setting out what care they proposed to buy for their populations. This meant, in theory at least, being explicit about their priorities: setting out both what they were going to buy and what they were not going to buy. In practice, the implications of the priorities for service provision were usually fudged. But some health authorities did specify what they were not going to purchase, mainly marginal cosmetic surgery procedures – ranging from tattoo removal to buttock lift. Media interest was aroused and, once aroused, ensured that every example of rationing would be seized upon. In 1995 the case of Child B – refused possibly life-saving but very expensive treatment for her leukaemia by Cambridge and Huntingdon Health Authority – provided human drama for the newspapers and television.[124] The health authority's decision reflected medical advice to the effect that the proposed treatment had little chance of success and was inappropriate rather than it being rationed due to resource scarcity. It was therefore scarcely a typical or good example of rationing. Nevertheless it fuelled the debate about rationing, giving the issue ever greater salience – a debate that, as we shall see, continued under Labour. Increasingly it was argued that central government should decide what treatments should be available on the NHS, rather than leaving it to local decision-making.[125] 'Postcode rationing', i.e. geographical variations in the availability of services or treatment, was not acceptable: it offended against the equity principle.

Ministers, however, refused to entertain such a dangerous notion: dangerous because it implied that they would have to accept direct responsibility for the consequences of their budgetary policies rather than sheltering behind clinical judgements. For once, they proclaimed their faith in the devolution in decision-making – in effect, the devolution of blame. As the 1996 White Paper put it:

> Many commentators have argued that the Government should pre-scribe at national level what treatments the NHS should provide. The Government does not believe this would be right. No such list of treatments could ever hope to accommodate the range and complexity of different cases which individual clinicians face all the time. There would be a real risk of taking decisions out of the hands of clinicians treating patients and into the province of others who possess neither the experience of caring for patients or the expertise to make such decisions.[126]

The medical profession was, however, ambivalent in its attitudes. On the one hand, it strenuously fought to defend the primacy of clinical judgement. On the other hand, doctors were becoming increasingly unhappy about carrying the burden of decision-making: a burden, which as they saw it, was getting ever heavier since the opportunities for effective intervention appeared to be expanding faster than the available resources. In the five years of the Major administration expenditure on the NHS increased by almost 10 per cent, i.e. just about the 2 per cent annual rate of increase conventionally thought necessary. But the growth was unequally distributed across time. A generous financial splurge, designed to grease the introduction of the 1991 reforms, was followed by leaner times. In two years, the rise topped the 2 per cent target; in two others, it fell well below it.[127] It was not a record designed to dispel the medical profession's sense of resentment at being saddled with the responsibility for allocating what they perceived to be inadequate resources. The Royal College of Physicians, for example, called for the creation of a National Council for Health Priorities.[128] This was a situation which required the Government, once again, to manage its relationship with the medical profession carefully. Having proclaimed its dependence on the profession, it had to shape its policies accordingly.

There are therefore no further major changes of policy direction to note in the years leading up to the 1997 General Election. There was a range of initiatives designed to improve specific NHS programmes, like cancer services. The scope of the *Patient's Charter* was extended and some of the standards tightened up. Here the emphasis of Government policy (backed by the allocation of earmarked funds) switched from cutting waiting lists to reducing waiting times: for example, in 1995 the guaranteed maximum waiting time for hospital treatment was reduced from two years to 18 months.[129] The 1992 commitment to achieving the targets for improving the population's health, set out in *Health of the Nation*, was maintained though not reinforced. So, too, was progress towards achieving them, although it was not at all clear how much of this was attributable to Government policies.[130] These were all policies where the Government might be – indeed was – charged with pursuing its objectives with inadequate zeal. They were not, however, ideologically sensitive. The only issue that did raise ideological hackles was the Private Finance Initiative (PFI). This was part of a wider, across government, initiative designed to circumvent Treasury restrictions on capital spending by attracting private investment. In the case of the NHS this prompted the criticism that new hospitals were being designed to benefit the private firms building them, rather than to meet the needs of the population. However, the claim that the PFI initiative represented a covert move to subvert the principles of the NHS[131] hardly squared with the Government's overall, consensus-seeking strategy.

In summary, then, the Conservatives bequeathed a mixed legacy to the successor Labour Government. The 1991 reforms disappointed their advocates and opponents alike, producing neither a transformation nor catastrophe.[132] They appeared to have improved the NHS's efficiency – i.e. the input/output ratio – so balancing the extra administrative costs of the new system. But they did not do much – if anything – to increase choice for patients or responsiveness to consumers, despite a stream of exhortations to health authorities to consult the views of the public (a sort of top-down consumerism). They did not, therefore, transform the NHS in the way intended by the architects of the 1991 reforms. However, the unplanned outcomes and by-products of the 1991 reforms generated changes in the NHS that proved more significant in the long term. The most obvious of these, the shift in the balance of power between GPs and consultants, has been explored above. But, perhaps equally important in the long term, the 1991 reforms gave much greater visibility to the activities of the NHS – exhuming some well-buried skeletons in the process. The NHS became a much more self-aware organisation. Even though information systems continued to be inadequate, even though the meaning of much of the data was often ambiguous, statistics and figures became part of the NHS vocabulary. In turn, this meant that the NHS inherited by Labour was a much more exposed (and politically vulnerable) organisation: its performance (and inadequacies) were much more open to public inspection – an effect compounded, as in the case of rationing, by greatly heightened media interest in the service.

It is this which explains a curious paradox: that criticism of the NHS increased even while it appeared to be delivering more to patients. The Conservative Government could claim that under their stewardship the NHS had succeeded in treating more people and had even reduced waiting times.[133] But, as so often in the past, such statistics did not persuade the public. In a 1996 survey, 50 per cent of those interviewed declared themselves to be dissatisfied with the NHS, as against 47 per cent at the beginning of the decade and a mere 26 per cent 10 years earlier. Conversely, the NHS emerged as people's top priority for extra spending, topping education by a large margin.[134] Such survey data are notoriously difficult to interpret since they do not indicate the intensity with which views are held or whether those views reflect personal experience as distinct from a constant dribble of media stories highlighting failings in the NHS. However, it does suggest one of the legacies bequeathed by the Conservative Government to its Labour successor was a growing gap between public expectations and public perceptions of the NHS's performance.

References

1. Secretaries of State for Health, Wales, Northern Ireland and Scotland, *Working for Patients*, HMSO: London 1989, Cm. 555.
2. Pascal, *Pensées*, Flammarion: Paris 1976, p. 95: 'Le nez de Cleopatre: s'il eut été plus court, toute la face de la terre aurait changé.'
3. Hugh Heclo, *Modern Social Politics in Britain and Sweden*, Yale UP: New Haven 1974.
4. John W Kingdon, *Agendas, Alternatives and Public Policies*, Little, Brown and Company: Boston 1984.
5. Nicholas Ridley, *My Style of Government*, Hutchinson: London 1991.
6. Nigel Lawson, *The View from No. 11*, Corgi Books: London 1993, p. 612.
7. Margaret Thatcher, *The Downing Street Years*, HarperCollins: London 1993, p. 608.
8. The notion of the implicit concordat between the State and the medical profession was originally put forward in the first (1983) edition of this book. However, it is said that the Prime Minister – who doubtlessly had not actually read this book and relied on garbled, second-hand versions – sent her civil servants scurrying in search of the contract in her anger with the Presidents of the Royal Colleges. It was, alas, not to be found.
9. Lawson, op. cit., p. 614.
10. Thatcher, op. cit., p. 608.
11. Sir Alec Merrison (chairman), *Royal Commission on the National Health Service: Report*, HMSO: London 1979, Cmnd. 7615.
12. Ken Judge and Michael Solomon, 'Public Opinion and the National Health Service: Patterns and Perspectives in Consumer Satisfaction', *Journal of Social Policy*, vol. 22, no. 3, 1993, pp. 299–327.
13. Social Services Committee Fourth Report, Session 1985–86, *Public Expenditure on the Social Services*, HMSO: London 1986, HC 387. The Minister concerned, Mr Barney Hayhoe, did not survive long in office.
14. Department of Health and Social Security, *Health Care and its Costs*, HMSO: London 1983.
15. Social Services Committee First Report, Session 1987–88, vol. 11, *Minutes of Evidence*, pp. 96–108.
16. Patricia Day and Rudolf Klein, 'Future Options for Health Care' in Social Services Committee, Third Report Session 1987–88, *Resourcing the National Health Service: Memoranda laid before the Committee*, HMSO: London 1988, HC 284–1V, pp. 48–51.
17. Organisation for Economic Co-operation and Development, *Financing and Delivering Health Care*, OECD: Paris 1987.

18. Ibid., pp. 13–14.
19. For an excellent contemporary account of events, see Nicholas Timmins, *Cash, Crisis and Cure*, The Independent: London 1988. For an academic retrospective on events, see John Butler, *Patients, Policies and Politics*, Open University Press: Buckingham 1992.
20. Central Committee for Hospital Medical Services, *NHS Funding: The Crisis in the Acute Hospital Sector*, BMA: London 1988.
21. DHSS evidence to the Social Services Committee, Third Report, Session 1987–88, *Minutes of Evidence*, op. cit., p. 105.
22. Karen Bloor and Alan Maynard, *Expenditure on the NHS During and After the Thatcher Years*, Centre for Health Economics: York 1993, Discussion Paper 113.
23. National Association of Health Authorities, *NHS Economic Review*, NAHAT: Birmingham 1987. See also, National Audit Office, *Financial Management in the National Health Service*, HMSO: London 1989, HC 566.
24. Sir Graham Wilkins (chairman), *Review Body on Doctors' and Dentists' Remuneration: Seventeenth Report 1987*, HMSO: London 1987.
25. The analysis of the Review is based on the accounts, rather different but not contradictory, given in Thatcher and Lawson, op. cit., supplemented by interviews with some of the participants in the process.
26. Patricia Day and Rudolf Klein, 'Constitutional and Distributional Conflict in British Medical Politics: The Case of General Practice, 1911–1991', *Political Studies*, vol. XL, no. 3, September 1992, pp. 462–78.
27. For an excellent review of the various proposals, on which this account draws, see John Brazier, John Hutton and Richard Jeavons (eds), *Reforming the UK Health Care System*, Centre for Health Economics: York 1988, Discussion Paper 47.
28. 'Evidence to the Government Internal Review of the National Health Service', *British Medical Journal*, vol. 296, 14 May 1988, pp. 1411–13.
29. David Green, *Everyone a Private Patient*, Institute of Economic Affairs: London 1986.
30. Richard Cockett, *Thinking the Unthinkable*, HarperCollins: London 1994.
31. Leon Brittan, *A New Deal for Health Care*, Conservative Political Centre: London 1988.
32. Alain C Enthoven, *Reflections on the Management of the National Health Service*, Nuffield Provincial Hospitals Trust: London 1985.
33. Social Services Committee, Fifth Report, Session 1987–88, *The Future of the National Health Service*, HMSO: London, HC 613.
34. Rudolf Klein, 'Health Care Reform: The Global Search for Utopia', *British Medical Journal*, vol. 397, 27 September 1993, p. 752.
35. Lawson, op. cit., p. 616.
36. Thatcher, op. cit., p. 609.
37. In this stress on independence, an important – if indirect – influence appears to have been a book published several years earlier: John Vaizey, *National Health*, Oxford: Martin Robertson 1984.
38. Robin Cook, *A Fresh Start for Health*, The Labour Party: London December 1990.
39. Thatcher, op. cit., p. 614.
40. The paternity of the notion of GP fundholding is much in dispute. A strong candidate is Alan Maynard. See, for example, 'Performance Incentives in General Practice' in George Teeling Smith, (ed.), *Health, Education and General Practice*, Office of Health Economics: London 1986.
41. Calculated in real terms, the NHS budget had been growing at a fairly rapid rate since the mid-1980s. But, because the NHS price index was increasing at a faster rate than prices generally (largely because of wage and salary rises), this translated into a negligible increase in volume terms, i.e. the volume of goods and services that the NHS budget could buy. In the three years from 1985–6 to 1988–9, the NHS budget rose by a total of 1.8 per cent in volume terms. In contrast, in the years from 1989–

90 to 1991–2, the increase was 10.4 per cent. Bloor and Maynard, op. cit., Table 1, p. 3.

42. Parliamentary Debates, vol. 152, no. 103, 11 May 1989, col. 1035.

43. 'BMA Launches Campaign against White Paper', *British Medical Journal*, vol. 298, 11 March 1989, pp. 676–9.

44. Daniel M Fox, *Health, Policies, Health Politics*, Princeton UP: Princeton 1986.

45. Peter Self, *Econocrats and the Policy Process*, Macmillan: Basingstoke 1975. See also Daniel M Fox, *Economists and Health Care*, Prodist: New York 1979.

46. Alan Williams, 'Health Economics: The End of Clinical Freedom?', *British Medical Journal*, vol. 297, 5 November 1988, pp. 1183–6.

47. For an acute analysis of the new 'ideology' of managerialism and economism, and its impact on policy, see Peter Self, *Government by the Market?*, Macmillan: Basingstoke 1993.

48. Patricia Day and Rudolf Klein, 'NHS Review: The Broad Picture', *British Medical Journal*, vol. 298, 11 February 1989, pp. 339–40.

49. Rudolf Klein, 'From Status to Contract: The Transformation of the British Medical Profession' in Hugh L'Etang (ed.), *Health Care Provision Under Financial Constraint*, Royal Society of Medicine: London 1990.

50. Susan Kerrison, Tim Packwood and Martin Buxton, *Medical Audit: Taking Stock*, King's Fund Centre: London 1993. Subversion through indifference was nothing new: lack of enthusiasm effectively killed the Cogwheel machinery introduced in the 1960s with the aim of persuading consultants to review their practice (see pages 77–8).

51. Audit Commission, A *Short Cut to Better Services: Day Surgery in England and Wales*, HMSO: London 1990; *Lying in Wait: The Use of Medical Beds in Acute Hospitals*, HMSO: London 1992; *A Prescription for Improvement: Towards More Rational Prescribing in General Practice*, HMSO: London 1994.

52. For a before and after review, see Lynn Ashburne and Liz Caimcross, 'Membership of the "New Style" Health Authorities: Continuity or Change?', *Public Administration*, vol. 71, Autumn 1993, pp. 357–75. The analysis concludes that there was a strong element of continuity in the membership but a significant increase in the proportion of non-executives from the private sector.

53. Eleven Working Papers were published by the Department of Health. These included No. 1, *Self-Governing Hospitals* and No. 2, *Funding and Contracts for Hospital Services*, HMSO: London 1989.

54. Social Services Committee, Fifth Report, Session 1988–89, *Resourcing the National Health Service: The Government's White Paper – Working for Patients*, HMSO: London 1989, HC 214.

55. Ray Robinson and Julian Le Grand, *Evaluating the NHS Reforms*, King's Fund Institute: London 1994.

56. Giandomenico Majone, *Evidence, Argument and Persuasion in the Policy Process*, Yale UP: New Haven 1989. The argument that policy-making should be seen as the experimental testing of theories is also very much associated with Aaron Wildavsky.

57. Patricia Day and Rudolf Klein, 'The Politics of Modernization', *The Milbank Quarterly*, vol. 67, no. 1, 1989, pp. 1–34.

58. General Medical Services Committee, *Report to a Special Conference of Representatives of Local Medical Committees on 21/22 June 1989*, BMA: London 1989.

59. For an account of events by the civil servants in charge of the negotiations, see Bryan Rayner, 'The Development of Primary Health Care Policy in the 1980s: A View from the Centre' in Patricia Day (ed.), *Managing Change: Implementing Primary Health Care Policy*, Centre for the Analysis of Social Policy: Bath 1992.

60. General Medical Services Committee, *Report to a Special Conference of Representatives of Local Medical Committees on 21 March 1990*, BMA: London 1990.

61. 'Meeting Just Fails to Back Ballot on Sanctions', *British Medical Journal*, vol. 300, 31 March 1991, p. 880.
62. General Medical Services Committee, *NHS Regulations*, BMA: London 1989.
63. Bentley B Gilbert, *The Evolution of National Insurance in Great Britain: The Origins of the Welfare State*, Michael Joseph: London 1966.
64. Day and Klein (1992), op. cit.
65. John Warden, 'Peace in our Time', *British Medical Journal*, vol. 300, 26 May 1990, p. 1359.
66. Sir Trevor Holdsworth (chairman), *Review Body on Doctors' and Dentists' Remuneration Twenty-second Report 1992*, HMSO: London 1992, Cm. 1813.
67. East Anglian Health Authority, *The Rubber Windmill: Managing Better Health*, EAHA: Cambridge 1990. This is a report on a simulation exercise designed to explore the problems of managing the internal market.
68. Brian Edwards, *The National Health Service: A Manager's Tale*, Nuffield Provincial Hospitals Trust: London 1993. This is a useful source of basic information about the changes as seen by a regional manager.
69. Tim Packwood, Justin Keen and Martin Buxton, *Hospitals and Transition: The Resource Management Experiment*, Open University Press: Milton Keynes 1991.
70. 'Consultants Say No to Self-Governing Trusts', *British Medical Journal*, vol. 300, 16 June 1990, p. 1539.
71. Barbara Millar, 'Guy's – First Casualty of a Capital Blitz?', *Health Service Journal*, 9 May 1991, p. 14; Tony Sheldon, 'Is Bradford on the Road to Heaven or Hell?', *Health Service Journal*, 16 May 1991, p. 12.
72. Jenny Duckworth, Patricia Day and Rudolf Klein, *The First Wave: A Study of Fundholding in General Practice in the West Midlands*, Centre for the Analysis of Social Policy: Bath 1992.
73. See, for example, Donald Light, 'Bending the Rules', *Health Service Journal*, 11 October 1990, pp. 1513–15 for the argument that American experience suggests that sellers will always dominate health care markets.
74. Ellie Scrivens and Adrian Heath, 'Working for Patients: Making the Internal Market Effective', *Public Money & Management*, Winter 1989, pp. 53–7.
75. This classification follows Clive Smee, 'The Market in Health Care' in Anthony Hopkins (ed.), *Regulation of the Market in the National Health Service*, Royal College of Physicians of London: London 1994.
76. Frances Miller, 'Competition Law and Anticompetitive Professional Behaviour Affecting Health Care', *The Modern Law Review*, vol. 55, no. 4, July 1992, pp. 453–81.
77. The situation in London was analysed in a series of papers published by the King's Fund Commission on London. See, in particular, Sean Boyle and Chris Smaje, *Acute Services in London*, King's Fund Institute: London 1992; Michaela Benzeval, Ken Judge and Mike Solomon, *The Health Status of Londoners*, King's Fund Institute, London 1991.
78. John H James, *Transforming the NHS: The View from Inside*, Centre for the Analysis of Social Policy: Bath 1994. This monograph provides a unique insight – from the perspective of a Department of Health civil servant turned chief executive of a London district – into the process of change and has been heavily drawn upon in what follows.
79. *London Health Care 2010: Changing the Future of Services in the Capital*, King's Fund: London 1992.
80. Sir Bernard Tomlinson (chairman), *Report of the Inquiry into London's Health Service, Medical Education and Research*, HMSO: London 1992.
81. Department of Health, *Making London Better*, Department of Health: London 1993.
82. Robert J Maxwell, *What Next for London's Health Care?*, King's Fund Centre: London 1994.

83. Department of Health and Office of Population Censuses and Surveys, *Departmental Report*, HMSO: London 1992, Cm. 1913, Table 11. I have deducted from the total given the funding of extra consultant posts since this seems incidental rather than integral to the reforms.

84. Department of Health and Office of Population Censuses and Surveys, *Departmental Report*, HMSO: London 1994, Cm. 2512, Tables 13 and 24.

85. Secretary of State for Health, *The Health of the Nation: A Strategy for Health in England*, HMSO: London 1992, Cm. 1986.

86. A classic exposition of this view in Thomas McKeown, *The Role of Medicine*, Nuffield Provincial Hospitals Trust: London 1976. But for evidence that medicine does make a difference, see John P Bunker, Howard S Frazier and Frederick Mosteller, 'Improving Health: Measuring Effects of Medical Care', *Milbank Quarterly*, vol. 72, no. 2, 1994, pp. 225–58.

87. Secretary of State for Health, *One Year On: A Report on the Progress of The Health of the Nation*, Department of Health: London 1993.

88. Department of Health and Social Security, *Prevention and Health: Everybody's Business*, HMSO: London 1976.

89. Sir Douglas Black (chairman), *Inequalities in Health*, Department of Health and Social Security: London 1980.

90. Prime Minister, *The Citizen's Charter*, HMSO: London 1991, Cm. 1599.

91. Secretary of State for Health, *The Patient's Charter*, Department of Health: London 1991.

92. NHS Executive, *Hospital and Ambulance Services: Comparative Performance Guide 1993–1994*, Department of Health: London 1994.

93. NHS Management Executive, *Local Voices: The Views of Local People in Purchasing Health*, Department of Health: London 1992.

94. Calum Paton, 'Devolution and Centralism in the National Health Service', *Social Policy & Administration*, vol. 27, no. 2, June 1993, pp. 83–108.

95. Compare, for example, the priorities and planning guidance for the NHS for 1992–3 with those for 1994–5 (NHS Management Executive EL(91)103 and EL(93)54 respectively, published in 1991 and 1993). The former is a modest seven-page document. The latter is more than twice as long.

96. 'Duncan Nichol Answers Your Questions about the New NHS Management Executive and Policy Board', *NHS Management Bulletin*, no. 21, May 1989, pp. 2–3.

97. Department of Health, *Managing the New NHS*, Department of Health: London 1993.

98. Terri Banks, *Review of the Wider Department of Health*, Department of Health: London 1994.

99. One of the most contentious issues by the mid-1990s was the Government's attempt to introduce locally determined, performance-related pay. This was fiercely resisted by doctors and nurses on the grounds that it would give more control over the performance of professionals to managers. See, for example, 'Local Pay Will Harm Care, Warns BMA', *British Medical Journal*, vol. 309, 10 September 1994, pp. 625–6.

100. Secretary of State for Health, *The National Health Service: A Service with Ambitions*, HMSO: London 1996, Cm. 3425.

101. NHS Executive, *Priorities and Planning Guidance for the NHS: 1997/98*, Department of Health: London 1996.

102. Diane Dawson, *Regulating Competition in the NHS*, Centre for Health Economics: York 1995, Discussion Paper No. 131.

103. Peter West, 'Market – What Market? A Review of Health Authority Purchasing in the NHS Internal Market', *Health Policy*, vol. 44, 1998, pp. 167–83.

104. Rudolf Klein, 'Why Britain is Reorganizing its National Health Service – Yet Again', *Health Affairs*, vol. 17, no. 2, July/Aug. 1998, pp. 111–25.

105. M Goddard, R Mannion and B Ferguson, *Contracting in the UK NHS: Purpose, Process and Policy*, Centre for Health Economics: York 1997, Discussion Paper No. 156.

106. Sharon Redmayne, *Reshaping the NHS: Strategies, Priorities and Resource Allocation*, National Association of Health Authorities and Trusts: Birmingham 1995.

107. Alain C Enthoven, *In Pursuit Of An Improved National Health Service*, The Nuffield Trust: London 1999.

108. Donald Light, 'Is NHS Purchasing Serious? An American Perspective', *British Medical Journal*, vol. 316, 17 January 1998, pp. 217–20.

109. Audit Commission, *What the Doctors Ordered: A Study of GP Fundholders in England and Wales*, HMSO: London 1996.

110. Christine Ennew and David Whynes, 'GPs as Entrepreneurs', in *Choices and Beliefs: Newsletter of the ESRC Research Programme on Economic Beliefs and Behaviour*, Economic & Social Research Council: Swindon 4 April 1997.

111. Two major investigations were carried out: by the Audit Commission in 1996, op. cit., and by Howard Glennerster, Manos Matsaganis and Patricia Owens, *Implementing GP Fundholding: Wild Card or Winning Hand?* Buckingham: Open University Press 1994. This account draws mainly on Nicholas Goodwin, 'GP Fundholding', in Julian Le Grand, Nicholas Mays and Jo-Ann Mulligan (eds) *Learning from the NHS Internal Market*, King's Fund: London 1998. This provides a comprehensive critical analysis of the available evidence.

112. NHS Executive, *NHS Purchasing and GP Fundholding: Towards a Primary Care-Led NHS*, NHSE: London 1994.

113. Nicholas Mays and Jennifer Dixon, *Purchaser Plurality in UK Health Care*, King's Fund: London 1996.

114. Sharon Redmayne, *Small Steps, Big Goals: Purchasing Policies in the NHS*, National Association of Health Authorities and Trusts: Birmingham 1996.

115. Secretary of State for Health, *Primary Care: The Future*, NHSE: Leeds 1996.

116. Secretary of State for Health, *Choice and Opportunity*, HMSO: London 1996, Cm. 3390.

117. Richard Lewis and Stephen Gillam (eds) *Transforming Primary Care*, King's Fund: London 1999.

118. Susan Kerrison, Tim Packwood and Martin Buxton, 'Monitoring Medical Audit', Chapter 7, in Ray Robinson and Julian Le Grand, *Evaluating the NHS Reforms*, King's Fund: London 1994.

119. Graham Winyard, *Promoting Clinical Effectiveness*, NHS Executive: Leeds 1996.

120. Patricia Day, Rudolf Klein and Frances Miller, *Hurdles and Levers: A Comparative US–UK Study of Guidelines*, Nuffield Trust: London 1998.

121. Brian Salter, *The Politics of Change in the Health Service*, Macmillan: Basingstoke 1998.

122. Rudolf Klein, Patricia Day and Sharon Redmayne, *Managing Scarcity: Priority Setting and Rationing in the National Health Service*, Open University Press: Buckingham 1996. The following analysis of rationing draws on this. See also David J Hunter, *Desperately Seeking Solutions: Rationing Health Care*, Longmans: Harlow 1997.

123. Henry J Aaron and William B Schwartz, *The Painful Prescription: Rationing Hospital Care*, Brookings Institution: Washington 1984.

124. Chris Ham and Susan Pickard, *Tragic Choices in Health Care: The Case of Child B*, King's Fund: London 1998.

125. See, for example, Bill New and Julian Le Grand, *Rationing in the NHS: Principles and Pragmatism*, King's Fund: London 1996.

126. Secretary of State for Health, 1996, op. cit., p. 39.

127. John Appleby, 'Government Funding for the UK National Health Service', *Journal of Health Services Research and Policy*, vol. 4, no. 2, April 1999, pp. 79–89.

128. Royal College of Physicians, *Setting Priorities in the NHS: A Framework for Decision-making*, Royal College of Physicians: London 1995.

129. Secretary of State for Health and Chief Secretary to the Treasury, *Department of Health*

and Office of Population Censuses and Surveys: Departmental Report, HMSO: London 1995, Cm. 2812.

130. John Appleby, 'Feelgood Factors', *Health Service Journal*, 3 July 1997, pp. 24–7.

131. Declan Gaffney, Allyson M Pollock, David Price and Jean Shaoul, 'The Politics of the Private Finance Initiative and the New NHS', *British Medical Journal*, vol. 319, 24 July 1999, pp. 249–53.

132. For the most authoritative summary of the impact of the 1991 reforms, see Julian Le Grand, Nicholas Mays and Jo-Ann Mulligan, 1998, op. cit.; Enthoven, 1999, op.cit., endorses the conclusions drawn in this review of the evidence.

133. Secretary of State for Health and Chief Secretary to the Treasury, *Department of Health: Departmental Report*, HMSO: London 1996, Cm. 3212.

134. Jo-Ann Mulligan, 'Attitudes Towards the NHS and its Alternatives, 1983–1996', in Anthony Harrison (ed.), *Health Care UK 1997/98*, King's Fund: London 1998.

Chapter 7

The politics of The Third Way

The statistics of the 1997 General Election, which brought Tony Blair's Labour Party back into power after an 18-year exile, suggest that it represented as much of a shift in the political geology of Britain as the 1945 General Election, which had brought Clement Attlee's Labour Party into office and the NHS into being.

The swing of votes from the Conservatives to Labour was, at 10 per cent, the largest two-party shift since 1945.[1] With a total of 419 MPs, and a majority of 179, Tony Blair's Government was in a more commanding position than any other post-war administration – Labour or Conservative – and so able to carry out its programme without inhibitions. Not since 1906 had any Government achieved such a large majority; in 1979 Mrs Thatcher had only managed to scrape up a majority of 44. The election thus appeared to usher in a new political era with Labour replacing the Conservatives as the natural party of government. A second term in office, perhaps even a third one, seemed not only likely but almost inevitable. The policy course appeared to have been set for the next decade at the very least.

But what was that policy course? New Labour was to be sharply distinguished from Old Labour. Blair was not Attlee's intellectual heir, nor did he see himself as the guardian of the legacy of 1945. Indeed New Labour had been largely shaped in a series of battles with Old Labour. A succession of leaders – Neil Kinnock, John Smith and finally, and most ruthlessly, Tony Blair – had fought to distance the party from its ideological inheritance: what was dimissively referred to as 'the old left'. Symbolically, and painfully for the party's traditionalists, the commitment to the public control of the means of production – embodied in the celebrated Clause Four of the party's constitution – had been ditched. The belief in nationalisation, central planning and technocratic paternalism, which had provided the context and the rationale for the creation of the NHS in 1948, had been abandoned, even while the party remained committed to the NHS. 'We want to save and modernise the NHS' was how the 1997 General Election manifesto put it.[2]

This chapter explores what saving and modernising the NHS meant in practice during Labour's first three years in office. On 16 January 2000 there took place what became known as the most expensive breakfast in history. Appearing on a television programme, 'Breakfast with Frost', the Prime Minister pledged an increase in spending on the NHS designed to bring funding for the service up to the average of the European Union. The announcement marked the beginnings of a decisive shift in Government policy as emphasis switched over the following years from modernising the service to re-designing it: while policy goals remained the same and there were many continuities in policy themes, attention switched to the NHS's dynamics – the engine for driving change. The politics of re-design are the subject of the next chapter. This chapter takes the story of the NHS up to the time of the Prime Minister's announcement. But before doing so, it analyses the overall strategy guiding New Labour's policies: what came to be known as The Third Way.

The Third Way

> For Forms of Government let fools contest;
> Whate'er is best administr'd is best.
> > Alexander Pope, *Essay on Man*, 1733

> What counts is what works.
> > Tony Blair, *Labour Election Manifesto*, 1997

Like Thatcherism, The Third Way was a response to a new environment. The social and economic transformation of Britain (*see* p. 106) which had brought Mrs Thatcher to power and allowed the Conservatives to remain in office for 18 years – and which had been accelerated by their policies – meant that Labour had to rethink its philosophy and strategies if it was to have any hope of ever returning to office. The decline of Britain's traditional industries – coal, steel and manufacturing – was reflected in the dwindling membership of the trade unions. New technologies were creating a new social and economic structure based on services. Gender roles were changing. The Labour Party could no longer base its political strategy on an appeal to working-class solidarity and loyalty: the very concept of 'working class' seemed to be in the process of losing the meaning ascribed to it in the past. Consumer politics were replacing producer politics. Britain's external environment was also changing: a change encapsulated in the much used, if also contested, notion of 'globalisation' – shorthand for a more open and competitive international economy in which individual countries are increasingly exposed to external shocks and movements of capital.

The prescriptions of The Third Way largely flowed from its analysis of this transformed environment. They are driven, in short, not by political philosophy but by a diagnosis of what it takes to win elections and to govern successfully in the twenty-first century.[3] The key word – repeated again and again – is 'new'. A new environment called for a New Labour Party with a new agenda. And the twin of 'new' was 'modernisation'. Inherited institutions, like the NHS, had to be 'modernised', as we have seen. In all this, the emphasis was on distinguishing The Third Way from both the old or fundamentalist left and the New Right, both of which were presented (in a somewhat over-simplified version of history) as prisoners of outworn dogma. The Third Way promised to reconcile and transcend themes that were seen as antagonistic in the past:[4] 'patriotism and internationalism; rights and responsibilities; the promotion of enterprise and the attack on poverty and discrimination'. It was, further, 'about traditional values in a changed world', about achieving social justice while promoting a dynamic market economy. To quote Blair at greater length, since one of The Third Way's defining characteristics was precisely its style and use of words:

> The grievous twentieth-century error of the fundamentalist Left was the belief that the state could replace civil society and thereby advance freedom. The New Right veers to the other extreme, advocating wholesale dismantling of core state activity in the cause of 'freedom'. The truth is that freedom for the many requires strong government.

A key challenge of progressive politics is to use the state as an enabling force, protecting effective communities and voluntary organisations and encouraging their growth to tackle new needs, in partnership as appropriate.

This passage identifies some of the key words and phrases that provide a thread through Third Way rhetoric: community, partnership and strong government (the last setting up a tension, as we shall see when turning to the specific case of the NHS, with one of the other themes: decentralisation and 'democratic self-governance'). Others that characterised it were responsibility and opportunity.[5] Rights should go hand in hand with responsibilities: 'an inclusive society imposes duties on individuals and parents as well as on society as a whole'. The role of the State was to go beyond handing out cash benefits by creating more opportunities to participate actively in society and work: 'effective access to the labour market is the key to personal prosperity'. There was more than a whiff here of Margaret Thatcher's admiration for the 'vigorous virtues', even though the State was given a larger and more positive role in promoting them.

Linguistic differentiation apart, what distinguished New Labour from Old? Both shaping and constraining the strategies of The Third Way was the perception of Britain as a vulnerable economy in a cruel world, reinforced by an awareness that the Labour Governments of the 1960s and 1970s had begun by spending generously to implement election pledges and had ended up retrenching drastically. The Third Way accepted the discipline of the international market-place. What is more, it acknowledged that the engine of economic growth was the private sector: 'I fully recognise that the private sector, not government, is at the forefront of wealth creation and employment generation', in Tony Blair's words. Prosperity depended on creating 'a dynamic knowledge-based economy founded on individual empowerment and opportunity, where governments enable, not command, and the power of the market is harnessed to serve the public interest'. From this flowed also the emphasis on education, New Labour's 'overriding priority': on equipping the labour force with the skills needed to compete in a high-technology world 'where the most valuable assets are knowledge and creativity'.

Two linked conclusions, with important implications for public programmes and services like the NHS, followed from this diagnosis. Taxation and public spending had to be kept under tight control: a Labour Chancellor of the Exchequer had to be lashed to the mast of fiscal austerity, deaf to the siren voices tempting him to spend more than the economy could bear. Not only had the election manifesto committed the party to maintaining the public expenditure programme inherited from the Conservatives for its first years in office, but it had also pledged the party not to increase income tax and, indeed, to reduce it if possible. The political calculations driving these commitments and pledges are obvious enough: the assumption was that Labour had to shed its 'spend and tax' image if it was to become electable again. But the emphasis on fiscal and monetary discipline represented more than political expediency. When Tony Blair proclaimed that 'Taxation goes to the heart of The Third Way', it reflected the conviction that keeping taxes down was the only way of managing the economy successfully. And only by managing the economy successfully could New Labour hope to achieve its aim, which was to win not just one but a series of General Elections.

Old Labour, Blair argued, had 'seemed to want to throw money at every problem, with little if any concern for the efficiency with which public resources were spent'. New Labour would not make the same mistake. There would indeed be investment, but it would be investment conditional on achieving results and reforms. There would be a drive to 'reinvent' government, to 'improve its image and effectiveness'. The emphasis would be on goals not rules, and on monitoring achievements not processes. In the case of the NHS, there would be 'no return to the old centralised command and control system'. Instead there would be 'partnerships at local level, with investment tied to targets and measured outcomes, with national standards but local freedom to manage and innovate'. And there would be a new 'pragmatism . . . in the relations between the public and private sectors'.

Pragmatism was indeed the hallmark of The Third Way. Asking himself rhetorically 'What of policy?', Tony Blair answered his own question as follows: 'Our approach is "permanent revisionism", a continual search for better means to meet our goals, based on a clear view of the changes taking place in advanced industrialised countries.' If some of those means appeared to be the same as those propounded by Mrs Thatcher – promoting entrepreneurship and innovation, developing further the managerial techniques introduced in the public sector in the 1980s and early 1990s – no matter. Some of the Thatcher Government's reforms were indeed seen, in retrospect, as 'necessary acts of modernisation'. Provided that the policy tools could be made to serve New Labour's goals, they were acceptable. They would be used not out of ideological conviction (contra the New Right) but because they 'worked'. It was in the goals that New Labour sets itself, rather than in the means used, that it distinguished itself from both the Thatcher era and from the diluted Thatcherism of her successor, John Major: in its commitment to promoting a fair and open society, in addressing social exclusion and promoting opportunity for all.

New Labour in office

This section sketches, briefly and selectively, aspects of the Blair Government's first three years in office most relevant to understanding the context in which policies for the NHS were developed. First, and foremost, the Government's prudent economic strategy was successful in combining low inflation with a rate of economic growth that was high by historical standards. Second, the Government maintained its commitment to working within the public expenditure plans inherited from the Conservatives, though relaxing its attitude of fiscal austerity somewhat in the case of the NHS and education: a point which is elaborated below. Third, income tax rates did not increase and were, indeed, shaved at the edges (although, as the Conservatives pointed out, some less visible forms of taxation rose). Fourth, reform of the social security programme began, introducing 'work tests' for some benefits – in line with the emphasis on promoting participation in the labour force – and increasing support for working families and children. Fifth, the overall effect of the changes was to bring about a modest degree of income redistribution.

Equally important, particularly for placing the NHS in the wider context of New Labour's style of administration, were a battery of initiatives designed to 'modernise' Government. Much emphasis was put on co-ordinating different streams of Government policies in order to address specific problems: so, for example, a Social Exclusion Unit was set up in the Cabinet Office to bring together the various strands of policy bearing on problems of poverty. Similarly, there was much stress on promoting 'active communities' – the New Deal for Communities – with grants going to the most deprived neighbourhoods in order to tackle crime, worklessness, health and educational under-achievement: one of a clutch of similar initiatives. Overall, the proclaimed aim was to promote 'responsive public services to meet the need of citizens, not the convenience of service providers' to deliver quality services.[6] There was an explicit recognition that in a consumer society, public expectations were changing. 'People are exercising choice and demanding higher quality in the private sector', New Labour's White Paper on modernising government argued. 'People are now rightly demanding better service not just from the private sector, but from the public sector too.'

Policy praxis, however, revealed some tensions in New Labour's programme. The commitment to decentralisation was reflected in the legislation for devolved government in Scotland, Wales and Northern Ireland. But at the same there was a movement in the opposite direction. Modernising public services took the form of ever tighter control by the centre. In 1998 the Treasury introduced Public Services Agreements (PSAs) as part of a comprehensive spending review,[7] so launching the target culture which was to have significant implications for the NHS and other government programmes. PSAs set a battery of targets for individual government departments and services, as well as a timetable for achieving them; in theory at least, Treasury funding was contingent on departments achieving these targets. Examples of targets ranged from cutting class sizes for the under-sevens to 30 or less by September 2001 to halving the time taken from arrest to sentence for young offenders. In the case of the NHS, as we shall see, the result was to set off an avalanche of target-setting. At the same time, central government strengthened its hold over local authority services: moving in when local authority services were seen to be failing and, if need be, insisting that those services should be contracted out. The powers of the school inspectorate were strengthened; a new inspectorate for local government was introduced.

There were other inconsistencies, too. There appeared to be a contradiction between the Government's proclaimed aim of strengthening democracy and the streak of command-and-control authoritarianism apparent in some of its policies. On the one hand, there were initiatives like the People's Panel – a 5,000 strong nationally representative group – 'to tell us what people really think about their public services'. On the other hand, there was the policy of being 'tough on crime', which included such measures as introducing curfew orders and codifying parents' duty to discipline their children. On the one hand, the Government seemed dedicated to transparency, publishing more information about its activities than ever before. In its first term of office the Blair administration produced an average of one press release every four minutes – 32,766 in all[8] – quite apart from a stream of lavishly illustrated, and often self-congratulatory, reports on its plans and activities. On the other hand, the flow of information and (even more importantly) its presentation was tightly controlled. So, for example, in 1998 a Strategic Communications Unit accountable to Alastair Campbell, the Prime Minister's Chief Press Officer, was set up in order to co-ordinate activity across Whitehall.[9]

There was also centralisation *within* Whitehall. Blair emerged as 'the most commanding post-war premier'.[10] In effect, a Prime Minister's Department was created. The Social Exclusion Unit set up in 1997 was joined by the Performance and Innovation Unit the following year. The number of special advisers at No.10 – political appointees brought in from outside – trebled between 1997 and 2000, rising from eight to 24: part of a more general trend across the Government, challenging the traditional role of civil servants as the virtual monopolists of policy advice. The network of special advisers, in turn, exercised considerable influence across Whitehall. In the case of the NHS, the Secretary of State for Health's special adviser, Simon Stevens, and his counterpart at No.10, Robert Hill, played a significant part in shaping policy; when Hill left Whitehall, Stevens was subsequently to move to No.10 to become the Prime Minister's adviser on health policy. Departmental civil servants winced when yet another note starting 'The Prime Minister thinks . . .' landed on their desk, as it all too frequently did.

In one respect, however, the story of the concentration of power at No.10 must be qualified. Blair's administration was, in effect, bi-polar: the Treasury, under the Chancellorship of Gordon Brown, was a rival, competing centre of power. Government departments were classified by insiders according to whether they looked to the Prime Minister or to the Chancellor of the Exchequer. The Department of Health was seen as belonging firmly in the former category.

In summary, three conclusions follow from even this brief analysis of The Third Way in theory and action. First, New Labour was a highly active – indeed hyperactive – Government: hardly a day went by without the announcement of a new working party, the appointment of a 'czar' to tackle some issue of social concern (be it drugs or cancer) or some other initiative. This was a Government determined to dominate the headlines and, it is tempting to conclude, at least as concerned with how its policies looked as with what they were. Second, New Labour was in many respects building on and developing the policies of its predecessors: witness the emphasis on outcomes rather than inputs and on improved managerial techniques. Despite the constant invocation of the word 'new', there was in fact a large element of continuity. Third, there were strains and stresses between the various strands of New Labour thinking: Tony Blair was strengthening the grip of central government even while acknowledging the need for devolution and more democracy. Strong government, it seems, was needed to make people act as the responsible, active citizens required by Third Way theory – just as strong government was needed by Mrs Thatcher to make markets work. All these themes and tensions are evident in the history of the NHS under the Blair Government.

Strategy for the NHS

Devising a strategy for the NHS posed some peculiar problems for New Labour in government. Here the tactics of symmetrically distancing the Blair regime from both Old Labour and the New Right could not be applied. The NHS had to be embraced as a gesture to the party faithful, while denouncing the Conservative legacy. But even while denouncing the Conservative record the Government was preparing to build on it. The exercise called for great skill in navigating through the rhetorical rapids. The 1997 election manifesto duly denounced the Conservatives for creating the internal market, thereby creating (among other evils) a bloated bureaucracy. So the internal market was to go, though the separation of purchasers and providers would remain. Again, fundholding was criticised for creating a two-tier system, though its role in changing the balance of power was acknowledged. So fundholding would be abolished but the lead role for primary care would be retained. Specifically, the manifesto promised to take 100,000 people off the waiting-list, to end waiting for cancer surgery and to set 'tough quality standards' for hospitals. Improvements were to be funded by cutting management costs by £1 billion, so echoing Margaret Thatcher's 1979 election manifesto promise to 'cut back bureaucracy'[11] – a promise cheerfully made by just about every incoming Government in the history of the NHS even while relying on those parasitic bureaucrats to carry out their policies.

Fiscal prudence, however, shaped New Labour's spending commitments for the NHS – in line with the Government's overall emphasis on discipline in spending and taxing. Unlike Old Labour it would not just throw money at problems. No attempt was to be made to exploit the apparent willingness of a majority of the public, revealed in a succession of surveys, to pay higher taxes to fund the NHS. The only promise made in 1997 was that 'We will raise spending on the NHS in real terms every year'. So, too, had the Conservative administrations of Mrs Thatcher and John Major.[11] The real question therefore was – by how much? And on this point, there was silence. Significantly, New Labour made little or nothing of the widespread assertion that the NHS was under-funded, particularly when compared to the spending levels of other European countries – an assertion which had punctuated the politics of the NHS throughout its history.

It was against the background of these commitments and constraints that the ministerial team chosen to run the NHS took office. They combined, in their persons, reassurance with radicalism. Frank Dobson, the Secretary of State for Health, was reassuringly Old Labour in style, a veteran of many bruising onslaughts on the Conservatives; Alan Milburn, his deputy and in 1999 his successor, was a New Labour man who had not even been in the House of Commons at the time of the 1991 reforms. And within months of taking office, the new Ministers unveiled their plans for the NHS. The White Paper published in December 1997 was entitled, drawing on standard New Labour vocabulary, *The New NHS: Modern–Dependable*.[12] In true Third Way style, it sought to mould themes which might appear to be contradictory into a new policy synthesis. It combined tributes to Old Labour's achievements with a new vision for the future, denunciation of the Conservatives with a willingness to build on their achievements. On the one hand, the creation of the NHS was held out 'as the greatest act of modernisation ever achieved by a Labour Government'. Nevertheless, there would be 'no return to the old centralised command and control systems of the 1970s'. On the other hand, 'the internal market was a misconceived attempt to tackle the pressures facing the NHS . . . it created more problems than it solved'. Nevertheless 'not everything about the old system was bad'. Enter pragmatism: 'If something is working effectively then it should not be discarded purely for the sake of it'. So back to the central theme of The Third Way: 'what counts is what works'.

So while the internal market was abolished, the separation of purchasers and providers was maintained, although the former word was effectively expunged from the new vocabulary. And while fundholding was also abolished, the role of GPs as purchasers was expanded. In effect, fundholding was universalised. The basic building bricks in the new NHS were to be Primary Care Groups (PCGs). These Groups were to bring together all the GPs and other primary care providers in a given geographical area: some 500 were to be set up, with an average population of about 100,000. PCGs would evolve over time, it was envisaged, from having devolved responsibility for managing the budget for health care for their patients but formally still part of the health authority to becoming free-standing trusts (PCTs) still accountable to the health authority but with added responsibility for providing community health services for their populations. In the outcome, PCGs were installed throughout the country by April 1999 and the first PCTs came on stream in April 2000.

The White Paper, inevitably, left many issues to be resolved in the process of implementation.[13] What precisely was to be the relationship between health authorities and PCGs and providers? 'Market style incentives' drove NHS trusts to compete, the White Paper argued, irrespective of whether this reflected local NHS priorities. In future, the emphasis would be on co-operation, not competition; on sharing information, not shielding it from prying eyes. Provider trusts would have to fit into local priorities and would have a voice in shaping them. Instead of annual contracts, there would be long-term agreements. But what sanctions were available, in the absence of 'market style incentives', should partnership by command fail to produce agreement and trusts fell short of delivering the required level and quality of services? The White Paper gave no clear answer.

There was a similar ambiguity about the relationship between health author-ities and PCGs. The latter were to be 'in the driving seat in shaping local services in the future'. But the former were to be responsible, in partnership with the PCGs, for drawing up three-year Health Improvement Programmes, i.e. for 'deciding on the range and location of health care services'. In practice, therefore, the ability of PCGs to use their budgetary power might be severely constrained. If the Health Improvement Programme revolved around developing services at a local hospital, a PCG dissatisfied with the services of that hospital might find that its health authority would not allow it to switch to another provider (to take an example from the first-year experience of one PCG). Thus PCGs might be in the 'driving seat' but their freedom to choose the route to be followed appeared to be limited. Other factors further reinforced the doubts about the ability of PCGs to set an independent course. The experience of the Total Purchasing Pilots (*see* previous chapter) had suggested that effectiveness depended on adequate managerial resources.[14] But the Government's insistence on cutting management costs meant that PCGs were put on short rations on this count. Moreover, PCGs were to be accountable to the health authorities, which also determined their budgets. The future balance of power within the NHS, as between health authorities and PCGs, therefore remained to be determined in the process of implementation.

On one crucial point, however, the White Paper was very clear. This was that PCGs would work within a 'single cash-limited envelope'. That is, their budgets would be calculated to cover their population's share of all NHS services, including prescribing. So was closed the one loophole in the NHS's otherwise tight system of controlling expenditure. For prescribing had always been excluded from the NHS's own overall cash limits, on the grounds that it was demand driven and thus uncontrollable. But fundholding had shown that it could be controlled: prescribing costs had been included in the budgets set for fundholders. Universalising fundholding thus allowed the Government – no doubt to Treasury cheers – to universalise this budgetary discipline. But closing this loophole also opened up a large, new question. Fundholding involved budgetary self-discipline by a team of doctors who had chosen this status. PCG budgets assumed that GPs would be willing and able to discipline their fellow practitioners, who might well be resentful conscripts rather than volunteers in this new enterprise. If individual GP practices put the budgetary viability of a PCG at risk – by overspending on prescribing or by referring too many patients to hospital – what sanctions did their colleagues have to bring them into line? Conversely, what incentives did individual GPs have to adapt their practices to the corporate plans of the PCG?

In one significant respect, however, the introduction of PCGs was more than an exercise in rationalising the Conservative legacy and giving it a new ideological twist (if only at the level of rhetoric). By accepting the introduction of PCGs, the medical profession was also accepting a collective responsibility for controlling the activities of its members – an acceptance all the more remarkable given that GPs had always prided themselves on their small shopkeeper status and fiercely opposed any threats to their independence. Yet, in striking contrast to its outraged hostility to the 1991 reforms, the BMA welcomed the 1997 White Paper. The welcome was all the more surprising given that the White Paper also included a raft of measures which appeared to threaten medical autonomy as traditionally defined by the profession. These measures, designed to strengthen control over the way in which doctors practised their craft, are examined in the next section. Here it is sufficient to note, and stress, that the dog did not bark – let alone bite. There were a variety of reasons for this. In part, it reflected the BMA's sense of satisfaction that its opposition to Mrs Thatcher's package had been vindicated: why quarrel about the small print when a major victory had been won? In part, it reflected changes in the composition and aspirations of the profession. In part, it reflected a lack of awareness about the full implications of the White Paper proposals: rank-and-file criticism only began to emerge during the process of implementation. Whatever the reasons, a new and more amicable era in the relations between the State and doctors appeared to have begun, although it was not to last.

The 1997 White Paper, however, went beyond carrying out the manifesto pledge of abolishing the internal market and fundholding. It was notable for developing two themes. The first was the emphasis on improving the health of the population and reducing inequalities. The second was the stress on devising new instruments for promoting efficiency and quality – two words which provide a refrain running through the text of the White Paper. Neither theme was entirely novel. Once again New Labour was building on previous developments. But if the aims of policy suggested continuity with the past, there were also some significant changes both in the rhetoric and in the means chosen to achieve the objectives.

Already under the Conservatives there were signs of a new policy paradigm emerging with the recognition that the care provided by the NHS was only one factor, and not necessarily the most important one, in determining the population's health. The 1997 White Paper, and a succession of subsequent policy statements, developed the theme further and *fortissimo*. In line with precedent, new 'tough and challenging' targets were set for reducing deaths from cancer, coronary heart disease, accidents and suicide.[15] The NHS was, in effect, given a wider role as part of a social engineering enterprise. The aim was to tackle 'the roots of ill health'.[16] To do so, the NHS had to engage with other agencies to address wider social problems. A statutory duty of partnership was imposed on health authorities to work with local government in promoting the economic, social and environmental well-being of their areas, in line with the new emphasis in Whitehall on promoting 'joined-up government', i.e. co-ordinating policies across departmental boundaries. Health Action Zones were introduced with the intention of bringing together organisations within and beyond the NHS to develop and implement strategies for improving the health of the local people.

Above all, distinguishing New Labour from its predecessor but echoing some of the preoccupations of Old Labour, there was much emphasis on reducing inequalities in health status and acceptance of the fact that this would require changes not just in the NHS but in governmental policies across the board. Following the example of the Labour Government of the 1970s, a committee to examine inequalities was set up under a former Chief Medical Officer of Health, Sir Donald Acheson.[17] It was a report that was generous in its recommendations for social action without any inhibitions about the budgetary implications of its recommendations (like raising social security benefits and free travel for pensioners) even though its own review of the research evidence gave cause for agnosticism about the likely impact on health inequalities, let alone the cost-effectiveness, of some of the interventions.[18] The Government's response underlined its anxiety to demonstrate that New Labour – however modern, however hard-nosed about budgetary restraint – remained faithful to the Party's concern for social justice. Without committing itself to any of the Acheson recommendations, it argued that they fitted into the Government's overall strategy for creating a 'fairer society': in effect, its response was a litany of policies already in place for improving education, housing and so on.[19] Reducing health inequalities was seen, in effect, as the by-product of policies desirable in their own right: a sensible enough stance but one that gave a hostage to the future. What if health inequalities were to persist even in a fairer society?

If the emphasis on public health and inequalities represented Old Labour concerns, the emphasis on efficiency and quality was one of the hallmarks of New Labour. The new NHS was to deliver fast, high-standard services to all. But how was this to be brought about? If competition was no longer to drive change, and could no longer be relied upon as the spur to efficiency, what would be the dynamics of the new NHS? The answer turned out to be a mixture of improved performance measurement backed by the threat of central intervention if performance fell short of expectations. In effect, the managerial strategy of the early and middle 1980s was resurrected. An expanded, more sophisticated set of performance indicators was produced,[20] designed to measure the various dimensions of NHS performance: fair access, the effective delivery of appropriate health care, efficiency, patient perceptions of the service offered and outcomes – the start of what was to become the contentious annual 'star rating' exercise discussed in the next chapter. And there was to be a hierarchic structure of accountability for performance with sanctions for failure. Health authorities would have the power to 'withdraw freedoms' from PCGs if the latter's performance was not up to standard. And the NHS Executive would be able, the 1997 White Paper stressed, 'to intervene to rectify poor performance in any part of the NHS'.

Moreover, the centre was to play a more active role in shaping performance at the periphery.[21] National Service Frameworks were to be produced, drawing on the best available evidence, to provide templates for the organisation of services. A series of expert groups was set up to produce such frameworks for cancer, coronary, diabetes and other services: their reports, reflecting the professional consensus about best practice, were to be published over the next few years.[22] A National Institute for Clinical Excellence (NICE) was to be set up to promote, bring together and diffuse evidence about good practice. A Commission for Health Improvement, an inspectorate for the NHS in all but name, was to monitor progress towards achieving the Government's programme for quality. The roles of the Institute and the Commission are analysed in more detail in the next section dealing with the regulation of professional activities. Here the main point to stress is that they formed part of a central element in the New Labour strategy for the NHS: a determination to make the NHS live up to its claim to be a *national* service. If the 1970s had seen the start of a drive to achieve equity in the geographical distribution of resources, New Labour was committed to achieving equity in the way resources were used locally. Geographical variations in the level and quality of services offered – the norm throughout the history of the NHS – were no longer seen as acceptable. The same degree of access, the same standard of care, should be available to people irrespective of where they lived.

It was a bold re-assertion of the NHS's founding principles. Bevan would, no doubt, have applauded. It also represented a re-assertion of the technocratic rationalism which had helped to shape the NHS in the first place. If the configuration of NHS services was to be evidence based, if experts were to determine the pattern of provision, what scope was left for those local variations which reflected local preferences? The dilemma was as old as the NHS itself. But whereas in the past variations largely reflected the inability as well as the unwillingness of the centre to impose a uniform pattern – and were rationalised as showing sensitivity to local needs – the new battery of instruments sought to make this a deliverable aim of policy. But if deliverable, was it desirable? It was not self-evident that evidence always spoke with a clear, unambiguous voice. Nor was it self-evident that there would be general acquiescence in the notion that technical expertise should have a dominant voice: the NHS could no longer draw on the unquestioning faith in, and deference to, expertise that had been a feature of the decades immediately before and after its birth. Moreover, there appeared to be a tension between this emphasis on national standards and national service patterns and the decision to put GPs in the driving seat on the grounds that they had a special understanding of patient needs. If there was a clash between top-down decisions and bottom-up preferences, it was not clear who would (or should) prevail.

There was a further tension also. The Third Way rested largely on the assumption that consumer politics had displaced producer politics. In turn, New Labour recognised, as we have seen, that people were demanding choice not only in the private sector but also in the public sector. But choice, like competition, had been expunged from the new vocabulary, 1997 version, of NHS policy-making. So it would not be the ability of consumers to switch their custom that would drive the new NHS, any more than it drove Mrs Thatcher's model, whatever the initial aspirations might have been. The NHS had to be modernised, the Prime Minister wrote in his foreword to the 1997 White Paper, 'to meet the demands of today's public'. But how were those demands to be articulated? One answer given was to launch a new national patient survey: patient views about the services provided were to be one of the new set of PIs. It was not an entirely convincing answer: essentially it was a top-down form of consumerism, using surveys as an input into managerial decision-making. It is therefore difficult to escape the conclusion that the Government's policies represented a gamble. The gamble was that the public valued choice of GP or consultant less than they did ready access to good quality services.[23] If the new NHS could deliver the latter, then lack of choice would not necessarily count against the Government. It was, as we shall see in the next chapter, a judgement that was to be reversed in the new century.

The 1997 White Paper thus left many questions unanswered and many tensions to be resolved. The Government was taking the first steps in a process of learning by doing or, to put it more brutally, devising policies without knowing precisely how they would work out or what problems would be thrown up in the course of implementation. It was a pattern which, as we shall see, was to characterise policy-making in the NHS not only in the first three years of the Blair regime but subsequently as well. It reflected the impatience of Ministers, taking their cue from Tony Blair, to get things done. As Alan Milburn was to put it later: 'There was a sense of expectation about us being able to put the NHS right . . . when you come into Government having been out for so long, you want to put it right, you want to get on with it, and get your hands dirty and get your sleeves rolled up and get on with the job.'[24] Ministerial impatience, in turn, reinforced a trend already evident in the Thatcher years. Across Whitehall, civil service culture was changing.[25] The emphasis increasingly was on the primacy of managing policy delivery rather than crafting policy advice. The traditional civil service role of tempering political enthusiasm with administrative scepticism appears to have been less valued, indeed resented, by Ministers. In the case of the Department of Health, as noted in the previous chapter, the preoccupation with service delivery had resulted in the creation of the NHS Management Executive, largely composed of NHS managers, to complement the civil service hierarchy headed by the Permanent Secretary. And early in 2000 the posts of Permanent Secretary and Chief Executive were merged. The new post went to Nigel Crisp (subsequently knighted), promoted from a regional directorate. If only at a symbolic level, managers appeared to have triumphed over civil servants.

Regulating the medical profession

In October 1997, two months before the publication of the Government's White Paper, the Professional Conduct Committee of the General Medical Council (GMC) began the hearing of a case that transformed the policy landscape as far as relations between the State and the medical profession were concerned.[26] The case revolved around the deaths of 15 small children while or after undergoing cardiac surgery at the Bristol Infirmary. At its conclusion the two surgeons involved were found guilty of serious professional misconduct. So, too, was the medically qualified chief executive of the trust. Two out of the three were struck off the medical register. The case was not only highly charged emotionally, attracting an unprecedented degree of media attention, it also, in effect, put the medical profession on trial. For what became clear as the story unfolded before the GMC was that there had been a collective, institutional failure at Bristol. At issue was not just the competence of the two surgeons to carry out the very fraught and unforgiving operations concerned and their failure to examine their own performance or to seek advice. At issue, too, was the failure of their colleagues as well as the chief executive to take action, although they had been alerted to the concerns felt by some doctors and nurses. The audit system had failed to pick up the problem; a whistle-blower had been ignored. In short, professional self-regulation had only worked after the event, when the GMC stepped in as a result of an article in *The Times*. Rightly or wrongly, the Bristol case was thus widely seen as showing that the medical profession was more concerned to shield its members than to protect the public.

It was against this background that the Government launched its own proposals for putting quality at the heart of the new NHS. The Bristol case may not have directly prompted these proposals, but it strengthened the Government's resolve and created a reservoir of public support for radical measures. Conversely, it put the medical profession on the defensive, all the more so since the Secretary of State's decision to set up a public inquiry into the Bristol case ensured that the issues raised would remain in the headlines. The result was that the profession acquiesced in a series of proposals which, in theory at least, exposed the performance of individual doctors to a degree of scrutiny unprecedented in the history of the NHS.

The first building block in the Government's strategy was the introduction of clinical governance.[27] All trusts were required to set up a system for monitoring standards and identifying poor performance. They were further charged with ensuring the implementation of the clinical standards of the National Service Frameworks and the recommendations of the National Institute. All doctors were required to take part in audit; no longer was participation voluntary. The trust's chief executive was to be made accountable for assuring the quality of the services provided. The trust's Board was to receive regular reports on the quality of clinical care. The aim in all this was not only to seek to prevent the recurrence of a Bristol-type scandal – inasmuch as any organisational mechanism can do so – but to ensure a continuous improvement in quality.[28]

The second building block in the Government's strategy was the creation of the Commission for Health Improvement. The functions of the Commission, as set out in the legislation,[29] were wide. They were to monitor the way in which clinical governance was implemented, to carry out investigations into the management, provision or quality of the health care provided by trusts, and to review the availability and quality of specific types of health care. And although the Commission was quasi-independent (a non-departmental public body), with its own Board, there was no doubt as to whose creature it was. 'The Secretary of State may give directions with respect to the exercise of any functions of the Commission.' Every trust in the country was to be reviewed by multi-disciplinary teams – doctors, nurses and other health professionals as well as lay members – within four years. The results of the reviews were to be published, and it would be the responsibility of the NHS Executive's regional offices to follow them up. In addition, the Commission would act as the Secretary of State's troubleshooter. Acting on the Commission's report, the Secretary of State could – under the 1999 Health Act – demand an immediate action plan, issue directives to the NHS bodies concerned and, in the last resort, sack the Board of the trust.

There were some subtle modulations in the way the Commission was pre-sented. The Commission itself was anxious to reassure doctors that it did not propose to model itself on OFSTED, the educational inspectorate whose 'hit squads' had evoked terror and resentment among teachers. Indeed the word 'inspectorate' was carefully avoided. But Ministers put a rather different, less emollient gloss on the new institution. At the launch of the Commission, the Prime Minister (no less) proclaimed: 'As OFSTED is playing a crucial role in driving up standards in schools, so the Commission will drive up standards in health care.' The Bristol case, he argued, had shown that such a new body was 'not just desirable but essential'. It was essential in order to ensure 'peace of mind for patients' and to make sure that 'treatment is excellent throughout the country'.[30] The Commission was thus presented as a crucial element in New Labour's project of modernising the NHS.

In 1999 yet a further initiative was announced to deal with a long-standing source of disquiet: the difficulties faced by health authorities and trusts when seeking to deal with doctors with performance problems. The consultative document[31] pointed out that 'present NHS procedures for detecting and dealing with poor clinical performance are fragmented and inflexible'. Accordingly it proposed reforming the NHS's disciplinary procedures, annual appraisals for both consultants and GPs, and the setting up of a scattering of Assessment and Support Centres to which doctors could be referred. Further momentum for the drive to scrutinise the activities of the profession came in January 2000 when a GP, Dr Harold Shipman, was convicted of murdering 15 of his patients.[32] Nor, as we shall see in the next chapter, was this the end of the story: pressure to identify and deal with inadequate or dangerous doctors increased, if anything, over the following years when the inquiries into the Bristol tragedy and the Shipman case reported.

Whatever the private reservations of members of the medical profession about some of these developments, there was no public opposition to the Government's policies. On the contrary, the Government's radical programme strengthened the position of those within the profession who had been urging change: who argued with Sir Donald Irvine, the President of the GMC, that a 'revolution' in medicine called for a re-definition of professionalism and a more active role in self-regulation.[33] In the wake of the Bristol case, the Royal Colleges and the GMC accepted the principle of revalidation – the notion that the continued competence of consultants should be regularly tested – though the process of translating the concept into practice proved to be highly contentious. In short, the medical profession recognised that self-regulation was a precarious privilege which could no longer be asserted but had to be earned. Self-regulation had survived but it had been made accountable; collegial control over the performance of doctors had largely been maintained but at the cost of limiting the autonomy of individual doctors. Once again, it was apparent that there had been a shift in the balance of power between the State and the profession. Mrs Thatcher had ignored the medical profession and then battered it into submission. Tony Blair flattered it into acquiescence, with the threat of a battering held in reserve. Either way, the profession could no longer reckon on dominating the policy agenda.

Resources, rationing and crisis

The public expenditure plans that the Labour Government inherited from the Conservatives[34] suggested that the NHS would have to expect hard times. The projected rise in spending, in real terms, was to be a mere 1.1 per cent in the 1997/98 financial year, falling still lower in the subsequent two years. Not surprisingly the new Government, while anxious to remain faithful to its manifesto pledge to stick to the Conservative *overall* expenditure plans for its first two years, abandoned its commitment to fiscal chastity in the case of the NHS. It started drip-feeding the NHS with extra funds almost from the moment that it took office. Quite possibly the Conservatives, had they remained in power, would have done the same. An extra £1.2 billion was ploughed into the NHS almost immediately and the expenditure plans were revised upwards.[35] In the first two years of the Labour Government spending on the NHS rose, in real terms, by just over 2 per cent annually. More was to come. As part of the Government 1998 Comprehensive Spending Review, setting out a new set of expenditure plans reflecting a new set of priorities,[36] the Government announced that the average annual increase for the NHS would be 4.7 per cent over the following three years. As always there was much questioning of the calculations behind the figures and some doubt as to whether they could be taken at face value.[37] But, in the context of a public expenditure settlement that was generally austere, they represented a relatively generous deal for the NHS.

In total, the effect of these changes was that in the two years leading up to the Prime Minister's television pledge on 16 January 2000 expenditure was increasing at the rate of 4 per cent in real terms.[38] This was higher than at any time in the decade, save for one year when the Conservatives were pouring in extra money to grease the path of the 1991 reforms. It was double, furthermore, than the 2 per cent a year rise that, according to conventional wisdom (*see* p. 142), was required to cope with demographic and technological change. Yet the Prime Minister's statement was precipitated by a general sense of crisis. Once again, as so often in its history, the NHS appeared to be on the point of collapse. Why?

One answer to this puzzle stems from Labour's election manifesto commitment to bringing down waiting-lists. It was a commitment that gave high visibility to this issue and a series of Government initiatives further reinforced its salience. A £500 million package of measures specifically designed to address the waiting-list problem was followed by a series of further injections of funds earmarked for this purpose. But, as the Government was to discover – like so many of its predecessors who had embarked on the same enterprise[39] – in doing so it had committed itself to the politics of Sisyphus. In 1997 the Labour Government had inherited, and made much of, waiting-lists of 1,160,000. But in March 1998 they were 1,297,000. No sooner had Ministers pushed the rock uphill than it rolled back again. After March 1998, there was a steep fall, and by the General Election of 2001 the Government could claim to have met its pledge of cutting waiting-lists by 100,000. But this was not quite the success story that it appeared at first sight. No sooner did waiting-lists for hospital treatment shrink, when it turned out that this had only been achieved by increasing the number of patients waiting for their first outpatient appointment, i.e. the queue for getting onto waiting-lists had become longer.[40] And the price of apparent success was to skew the NHS's priorities towards elective surgery, as many clinicians complained, even though high political visibility did not necessarily accord with other indicators of medical need.

The saga of waiting-lists was not only an example of a Government creating a problem for itself, it also illustrated the complexity and frustrations of attempting to direct the activities of the NHS from the centre. Waiting-list initiatives were indeed successful in increasing the number of operations carried out and, eventually, in cutting the headline numbers. But they did not necessarily ease the pressures on the NHS. On the contrary, they may have added to them. As the Department of Health's former Principal Finance Officer pointed out,[41] pouring more resources into reducing waiting-lists was 'rather like offering to reduce road congestion in London by building more roads. The better the roads, the more people travel; the better the hospital service, the more patients are referred to hospital'. If the lists went down, GPs were encouraged to refer more patients to hospital: the threshold for referral is lowered. Moreover, trusts and consultants had an incentive to maintain waiting-lists at a high level: trusts because they otherwise risk losing out from the extra funding that regularly becomes available for reducing the lists, consultants because the lists encourage patients to seek private treatment. Far from being an accurate measure of unmet demands, waiting-lists are to a large extent the product of myriad decisions taken by people working in the NHS for reasons which may be at odds with the Government's intentions. Nor is it self-evident that the length of waiting-lists – as distinct from the time taken between seeing their GP and receiving treatment in hospital – is what matters most to patients: which is why the Conservative administration had sought to switch attention to waiting times, an example the Labour Government was increasingly to follow by setting targets for waiting times.

But having nailed itself to the cross of reducing waiting-lists, the Labour Government was in effect advertising the NHS's shortcomings. No matter that the lengths of the lists were an ambiguous indicator of performance. No matter that they were, if anything, a misleading measure of the NHS's ability to meet demands. Waiting-lists were confirmed as the symbol of the NHS's inability to meet public expectations of quick and ready access to treatment. They represented rationing by delay. The issue thus fed into the wider debate about rationing in the NHS, a debate which continued under the Labour Government much as it had done under its predecessor – if at a higher temperature. Like their Conservative predecessors, Labour Ministers shied away from the word. As before, responsibility (and blame) for taking decisions about who should receive expensive new drugs like Beta Interferon or be eligible for costly treatments like *In Vitro* Fertilisation (IVF) was diffused to individual health authorities and clinicians. The new element in the situation was that, once sensitised to the issue, the media relentlessly pursued examples of variations in policy and practice to draw attention to 'postcode rationing'.[42] Nor was it just a matter of new drugs or new forms of treatment. Similar geographical variations were identified in the availability of specialist treatment in mainstream programmes, like those for the treatment of heart disease and cancer. And not only were there seemingly arbitrary variations within the NHS. Compared to most West European countries, the NHS as a whole appeared to fall short in terms of specialist provision (and outcomes) in these key services.[43] The conclusion appeared to be as clear as it was dismal: people were dying and suffering unnecessarily.

The Government itself reinforced the indictment. Its new set of performance indicators, published in 1999, further documented the extent of variation in access to services.[44] These showed a 3:1 variation in the rate of hip replacements as between health authorities and a similar ratio for cataract replacements. The figures may, in part, have been a statistical artefact; they certainly did not allow for differences in need. But, fine-print reservations apart, they once again gave visibility to the NHS's failure to achieve anything like common standards of service across the country. In doing so, they reinforced the case for striving to achieve such common standards. However, this goal could not – as Ministers reiterated – be achieved overnight. In the meantime, as in the case of waiting-lists, the flood of statistics continued to advertise the NHS's shortcomings. Statistical transparency – in the service of public accountability for the performance of the NHS – meant political vulnerability. So, too, did the targets set for the NHS under the 1998 Public Service Agreement with the Treasury.[45] If priorities were the language of Socialism (according to Aneurin Bevan), targets were the language of New Labour. The 1998 set ranged widely: they included ensuring that everyone suspected of cancer should be seen by a specialist within two weeks of a GP referral, reducing the death rate from heart disease and stroke (among other causes of mortality) and improving the responsiveness of the NHS by means of surveys of patient experience. The list of targets was to grow over time, adding both to the pressures on NHS managers and to the political risks involved should they not be achieved.

The emphasis on working towards common standards raised a further issue. Could the goal be achieved without Ministers determining who should get what, thus abandoning the strategy of blame diffusion? Would they not inevitably be drawn into defining the criteria of eligibility for treatment and determining what should be available to whom, so in effect taking responsibility for rationing even while repudiating the notion? Enter the National Institute for Clinical Excellence. If in the past politicians had sheltered behind the doctrine of clinical autonomy – i.e. leaving it to clinicians to determine how to use resources – in future they would shelter behind the dictates of evidence-based medicine. It would be NICE which would be responsible for laying down standards and determining the criteria for the use of new drugs and technologies in the light of the best available evidence about both clinical and cost effectiveness. The experts, not politicians, would take the difficult decisions; collegial decisions would guide individual consultants towards consistent ways of working and using resources.

The one example of an explicit rationing decision taken by the Secretary of State, Frank Dobson, suggests that expertise would not always trump other considerations. This was the case of Viagra,[46] a drug for the treatment of impotence or, to use the medical term, erectile dysfunction. The drug arrived on the scene before the creation of NICE. However, the Secretary of State did have expert advice from the Standing Medical Advisory Committee. After reviewing the evidence, the Committee concluded that Viagra was effective and saw 'no medical reason why it should not be available on the NHS . . . nor why it should not be prescribed by GPs'.[47] However, the views of medical experts apart, there was another consideration: affordability. The issue, as Dobson defined it, was to strike 'a sensible balance between treating men with the distressing condition of impotence and protecting the resources of the NHS to deal with other patients, for example those with cancer, heart disease and mental health problems'.[48] Impotence, he argued, caused neither pain nor death: the new definition seemingly of medical necessity. Accordingly GPs were only to prescribe Viagra to those suffering from a limited number of conditions – such as men with spina bifida or diabetes and men treated for prostate cancer or kidney failure. In other cases, they would have to refer men to hospital specialists. What is more, the Secretary of State laid down the precise quantity of Viagra to be prescribed: one treatment a week. It was an unprecedented decision and one which clearly demonstrated the limits of using expert evidence as the basis for, and justification of, rationing. The experts had spoken – but it was the politicians who had to decide, invoking a different set of values and using a different calculus.

Medical scandals, waiting-lists and rationing apart, there were other issues which kept the NHS in the headlines during the first years of the Labour Government. The searchlight of media attention was intense and cruel. There was a steady drip of stories highlighting NHS inadequacies, ranging from the failure of cervical screening services to diagnose women accurately[49] to surgical mistakes by individual clinicians. Whether or not this was the result of a deterioration in the NHS's performance or of a growing gap between expectations and what was being delivered is an open question. What is certain, however, is that it reflected the growing intensity of the scrutiny to which the NHS was exposed and the growing assertiveness of patients in seeking redress when matters went wrong. The explosion in the number of negligence claims against the NHS – a trend accelerated by the introduction of contingency fees which encouraged lawyers to trawl for custom – provides striking evidence of the latter. The total charge to the NHS for provision for settling claims rose sevenfold between 1995 and the end of the millennium. As of March 2000, there were 23,000 outstanding claims, with a potential cost of £2.6 billion.[50]

Throughout 1999 the headlines proclaimed the parlous state of the NHS. The Chief Executive of the NHS Confederation, representing provider trusts, warned that the service was facing cuts because of financial problems; the Audit Commission reported a growing NHS financial deficit, a warning reinforced by the Association of NHS Finance Officers. In the months leading up to the Prime Minister's January 2000 statement the exposure of the NHS's weaknesses through the media megaphone reached a crescendo. Adding to the trouble came an outbreak of influenza. Hospital accident and emergency departments were flooded with patients. Stories of elderly patients waiting for 20 or more hours on trolleys in the A & E departments before being found a bed in a ward multiplied. A national shortage of intensive care beds was proclaimed, as these filled with the elderly victims of flu. Pressure on the service sometimes led to tragedy: one woman, Mrs Mavis Skeet, had her operation for cancer cancelled four times with the result that her condition became inoperable. The NHS, it seemed, had too few beds, too few doctors and too few nurses. The picture may have been exaggerated; some of the problems may have reflected poor use of existing resources rather than inadequate funding.[51] But the impression of a service unable to cope with demands was overwhelming.

The media message received authoritative reinforcement, not for the first time, when the medical profession proclaimed the NHS to be in crisis. This time it was Lord Winston, a Labour peer as well as a distinguished consultant, who provided the drama. The NHS, he argued in an interview in the *New Statesman*,[52] was 'gradually deteriorating because we blame everything on the previous government'. In putting his case, he cited the experience of his 87-year-old mother: 'She waited 13 hours in casualty before getting a bed in a mixed-sex ward – a place we said we would abolish. None of her drugs were given on time, she missed meals and she was found lying on the floor when the morning staff came on. She caught an infection and she now has an ulcer on her leg.' Nor was this an exceptional case: 'It is normal. The terrifying thing is that we accept it.' The interview was taken up, and headlined, by the newspapers on January 15. The following day Tony Blair announced his new package of funding for the NHS. If the Winston interview did not precipitate the Prime Minister's pledge directly, it helped to concentrate his mind – much as the statement by the Presidents of the Royal Colleges had helped to push Mrs Thatcher over the brink in 1987.

Tony Blair's statement came as a surprise to Department of Health officials, as well as to the Cabinet. January 16 was a Sunday and the Department's Chief Economic Adviser was caught at home when he was asked to work out the annual rate of growth required to implement the Prime Minister's promise to bring spending up to the European Union average; he records that his daughter's boyfriend did most of the calculations since the latter knew how to work the compound interest function on his calculator.[53] However, the NHS had, in line with the headlines, been moving up Tony Blair's consciousness and agenda for some time. Individual scandals, such as that of Mrs Mavis Skeet, made a great impression on him. So did a memorandum from Philip Gould, the Prime Minister's influential adviser on public opinion, which stressed that the Government continued to be vulnerable on the issue of the NHS.[54]

Anger, rather than surprise, was the reaction of the Chancellor of the Exchequer. The Treasury had indeed been examining the case for increasing funding for the NHS, spurred on by Alan Milburn, who spent some time there as Chief Secretary in between being Minister and then Secretary of State at the Department of Health. But Gordon Brown was reported to be 'furious' at being upstaged, without consultation, by the Prime Minister. His hand had been forced, and in his 2001 March Budget he announced a 35 per cent real-term rise, partly financed by an increase in National Insurance contributions, over the coming five years: an average annual rise of 6.1 per cent. At the same time, he commissioned a review into the future funding needs of the NHS, the Wanless Inquiry. Two years later the Wanless report (*see* Chapter 8) was to mark a decisive turning point in the long debate about whether there was any objective way of determining those 'needs', a debate which has provided one of the themes running through the history of the NHS and this book. In effect, it was to provide an after-the-event rationalisation of the January announcement.

For the Prime Minister's January announcement did not, of course, rest on any precise calculations about the 'needs' of the NHS. The goal of achieving the European Union average was essentially arbitrary, conveniently ambiguous enough to allow for flexibility in interpretation.[55] It was a target designed to make the maximum impact on the media and the public. But its impact was also felt within Government. 'A step change in resources must mean a step change in reform', the Prime Minister insisted.[56] A Cabinet Committee, chaired by the Prime Minister and including the Chancellor of the Exchequer, was set up to monitor the NHS. The process of rethinking New Labour's policies for the NHS had begun, a process that was to become ever more radical over the next five years. The next section summarises, in conclusion, the stresses, tensions and contradictions that made such a rethink necessary.

Commanding but not controlling?

In the period between 1997 and 2000, the Labour Government's policies for the NHS faithfully reflected the aspirations and ambitions of the new Third Way public philosophy, if adapted to the idiosyncratic characteristics of the service. On the one hand, there was the attempt to create a new synthesis, reconciling seeming opposites. Thus fundholding was abolished but reincarnated in Primary Care Groups; the internal market was abolished but the purchaser–provider split was maintained. In both cases the new synthesis both built on and adapted the Conservative legacy, itself the product less of ideology than of a process of experimentation. On the other hand, there was a great deal of pragmatism: witness, for example, the continued reliance on the ideologically suspect Private Finance Initiative scheme to raise capital for the NHS. On the one hand, there was much invocation of Old Labour themes. The emphasis on promoting the health of the population and on achieving Bevan's aim of uniform, national standards of excellence were both calculated to warm Old Labour hearts. On the other hand, there was the continued stress on the need for the NHS to change and to be more accessible to patients now transformed into consumers. NHS Direct was introduced: a national, 24-hour service, manned by nurses, to dispense advice and perform triage (and to lessen the pressure on primary care). The potentials of information technology (IT) were to be fully exploited. New ways of working were to be introduced, demarcation lines between professions were to be redrawn. Overall, then, the principles that had shaped the NHS in the first place were to be faithfully implemented but the service, like Government generally, had to be modernised.

The means chosen to modernise the NHS underlined, however, a central tension within The Third Way. While The Third Way put much stress on enlarging the role of local communities and on individual responsibility, its modernisation project for the NHS could only be achieved by strengthening the power of the centre. In this respect, policies for the NHS followed the pattern set in other spheres of public policy, notably education. If the NHS was to deliver a service of uniform excellence, if national standards were to be achieved throughout the country, if 'postcode rationing' was to be eliminated, new instruments had to be devised for controlling the activities of health authorities, trusts and doctors. Hence the increased prominence given to the use of performance indicators, the creation of new institutions for defining and inspecting standards, and the strengthening of the mechanisms for ensuring the competence of doctors.

All this appeared to be at odds with Tony Blair's insistence (*see* above) that there would be 'no return to the old centralised command and control system' in the NHS. And in one sense, the changes introduced did not represent a 'return' to such a system. For such a system had never existed. The system in the first few decades of the NHS's existence can more accurately be described as one of 'exhort and influence' (*see* Chapter 2). It gradually evolved and tightened with the introduction of performance indicators in the 1980s and the creation of a more hierarchical managerial system in the 1990s. But to a large and stubborn extent, the NHS had largely remained a conglomerate of local services rather than a national one. If the Labour Government was to change this – as it was committed to doing – then new, more powerful instruments of central control had to be created. So they were: in effect, the reinvention of the NHS meant inventing a command and control system for the first time in its history. The new strategy was not wholly consistent. Putting Primary Care Groups and trusts 'in the driving seat' might seem to promise a new era of devolved decision-making.[57] But in practice their freedom would have to be severely constrained if the Government's principal objectives were to be achieved: freedom lay in the knowledge of necessity – the necessity of meeting the targets set by the centre.

In all this, New Labour's policies can thus be seen as an attempt, for the first time ever, to apply the full logic of the values and constitutional principles that had shaped the NHS in 1948. If uniform standards of excellence were to be achieved, central control had to be exerted. If Ministers were to be accountable to Parliament for everything that happened in the NHS, then they had to be in a position to monitor and shape activities at the periphery. Only so could New Labour make a reality of Old Labour's vision. To do so the authority of technical expertise – so dominant in 1948 but in decline through the 1970s and 1980s – had to be resurrected and institutionalised. And the full potential of IT – in making the activities of the NHS more transparent and more rapidly accessible – had to be exploited. If previous governments (Conservative as well as Labour) had been inhibited by their fears of antagonising the medical profession or held back by the lack of an adequate information system in their centralising strategies, Blair's Government had no such inhibitions and was determined to create the necessary means. The aims of the founding fathers would thus at long last be achieved by their Third Way descendants: radicalism in the service of traditional values.

The strategy carried one major political risk, however. The Prime Minister and the Secretary of State might stress, as they did again and again, that they were only at the beginning of a 10-year modernisation programme for the NHS. But the constant flow of new initiatives, the reiteration that the NHS had moved into a new era, were calculated to excite public expectations rather than to dampen them. In short, the danger was that expectations would rise even faster than before, outpacing the Government's capacity to deliver. Rather than closing the gap between expectations and the NHS's ability to satisfy them, the Government's policies might widen it. Compounding the danger was a further factor. Already under the Conservatives, as noted earlier in this chapter, the NHS was subjected to an ever more intensive public and media scrutiny. If anything, Labour's policies seemed designed to reinforce this trend. With performance indicators and targets multiplying, with the Commission for Health Improvement's inspectors identifying shortcomings, with the activities of the medical profession subject to ever more rigorous examination, the NHS was becoming transparent to the point of nakedness. The veils of deference and ignorance were being stripped away. If there were shortcomings, if there were failures in the quality of treatment offered, if waiting-lists and variations persisted, they would be exposed to the public gaze.

At the same time, by forging new instruments of control and accountability, Ministers were also increasing their own political vulnerability if they did not deliver. Centralising power implied, in turn, centralising blame if the NHS's performance fell short of the promised goals. Yet reaching those goals was certain to prove difficult. Over the decades the NHS, a uniquely complex, heterogeneous and intractable organisation, had proved remarkably resistant to attempts to steer it from the centre. Central policy initiatives were aborted, adapted or modified in the process of implementation, most conspicuously so in the case of Mrs Thatcher's 1991 reforms. The NHS marched to the tune of developing professional practices and expanding technological possibilities, with individual professionals free to indulge in their own improvisations. If the medical profession and other NHS staff were to play from a score prepared by central government, there would have to be a remarkable transformation: a free-wheeling jazz group would have to be turned into a disciplined symphony orchestra conducted by the Secretary of State for Health. In attempting to bring about precisely such a transformation, the New Labour Government was thus taking on a peculiarly challenging task.

The January 2000 announcement meant that the economic costs to the Government of addressing this challenge would be high. If the political benefits were to be commensurate then not only did the NHS have to deliver on the promise that it would once again become 'the envy of the world' – in Tony Blair's words when introducing the 1997 White Paper – but it had to be seen to do so: performance and expectations had to be brought into line. And over the next five years this meant substantially rethinking some of the assumptions that had shaped policy in the first period in office, as we shall see in the next chapter.

References

1. David Butler and Dennis Kavanagh, *The British General Election of 1997*, Macmillan: London 1997.
2. Labour Party, *New Labour Because Britain Deserves Better*, Labour Party: London 1997.
3. Alan Finlayson, 'Third Way Theory', *The Political Quarterly*, vol. 70, no. 3, July–Sept. 1999, pp. 271–9.
4. Tony Blair, *The Third Way: New Politics for the New Century*, The Fabian Society: London 1998, Pamphlet No. 588. The quotations that follow are all taken from this pamphlet. For a longer and intellectually more ambitious exposition, see Anthony Giddens, *The Third Way: The Renewal of Social Democracy*, Polity Press: Cambridge 1998. For a critique of both, see Rudolf Klein and Anne Marie Rafferty, 'Rorschach Politics: Tony Blair and The Third Way', *The American Prospect*, No. 43, July–Aug. 1999, pp. 44–50 and Martin Powell, 'Something Old, Something New, Something Borrowed, Something Blue: The Jackdaw Politics of The Third Way', *Renewal*, vol. 8, no. 4, Autumn 2000, pp. 21–31.
5. Julian Le Grand, 'The Third Way Begins with Cora', *New Statesman*, 6 March 1998, pp. 26–7. Cora stands for: community, opportunity, responsibility and accountability. Substitute authoritarianism for accountability and the acronym is a fair summary.
6. Prime Minister and the Minister for the Cabinet Office, *Modernising Government*, The Stationery Office: London 1999, Cm. 4310.
7. Chief Secretary to the Treasury, *Public Services for the Future: Modernisation, Reform, Accountability*, The Stationery Office: London December 1998, Cm. 4181.
8. Andrew Marr, *My Trade*, Pan Books: London 2005, p. 180.
9. Anthony Seldon, *Blair*, Free Press: London 2005, p. 302.
10. Peter Hennessy, *The Prime Minister: The Office and its Holders since 1945*, Penguin Press: Harmondsworth 2000. See Chapter 18 for an account of Tony Blair's style of government. I have drawn heavily on this and on Hennessy's other, subsequent 'overflights', i.e. his regular reviews of how that style evolved.
11. Conservative Party, *The Conservative Manifesto, 1979*, Conservative Central Office: London 1979.

12. Secretary of State for Health, *The New NHS: Modern–Dependable*, The Stationery Office: London 1997, Cm. 3807.
13. Rudolf Klein (ed.), *Implementing the White Paper: Pitfalls and Opportunities*, King's Fund: London 1998.
14. Total Purchasing National Evaluation Team, *Developing Primary Care in the New NHS*, King's Fund: London 1999.
15. Secretary of State for Health, *Saving Lives: Our Healthier Nation*, The Stationery Office: London 1999, Cm. 4386.
16. Department of Health, *Modernising Health and Social Services: National Priorities Guidance 1999/00–2001/02*, DoH: London September 1998.
17. Independent Inquiry into Inequalities in Health (Chairman: Sir Donald Acheson), *Report*, The Stationery Office: London 1998.
18. Sally Macintyre, Iain Chalmers, Richard Horton and Richard Smith, 'Using Evidence to Inform Health Policy: A Case Study', *British Medical Journal*, vol. 322, 7 Jan. 2001, pp. 222–5.
19. Department of Health, *Reducing Health Inequalities: An Action Report*, DoH: London 1999.
20. NHS Executive, *The New NHS – Modern and Dependable: A National Framework for Assessing Performance*, DoH: London 1998.
21. Secretary of State for Health, *A First Class Service: Quality in the New NHS*, DoH: London 1998.
22. See, for example, Department of Health, *National Service Framework for Coronary Heart Disease*, DoH: London March 2000. This was produced by an expert group headed by Sir George Alberti, President of the Royal College of Physicians.
23. The first national patient survey carried out provided some support for the Government's view: see *National Surveys of NHS Patients: General Practice 1998*, DoH: London 1999. Only 17 per cent of patients referred by GPs to hospital were given a choice of clinics, but 75 per cent of patients declared themselves to be happy with leaving it to the GP to decide and a mere 7 per cent said that they would have liked a choice.
24. Interview with Alan Milburn, January 2004, in Brian Edwards and Margaret Fall, *The Executive Years of the NHS*, Radcliffe Publishing: Oxford 2005, p. 157. Edwards and Fall provide an authoritative account of the changing institutional governance of the NHS and the Department of Health between 1985 and 2003.
25. Patricia Day and Rudolf Klein, *Steering But Not Rowing? The Transformation of the Department of Health*, Policy Press: Bristol 1997.
26. Rudolf Klein, 'Regulating the Medical Profession: Doctors and the Public Interest', in Anthony Harrison (ed.), *Health Care UK 1997/98*, King's Fund: London 1998.
27. Secretary of State for Health, 1998, op. cit. For a subsequent elaboration of this, see NHS Executive, *Clinical Governance in the New NHS*, NHSE: Leeds 16 March 1999, Health Service Circular HSC 1999/065.
28. The emphasis on continuous quality improvement very much reflected the views of the Chief Medical Officer, Sir Liam Donaldson. See G Scally and LJ Donaldson, 'Clinical Governance and the Drive for Continuous Quality Improvement in the New NHS in England', *British Medical Journal*, vol. 317, 1998, pp. 61–5. For a sceptical medical view, see Neville W Goodman, 'Clinical Governance', *British Medical Journal*, vol. 317, 1998, pp. 1725–7.
29. Section 19 of the Health Act, 1999.
30. Tony Blair, *Speech by the Prime Minister at the Launch of the Commission for Health Improvement*, 10 Downing Street Press Office: London 28 October 1999.
31. Department of Health, *Supporting Doctors, Protecting Patients*, DoH: London 1999.
32. Bill O'Neill, 'Doctor as Murderer', *British Medical Journal*, vol. 320, 3 Feb. 2000, pp. 329–30.

33. Donald Irvine, 'The Performance of Doctors: The New Professionalism', *The Lancet,* vol. 353, April 1999, pp. 1174–7.

34. Secretary of State for Health, *Departmental Report,* The Stationery Office: London 1997, Cm. 3612.

35. Secretary of State for Health, *Departmental Report,* The Stationery Office: London 1998, Cm. 3912.

36. Chancellor of the Exchequer, *Modern Public Services for Britain: Investing in Reform,* The Stationery Office: London 1998, Cm. 4011.

37. An increase in real spending, i.e. ironing out the effects of inflation, does not necessarily translate into an equivalent increase in the input of resources into the NHS. If the price of inputs into the NHS (pharmaceuticals, wages and salaries etc.) goes up at a faster rate than prices generally, then the increase in the volume of these inputs will be less than the increase in real spending.

38. Secretary of State for Health, *Departmental Report,* The Stationery Office: HMSO 1999, Cm. 4203.

39. Almost 40 years previously, Enoch Powell had described his own attempts as Minister of Health to reduce waiting-lists as being 'as hopeful as filling a sieve'. See J Enoch Powell, *Medicine and Politics,* Pitman Medical: London 1966, p. 40.

40. Anthony Harrison and Bill New, *Access to Elective Care,* King's Fund: London 2000.

41. Geoffrey Hulme, 'What to Read into NHS Waiting-Lists', Letter in *The Times,* 25 Feb. 1998, p. 19.

42. See, for example, Vanora Bell, 'IVF Treatment and the Lottery by Postcode', *The Times,* 23 Feb. 1999, pp. 16–17.

43. David G Green and Laura Casper, *Delay, Denial and Dilution: The Impact of NHS Rationing on Heart Disease and Cancer,* Institute of Economic Affairs Health and Welfare Unit: London 2000.

44. NHS Executive, *Quality and Performance in the NHS: High-Level Performance Indicators,* NHSE: Leeds 1999.

45. Chief Secretary to the Treasury, 1998, op. cit.

46. Steve Dewar, 'Viagra: The Political Management of Rationing', in John Appleby and Anthony Harrison (eds), *Health Care UK 1999/2000,* King's Fund: London 1999.

47. Department of Health, *Advice from the Standing Medical Advisory Committee on the Use of Viagra (Sildenafil) in the Treatment of Impotence (Erectile Dysfunction),* DoH: London 1998.

48. Department of Health, *Impotence Consultation – Dobson Announces Final Decision,* DoH: London, Press Release 7 May 1999.

49. Sir William Wells (chairman), *Review of Cervical Screening Services at Kent and Canterbury Hospitals NHS Trust,* NHSE South Thames: Eastbourne October 1997.

50. Comptroller and Auditor General, *Handling Clinical Negligence Cases in England,* The Stationery Office: London 2001, HC 403.

51. For evidence about inefficiencies in the use of resources in critical care, see Audit Commission, *Critical to Success,* Audit Commission: London 1999.

52. Mary Riddell, 'Robert Winston: He May Be Held in Awe at No.10 but God's Imitator Thinks New Labour Has Made a Hash of the Health Service', *New Statesman,* 17 Jan. 2000, pp. 14–15.

53. Clive Smee, *Speaking Truth to Power,* Radcliffe Publishing: Oxford 2005, pp. 24–5.

54. Arthur Seldon (2005), op. cit., pp. 434–5. See also Mary Ann Sieghart, 'How Blair Came Late to Reform of the NHS', *The Times,* 24 March 2000, p. 22.

55. Subsequently a more cautious gloss was put on the Prime Minister's pronouncement. Was it an unconditional pledge or contingent on continued growth in the economy? Was the target to be calculated as the arithmetic average of spending by the EU countries or weighted by the size of their economies? See Adrian Towse and Jon Sussex, 'Getting UK Health Expenditure Up to the European Union Mean – What Does it Mean?', *British Medical Journal,* vol. 320, 4 March 2000, pp. 640–2.

56. *Statement by the Prime Minister on the National Health Service,* Press Notice 22 March 2000, London: 10 Downing Street.

57. For the argument that Labour policies were not necessarily centralist, see Chris Ham, 'More on Reform of the NHS', *Health Affairs*, vol. 18, no. 2, March/April 1999, pp. 261–2.

Chapter 8

The politics of reinvention

This chapter takes the story of the NHS to the end of 2005, by which time it was clear that the service was travelling in a new direction even though the final destination was uncertain. For by 2005 Ministers had, in effect if not in intent, created a largely self-inventing institution whose trajectory they could influence but not control with precision. It was a trajectory which was not the product of some grand design, the careful implementation of a blueprint, but an evolving process of discovery as the realisation that previous policy decisions had failed to deliver the expected results – or had, indeed, created new problems – led to the invention of new instruments. The process started in 2000 with the January 16 announcement of more money for the NHS, a golden shower which created new opportunities and heightened expectations. To seize the opportunities and to meet the expectations, Ministers exercised ever greater central control over how the money was spent. The process ended in 2005 with the Government moving towards a pluralistic, mimic-market model whose dynamics were at odds with the command-and-control model which it had built up in its first years. It remained to be seen whether Ministers would follow through the full logic of their new course and whether it was compatible with their ideological goals.

For, even while radically changing the institutional dynamics of the NHS, the Labour Government remained faithful to the ideological foundations of the NHS. The commitment to a tax-financed system, with care free at the point of delivery, was maintained and reaffirmed. Similarly, the commitment to the aspirations of the founding fathers to 'generalise the best', in Aneurin Bevan's phrase, and to address health inequalities remained as firm as ever. The contention of Ministers, as we shall see, was precisely that radical changes were needed to achieve Old Labour goals. Absent such changes, so the argument went, popular support for the NHS and other public services would erode. To survive, these services had to adapt to the transformation of a producer society into a consumer society. They would have to be consumer driven, not producer driven. So, in the case of the NHS, the 1997 catchphrase of a patient-centred service had become the 2005 slogan of a patient-driven service: the passive role has been translated into an active one.

But while policies in the post-2000 phase of New Labour did not represent an abandonment of Old Labour ambitions for the NHS, they did reflect a remarkable change in the ideas driving policy across all public services: ideas about the means required to achieve traditional goals.[1] Choice and competition were to be harnessed in the service of equity and universalism; diversity and pluralism were to be welcomed. It was part of a larger transformation in the intellectual climate, a transformation that had begun in the Thatcher years. The language of markets, the acceptance that private production was compatible with public ends, had become part of the emergent conventional wisdom on which policy-makers drew. A 2005 survey of the publications of 'Think Tanks' across the political spectrum noted that there had been a 'mainstreaming of ideas which, only 15 years ago, would have been inconceivable or confined to the extreme edges of the political landscape'.[2] Before examining in detail the nature of the consequent policy revolution – no less a word will do, even though the process itself was evolutionary – the next section sets out the economic and political context in which it took place.

Economic success, political victory

Tony Blair's administration was the first Labour Government in history not to be driven off course by economic crisis and the first, too, to notch up three successive election victories. The two were, of course, connected: economic success brought political success. The economic record, as set out by Chancellor of the Exchequer, Gordon Brown, in December 2005 was indeed impressive,[3] even though some of the credit should perhaps have gone to his Conservative predecessor, Kenneth Clarke. The Labour Government, he pointed out, was the first of any party 'to achieve eight years of uninterrupted growth since 1805'. For the fifth successive year running, Britain's growth rate had been higher than those of France, Germany and Italy, among others. Inflation was low. So, too, was unemployment. From being the laggard among European economies, Britain had moved to being a leader. New Labour's model for economic success – market liberalism and fiscal discipline – appeared to offer an example to other countries.

Just as the NHS had been one of the victims of economic failure in previous decades, so in the new millennium it became the beneficiary of economic achievement. The extra billions ploughed into the service represented, in effect, the dividends of economic growth. The Chancellor followed up the Prime Minister's January 16 pledge by announcing that the growth in NHS funding would run at the rate of 6.1 per cent for the following four years. And in the 2002 Spending Review, he increased the rate to 7.3 per cent for the following five years – following the Wanless report (*see* below) – a figure confirmed in the 2004 Spending Review. So the NHS was assured of a historically unprecedented rate of growth until the end of the fiscal year 2007/8. Spending on the NHS, which had risen from £35 billion in the financial year 1997/8 to £44 billion in 2001/2, was set to soar to £92 billion by 2007/8, all in real terms (i.e. after allowing for general price inflation).

Economic growth provided the foundations of electoral victory. In the 2001 General Election, Labour's majority remained commanding, at 166. In the 2005 election, the majority fell to 66, in part at least because of anger and disillusionment over the Iraq war. In both cases, health care came top of the list of issues considered 'very important' by the public when deciding how to vote, just ahead of education. In both cases, too, the public thought that Labour, as against the Conservatives, had the best policies: by a margin of 49 per cent to 14 per cent in 2001 and by 36 per cent to 22 per cent in 2005.[4] But although health care featured prominently in both election campaigns, and although all parties tried hard to differentiate their policies from those of the others, there was in fact remarkably little that separated their proposals for the NHS. The political consensus about the NHS as a tax-funded, universal service was holding, though one crack was beginning to show.

Consider the 2001 manifestos. The Labour manifesto[5] predictably congratu-lated itself on the fact that the promised 100,000 fall in waiting-lists had been achieved and on the increase in the number of doctors and nurses coming on stream. It also pledged a cut in waiting times and more choice for patients: specially built surgical units, managed by the NHS or the private sector, would guarantee shorter waiting times. There would be 'greater decentralisation to the front line': Primary care trusts (PCTs) would control 75 per cent of NHS funding by 2004, and the number of health authorities would be cut to yield a saving of £100 million a year. The Conservative manifesto[6] made much of choice: 'We will give back to patients and their doctors the power to choose.' Hospitals would be rewarded for the operations they carried out so that good hospitals would attract more patients and more funding. Stand-alone surgical units, funded by the NHS and operated by either the NHS or private providers, would be encouraged. The role of the Secretary of State would be 'to agree to funding and to regulate standards of quality, not to micro-manage hospitals'.

Only in one respect was there anything like a challenge to the existing consensus. The Conservatives, picking up on one of Mrs Thatcher's favourite themes, promised to abolish taxes on private insurance policies 'when affordable'. Otherwise there was little to choose between the two prospectuses. If anything the Conservative manifesto was a better guide to the future than the Labour one, anticipating many of the changes to come.

The 2005 manifestos also suggested convergence rather than divergence. Labour[7] naturally made much of its achievements in increasing the NHS's capacity and improving access. Patient power and patient choice were to shape the future NHS: by the end of 2008 all patients would be able to choose from any hospital that could provide an operation to NHS medical and financial standards. The manifesto also promised, like its predecessors, to cut bureaucracy: the staff of the Department of Health was to be reduced by a third, and the number of quangos would be halved, providing a saving of £500 million. The Conservatives[8] promised to increase the NHS budget by 'at least as much as Labour' and 'to give power and responsibility to local professionals'. Funding would follow the patient, with patients being free to choose 'the hospital or care provider that is right for them'.

Again, only in one respect was there was divergence. Building on their 2001 theme of encouraging private insurance, the Conservatives proposed to provide a subsidy to patients using the private sector: they would be paid one half of the cost of the operation in the NHS. Some saw this as a repudiation of the consensus about the NHS as a universal service. Given that the proposal came in the context of a pledge to continue to increase funding for the NHS, it could perhaps more accurately be described as a crack in that consensus. If the Conservatives had won office and implemented their policies, that crack might well have widened enough to shatter the consensus. But that was not to happen. One of the first decisions of David Cameron – elected to the leadership of the Conservative Party at the end of 2005 – was to repudiate publicly his predecessor's commitment to subsidising the use of the private sector.[9]

Given the degree of policy convergence in the party manifestos, drawing on a common stock of ideas, there is a puzzle. Why in 2001 did the voters think, by a large margin, that Labour had the best policies? And why was that margin significantly smaller in 2005 when the performance of the NHS had improved quite considerably? Unfortunately, survey evidence provides few clues as to precisely what persuaded voters. It seems highly unlikely that many of them had studied and weighed up the policy proposals in detail. More plausibly, they were swayed by general considerations which had little or nothing to do with the small print of the manifestos or campaign speeches. Given that Labour could claim paternity for the NHS, given also that Labour had invested heavily to justify its claim as being the party with the NHS closest to its heart, it seems likely that voters judged (consciously or not) that it was more likely to deliver on its promises. In short, it was a judgement about comparative dedication and competence, not about the comparative merit of specific policy packages.

That, certainly, appears to have been the conclusion drawn by Tony Blair after the 2001 election. During the campaign he had been given a sharp reminder of his Government's vulnerability to criticism about the performance of the NHS – with individual grievances amplified through the megaphone of the media – when he was publicly berated by the partner of a cancer patient, complaining about poor treatment and bad conditions.[10] The capacity of the NHS to evoke strong public feelings was also underlined by the loss of a parliamentary seat to an independent candidate, Dr Richard Taylor, who had campaigned on the single issue of cuts in the hospital services in his constituency. Not surprisingly, therefore, Blair came back to Downing Street more than ever determined to improve the performance of the NHS and other public services, conscious that policy implementation was as important as policy formulation. Delivery was all.

The constellation of special units in the Cabinet Office, i.e. the Prime Minister's Department, expanded.[11] A Delivery Unit was set up to monitor progress against targets in the NHS and other public services; there were regular stock-taking meetings, presided over by the Prime Minister, to receive reports on progress. Another, subsequent innovation was the creation of an Office of Public Service Reform to drive change. The pressure on the NHS to justify its extra billions was not to relax. Indeed it was intensified every time the Prime Minister visited a hospital offering a model of good service or practice. Such visits fed his impatience: if one hospital could do it, why could not the NHS as a whole? For Tony Blair this was not just a matter of winning the votes needed to keep Labour in office but also of ensuring his place in history as the man who modernised Britain's public services. While the precise meaning of the incantatory word 'modernisation' was elusive – and indeed, in the case of the NHS, went through several incarnations – the Prime Minister's fervour did not falter. Addressing the Labour Party annual conference after the 2005 election, he declared: 'Every time I've ever introduced a reform in Government, I wish in retrospect I had gone further.'

The great transformation

The Government's strategy for spending the extra billions was unveiled in July 2000 when *The NHS Plan*[12] was published. By then Frank Dobson had been replaced by Alan Milburn as Secretary of State for Health, a switch from Old to New Labour.

Working with a small group of political advisers and civil servants and with both the Prime Minister and the Chancellor of the Exchequer looking over his shoulder, Milburn himself drafted the document on his office computer.[13]

Preparations for it had started four months earlier when 'modernisation action teams' were set up to identify issues and come up with solutions. 'Doctors, nurses and managers' were to be the 'key architects' in devising the plan.[14] And in a preface to the White Paper, a battery of dignitaries – including the presidents of various Royal Colleges and the chairman of the British Medical Association's Council – committed themselves to working with the Government in modernising the NHS. The launch of *The NHS Plan* was thus very much an exercise in creating a professional consensus and mobilising support for new ways of working within the service. Similarly, the new policy instruments introduced were designed to encourage, support and monitor changes in the practice and organisation of care, leaving the institutional architecture of the NHS intact. 'The principles of the NHS are sound', the document argued, reviewing and rejecting the case for moving towards a different system of funding. However, 'its practices have to be reformed'. As Milburn put it in his introduction to the document: 'At its heart the problem for today's NHS is that it is not sufficiently designed around the convenience and concerns of the patient.'

Not surprisingly, therefore, the Plan put much emphasis on increasing capacity and changing working patterns, both intended to produce better access and an improved environment for patients. More doctors and nurses were to be trained and recruited. More new hospitals were to be built. Bedside telephones and television sets were to be provided. Hospitals were to be cleaner, serving better food. More, much more, money was to be invested in information technology: what was to become a £6 billion programme was set in train, designed to bring about electronic prescribing of medicines and electronic personal medical records for patients. Staff were to receive better pay, better training and better conditions. New GP and consultant contracts would be negotiated. Traditional 'hierarchical ways of working' would give way to 'more flexible teamworking between different clinical professions': so, for example, nurses would be empowered to take on a 'wider range of clinical tasks'. Services were to be redesigned around the needs of patients. Waiting times would be cut. There would be 'a national framework for partnership between the private and voluntary sector and the NHS'.

But what was to be the dynamic that would drive the process? Here *The NHS Plan* spoke with forked tongues. On the one hand, there was to be 'a leaner and more focused centre with the Secretary of State devolving power'. There would be 'maximum devolution of power to local doctors and other health professionals'. On the other hand, *The NHS Plan* retained, and indeed strengthened, the command-and-control system introduced by the 1997 White Paper. The drive to set national standards continued: more National Service Frameworks were to be produced and the work programme of the National Institute of Clinical Excellence in providing guidance on best treatments and interventions was to be expanded. The Performance Assessment Framework was to be applied to all trusts which would then be classified as green (meeting all core national targets), yellow (meeting most core targets) or red (failing to meet a number of core targets). The better the performance, the greater would be their 'earned autonomy', i.e. lighter touch monitoring; the worse the performance, the greater would be the degree of intervention in their affairs – which might extend to drafting in a new management team to run them. Further, green trusts would draw their share of money from a newly created National Performance Fund as of right, while the others would have only conditional access. In terms of logic, Ministers could correctly claim that there was nothing incompatible between imposing a corset of control designed to ensure adequate standards throughout the NHS and allowing freedom within that constraint to those who met those standards. In terms of practice, however, everything depended on how tightly the corset was laced up and, consequently, the scope for freedom allowed. In the event, as we shall see, the corset was more in evidence than the freedom.

There were three other themes in *The National Plan* which require noting. First, there was the missionary theme. A Modernisation Agency was to be set up to spread the message of good practice. Its tasks would be 'to help local clinicians and managers to redesign local services around the needs and convenience of patients'. The chief executive would be accountable to a Modernisation Board composed of 'key stakeholders committed to the modernisation of a sustainable tax-funded NHS' for the implementation of the plan: in the event the line of accountability never ran through the Board, whose only visible activity was the publication of a glossy annual report. Second, there was the patient protection theme. The machinery of professional regulation, notably the General Medical Council, was to be overhauled; similarly, a National Clinical Assessment Authority was to be set up to review the performance of doctors thought to be falling short in their work. Third, there was the theme of giving patients more influence over the way in which the NHS worked. A Patient Advocacy and Liaison Service (PALS) was to be set up in every trust. So, too, would a Patient Forum 'to provide direct input from patients into how local NHS services are run', to take the place of Community Health Councils. There were to be regular surveys of patient views at every level of the NHS. Patient choice, too, would be strengthened. More information about GP practices would be made available so that patients could exercise informed choice. Finally, patients would have more choice in terms of being able to book their hospital appointments at times convenient to them, though they would have no choice about where they were to be treated: it would be PCTs which would decide where to place their contracts, taking account of 'published information about patients' views of hospital services'.

That was 2000. By the end of 2005 the policy picture had been transformed. The extent of that transformation was summed up in a document published by the Department of Health setting out the programme of reform[15] as it had evolved in the intervening years. The aim of the programme was to achieve a 'self-improving' NHS, i.e. a service with 'an inbuilt dynamic for continuous improvement'. The reforms, it was stressed, were 'not designed as a blueprint for *how* services should be delivered; they are a means to improvement not an end in themselves'. The professed aim was to move from a politician-led NHS to a patient-led NHS. 'In an environment as complex and changing as that of health care, for the NHS to improve and innovate on a sustainable basis, the system as a whole has to better support the motivation and aspiration of staff to provide good-quality services', the document argued. 'Targets alone, especially targets driven from the centre, cannot achieve this.'

The reform programme rested on four pillars. First, there were the demand-side measures. Here the key feature was patient choice: by 2008 all patients were to be offered a free choice on referral of any provider, public or private, who met NHS standards and prices. Second, commissioning hospital and other services would become the responsibility of GP practices. Third, there were the supply-side reforms designed to encourage more diverse providers with more freedom to innovate and improve. On the one hand, NHS providers would continue to be encouraged to transform themselves into Foundation Trusts (FTs) with more freedom from central performance management and greater accountability to local people. On the other hand, the introduction of more private and voluntary sector providers would 'bring more capacity, more innovation and new ways of working'. Fourth, money was to follow patients. The introduction of a payment by results system would reward the best and most efficient providers and give others the incentive to improve. Finally, the framework of system management would have to adapt, with the emphasis increasingly on regulatory functions such as setting the rules for competition between providers, setting standards and monitoring compliance with them, and setting prices.

In subsequent sections of this chapter, this outline will be filled out by analysing the main components of the new policy programme, as well as examining the elements of continuity. The point of summarising the reform programme, as encapsulated in the Government's 2005 document, is to underline the dramatic nature of the change that took place as well as to provide context for the more detailed discussion. In effect, the Labour Government had reinvented the Conservative internal or mimic market. It did so in a more sophisticated way, as we shall see, designed to avoid some of the pitfalls and perverse side effects of the original: an example of policy learning. It was also a market that dared not speak its name: Patricia Hewitt, who had become Secretary of State for Health in 2005, indignantly repudiated the notion that the Government had created a market.[16] But the main elements of a market were there: choice for consumers, money following the patient and competition between a plurality of diverse providers. So, too, was GP fundholding, in effect if not in name. There were important differences between the 1991 reform programme and the 2005 reform programme. But the family resemblance is unmistakable. No wonder that the political consensus about the NHS held.

The main landmark in the path to 2005 was the White Paper published in April 2002, *Delivering the NHS Plan*,[17] followed by a succession of policy papers filling in the outlines. In this, the Secretary of State set out the new direction. The emphasis was to switch from institutional structures – such as the gaggle of new agencies created – to the dynamics of the NHS. Patients (and not GPs, as in the 1997 model) were to be in the driving seat. Patient choice took centre stage: as NHS capacity increased, so the scope for patient choice of hospitals would grow. So, too, did the notion of incentives. And the link between the two was to be payment by results. 'In any health care system incentives shape performance', the document argued. 'The history of the NHS is that it has had weak or perverse incentives and as a result has relied on top-down instruction.' A payment by results system, reflecting the preferences of patients, would provide appropriate incentives by rewarding good performance. There was much emphasis also on devolution to the front line: so, for example, the new NHS foundation hospitals would enjoy greater independence and autonomy than existing trusts. Conversely, the Department of Health would be slimmed down, and concentrate on 'the core functions of determining standards, distributing and accounting for resources, and securing the integrity of the system', while the regulatory system would be strengthened. Finally, *Delivering the NHS Plan* embraced the principle of plurality and diversity, repudiating the Old Labour notion that collaboration with private finance or the private sector would somehow contaminate the NHS. The scope of the Private Finance Initiative was broadened; more use would be made of spare capacity in the private hospital sector and overseas providers of health care would be encouraged to set up shop in England. The organisation structure of the NHS was to be streamlined. Here, in sketch outline, was the new model. Subsequent policy papers added some extra features. For example, in 2004 the notion of practice-based commissioning – the new version of fundholding – was resurrected,[18] with a reminder that it had had a brief mention in the 1997 White Paper. The same year *The NHS Improvement Plan*[19] elaborated on the plans and reiterated, *fortissimo*, the theme of patient choice as a 'key driver of the system'.

So the decisive change of direction in New Labour's policy programme appears to have taken place by the beginning of 2002. What explains this 'tectonic' shift?[20] As in the case of Mrs Thatcher's 1989 reforms, there are a number of ways of telling the story. One way of constructing the narrative is to see the development of policy as a deliberate, step-by-step process, each step building on what had gone before. Increasing the NHS's capacity came first, as the necessary condition for improving access; next came creating the framework of targets, standards and inspection required to ensure high quality across the board; only then was it possible to move towards a system where choice in a competitive, pluralistic world of health care provision would provide the incentives required for both efficiency and responsiveness within the regulatory framework. On this interpretation the 'tectonic' shift can be seen as following a predetermined path and the product of rational analysis.

Equally, and more persuasively, it is possible to tell the story as a series of policy lurches, with policy-makers responding to a variety of pressures and learning from their mistakes, with some confusion (and even contradictions) between different and overlapping policy streams. There was the pressure from the Prime Minister, impatient for results and, like Mrs Thatcher, increasingly irritated by being confronted by individual cases at question time in the House of Commons: so, for example, in January 2002, the Leader of the Opposition raised the case of 94-year-old Mrs Rose Addis, whose family alleged that she had been left 'caked in blood' for three days in the casualty department of a London hospital.[21] A command-and-control system inevitably reinforced the centralisation of blame: the costs of political direction from the centre were once again being demonstrated.[22] At the same time Ministers were becoming aware of the limits of their own ability of bring about change from Whitehall, as well as of the perverse effects of some of their measures. As the Prime Minister's health policy adviser was subsequently to comment: 'The risk of relying principally on hierarchical strategies is that they centralise blame, undermine intrinsic motivation and produce a compliance culture in which only what gets measured gets done.'[23] By the beginning of 2002 the new mood was reflected in a series of speeches by Alan Milburn which took decentralisation, localism and diversity as their theme.[24] In 1997 Ministers had been concerned with the anatomy of the NHS; after 2001 their concern was with its physiology, as one policy-maker put it. The following sections examine the context for this dramatic conversion in more detail.

Present needs, future demands

Retrospective legitimation for spending many billions more on the NHS was provided by Sir Derek Wanless, a former Chief Executive of the National Westminster Bank, who in March 2002 had been asked by the Chancellor of the Exchequer to report on 'the resources required to ensure that the NHS can provide a publicly funded, comprehensive, high quality service available on the basis of clinical need and not ability to pay'. Following an interim report in 2001,[25] a final report was published in April 2002.[26] Both drew heavily on the work of the Department of Health analysts.[27] Those who had argued through the 1980s and 1990s that the NHS had been massively under-funded appeared to be vindicated.

In 1979 the Royal Commission on the NHS had concluded, in line with all previous inquiries (*see* Chapter 6), that 'There is no objective or universally acceptable method of establishing what the "right" level of expenditure on the NHS should be'. The Wanless Inquiry represented the first attempt to prove this contention wrong. Its starting point was that NHS standards had fallen below those of comparable European Union countries, in terms both of inputs (such as the number of doctors) and outcomes (such as survival rates for cancer) and that public expectations would drive increasing demands for more effective treatment, speedier access and a better equipped environment. But how was the cost of closing the gap between what the NHS was currently offering and what it should be offering if it was to provide a world-class service to be measured? Here National Service Frameworks came to the rescue. These appeared to embody 'objective' judgements, based on a clinical consensus, of what high-quality services should look like. And the cost of implementing them could be calculated. Further, the Department of Health analysts convinced the Wanless team that these costs could be extrapolated to other disease areas. The team's estimates also took account of other factors likely to fuel demands for more spending, including demographic changes, technological innovation and the costs of implementing Government commitments such as clinical governance. But the single most important element remained the NSF costings, and their extrapolation.

The message of the Wanless report was so welcome that its methods received remarkably little critical scrutiny. Comparisons with other countries tended to skate over the fact that discontent with health services was not a British monopoly and that even high spenders did not necessarily offer services of uniformly high quality. Inevitably, too, some heroic assumptions had to be made in the calculations. Similarly, the justification offered by Wanless for spending more money tended to overshadow the report's conclusion that radical changes in the NHS's ways of working would be needed if expenditure on health care was not to absorb an ever-increasing share of the national income in the longer term. And while there is no evidence that the Wanless report influenced policy directly, its emphasis on the need to increase the efficiency with which resources were used reinforced some already existing concerns.

Up to 2008, the Wanless reports took the Government's projected spending plans as read, as a necessary exercise in making up for decades of under-spending. Projecting spending needs a further 15 years into the future, however, Wanless provided three different scenarios. Each scenario had two components. On the one hand, there were public attitudes and behaviour affecting the demand for health care: a theme to which Wanless was to return in a subsequent report on population health. On the other hand, there was the NHS's own performance in terms of improving productivity by using IT more intensively, by changing the skill mix of its workforce and by organising clinical practice more effectively. The most optimistic scenario, assuming full commitment on both the demand and the supply sides of the equation, implied that public expenditure on the NHS would account for 10.6 per cent of the national income by 2022, only a modest increase on the 9.4 per cent figure projected for 2008. The least optimistic scenario, however, implied a figure of 12.5 per cent. The difference between the two long-term projections – the optimistic and the pessimistic scenarios – was £30 billion a year, or almost half the NHS's total budget in the year that the final Wanless report was published, a difference with significant implications for the level of taxation needed to support the service.

The Government was already committed to acting on the demand side of the equation, and the Wanless team were to produce two more reports on this theme (*see* below). 'Improving health is now a key priority for all government departments', *The NHS Plan* had proclaimed. And there was particular emphasis on reducing health inequalities. But what about the supply side? Here the Prime Minister's Strategy Unit sounded a warning note in its comments on Wanless.[28] It underlined the fragility of all projections of long-term resource requirements, and pointed out that 'lifestyle factors could make an appreciable difference to future health care costs but not a large enough difference to remove the need for very large increases in health care resources'. So productivity – the efficiency with which resources were used – was all-important. And on this score there certainly was cause for concern. The instrument conventionally used to measure productivity – the NHS efficiency index – showed a fall in the years after 1995.[29] Whatever else New Labour's policies were achieving, they appeared to be failing on this score. The message was subsequently reinforced by the Office of National Statistics[30] in a report on public service productivity. This concluded that, using a variety of different methods, the average annual change in NHS productivity between 1995 and 2003 had been between −1 per cent and zero per cent. The extra billions flooding into the NHS had, seemingly, not resulted in a commensurate increase in outputs.

One reason was that the extra billions did not automatically translate into extra resources. The Treasury figures, as already noted, were in real terms, i.e. allowing for general price inflation. But there was another factor: price rises unique to the NHS. Wage and salary levels in the NHS increased significantly faster than in the economy as a whole. The index of NHS pay, set at 100 for 1992/3, rose to 119.1 by 1997/8 but had shot up to 174.2 by 2003/4,[31] with the effects of generous new contracts for GPs and consultants (*see* below) still to work themselves through in subsequent years. Of the additional £6.7 billion flowing into the NHS in 2004/5, almost a third was needed to finance increases in the level of staff pay.[32]

In any case, the estimates of productivity were problematic in one key respect. Specifically, the output figures used did not capture improvements in quality, particularly as reflected in changing patterns of work. So much attention was given to producing more sophisticated estimates. And if the NHS's activities had increased at the same rate as the various attempts to improve the methodology, no doubt all doubts about its productivity would have been dispelled long since. Sir Tony Atkinson was asked to conduct a review of the measurement of productivity across the public sector. The Department of Health commissioned a study from York University, as well as continuing with its own work on methodology. Their combined efforts suggested that making a variety of quality adjustments would add about 0.8 per cent a year to the figure for productivity growth. Nevertheless, the Department conceded, the methodology remained 'far from perfect'.[33] So doubt remained about just how to measure NHS efficiency, let alone changes over time. But any doubt about the urgency of increasing NHS productivity – however measured – had been dispelled. If targets and ministerial pressure did not do the trick, necessary though these may have been in the first instance, might incentives and competition be the answer in the longer term?

Managing the performance of the NHS

The command-and-control model developed in the years after 1997 did not change with the turn of the millennium. On the contrary, it was strengthened. The system of monitoring progress towards central government targets, and dealing with laggards, was reinforced. The Performance Assessment Framework took centre stage. It changed in form but not in intent. The traffic light signals – green, yellow and red – were replaced by Michelin-type stars. The best performing trusts were awarded three stars; the worst performing ones got none. Three-star trusts qualified for 'earned autonomy'; no-star trusts were candidates for central government action, which could mean drafting in a new chief executive and team of directors. 'Performance management' became the NHS's dominant preoccupation.

The first set of performance ratings for NHS trusts was published by the Department of Health in September 2001, covering acute trusts. Subsequently, the scope of the exercise was extended to cover all trusts and responsibility for producing the ratings was transferred first to the Commission of Health Improvement and then to its successor, the Healthcare Commission. However, the methodology changed only marginally, though the Healthcare Commission is adopting a different approach after 2006 (*see* below). The main elements remained constant.[34] Trusts were rated in four dimensions, with variations according to the type of trusts. First, in the case of acute trusts, there was performance against key targets: these included A&E waiting times, the number of inpatients and outpatients waiting longer than the standard, financial management and hospital cleanliness. 'Key targets are the most significant factors in determining overall performance ratings this year', the 2003 publication noted. Second, there was performance against a number of clinical indicators: for example, deaths within 30 days of selected surgical procedures, emergency readmissions to hospital following discharge and thrombolysis treatment times. Third, there was performance against a number of 'patient focus' indicators: for instance, the quality of food, the results of surveys eliciting the experience of patients and inpatient waiting times. Fourth, there was the managerial capacity and capability dimension, using indicators such as the sickness absence rate, the proportion of consultants who had gone through an appraisal process and staff opinion surveys. Finally, the exercise produced – with much statistical ingenuity – a 'balanced scorecard' that determined the final rating.

Over time, the number of three-star acute trusts rose from 35 in the first year of the exercise to 58 in the 2005 round.[35] And the number of zero-star acute trusts fell from 12 to eight, with an upward blip to 14 in 2003. And much the same trend was evident in the ratings of other types of trust. The ultimate sanction on zero-rated stars – drafting in a new senior management team – was invoked in the case of six trusts following the 2001 ratings exercise, but only once the following year. Subsequently, less drastic forms of intervention were thought sufficient to put failing trusts back on track. The strategy appears to have been successful. Of the eight zero-rated acute trusts in the 2002 exercise, only one appeared in the sin bin in the 2005 round: three had achieved the respectability of two stars.

The exercise, and the managerial style that it represented, were widely criticised and much resented in the NHS. Both the criticism and the resentment were not confined, however, to the NHS or to the star ratings exercise. There was a more wide-ranging reaction against the reliance on targets and performance indicators that characterised the Labour Government's management of public services. Although the roots of this managerial style went back to the 1980s (*see* Chapter 5), under Labour the number of targets multiplied and the use of performance indicators intensified: a trend of which the star rating exercise was just one example. There was no dispute about the usefulness of these instruments of governance. They forced Ministers to be explicit about their goals. They gave transparency to the progress – or lack of it – towards achieving those goals. They provided a focus on delivering results. In all these respects, they reinforced the accountability of government. But everything depended on their design and the use to which they were put. While performance indicators had originally been designed as tin-openers – i.e. as prompts to further investigation – they were now being used as dials[36] supposedly giving an automatic reading of the performance of individual NHS trusts, schools and other public services. And this raised questions not only about their accuracy and appropriateness but also about the risk of perverse effects.[37]

Prominent in the chorus of criticism was the House of Commons Public Administration Committee in its 2003 report on the 'measurement culture'.[38] 'The Government hopes that target-setting will encourage service providers to apply creativity in making their activities contribute effectively to delivery', the report commented, 'but in some cases creativity is being directed more to ensuring that the figures are right than to improving services'. There was evidence of figures being massaged and outright cheating. Further, 'Another problem is the tendency for departments sometimes to appear to pluck targets out of the air in support of the latest initiative. Such targets will command neither respect nor credibility'. And it concluded that the Government should decentralise performance measurement, increase local involvement in target-setting and cut the number of targets. Many of these criticisms were echoed in a subsequent report from the Royal Statistical Society,[39] focusing more on the technical aspects of target-setting and measurement. There was the risk of the indicators 'identifying a unit as under-performing when in fact there is no significant difference between it and others judged as adequately performing', the report pointed out. Also, it was 'inept' to set targets such as 'no patient shall wait in A&E for more than four hours' because 'as soon as one patient waits in A&E for more than four hours, the target is foregone'. Avoiding extremes, the report pointed out, 'consumes disproportionate resources'.

It was no accident that both reports took many of their examples from the NHS. Nowhere was the 'measurement culture' more evident, as the star-listing exercise demonstrated. The Department of Health's PSA high-level targets negotiated with the Treasury were relatively modest in number: the first, 1998 set listed 23 targets for the NHS – ranging from reducing the death rate from cancer and heart disease to ensuring that everyone with suspected cancer should see a specialist within two weeks of their GP requesting an urgent appointment. Subsequent PSAs added or substituted a variety of other targets, with particular emphasis on waiting times but also including a requirement that there should be a 'year-on-year improvement' in patient satisfaction with standards of cleanliness and food. However, the number of targets proliferated as the Department translated the PSA 'high-level' list into more specific requirements for service providers: for example, the provision of single-sex accommodation in all NHS hospitals. At the peak of the target boom NHS managers claimed that they had to meet more than 300 targets, though Ministers insisted that there were only 60, a difference probably explained by disagreement about how the term should be defined: thus in the case of the PSA targets, a number of different performance measures are often subsumed under individual headings. And even if the claims of the managers were exaggerated, they accurately reflected the sense of oppression and frustration created within the NHS by the plethora of targets reaching deep into the housekeeping arrangements of hospitals. As the Audit Commission warned:[40] 'Targets that front-line clinicians and managers perceive to be unrealistic, inappropriate or not the real priorities can become obstacles to change . . . such targets risk being seen as an irritating distraction.'

A variety of factors appear to have driven this explosion of targets and the accompanying use of performance indicators. There was ministerial impatience with the failure of the NHS over the decades to pay attention to basics. 'Frankly, it should never have needed Ministers to tell hospitals that informed consent, clean wards and good food are basic requirements for a modern NHS', Alan Milburn argued. 'It is a salutary lesson for those who complain about too much central intervention that it was only this process which focused attention on getting some of the fundamentals of care right for patients'.[41] There was the dilemma of all target-setting systems. If targets are introduced parsimoniously, the risk is that all efforts will be concentrated on achieving them to the neglect of other policy goals. If, conversely, targets attempt to cover the whole range of policy goals, the risk is of overload and confusing signals. Finally, there was the persistent trickle of new initiatives – responding to public anxieties about new problems, such as an epidemic of hospital infections – each a candidate for a new target designed to monitor its implementation.

The NHS also provided plenty of examples of the perverse effects of the 'measurement culture'. There was evidence of cheating. In 2001 the National Audit Office found that waiting-list statistics had been 'inappropriately adjusted'[42] in nine trusts. In 2003 the Audit Commission reported on spot checks at 41 trusts. These found evidence of 'deliberate misreporting' at three trusts, and reporting errors in 30% of all waiting-list PIs examined.[43] And there was the evidence that the targets for waiting-lists and times distorted clinical priorities. Patients were being treated simply because delay would have imperilled achievement of the waiting-time target, clinicians complained, to the detriment of more urgent cases who had not yet reached the critical cut-off point. Further, hospitals were cancelling follow-up appointments in order to meet their waiting-time targets for new patients: giving evidence to the Public Administration Committee, an ophthalmologist cited the example of an elderly lady whose 'follow-up appointment for glaucoma was delayed several times' with the result that 'her glaucoma deteriorated and she became totally blind'. Such horror stories were, no doubt, exceptional but they helped to fuel the reaction against the 'measurement culture'. Conversely, there were the horror stories among NHS managers of aggressive telephone calls from ministerial offices and of 'bullying and harassment',[44] forcing them to concentrate on the politically sensitive issue of the day and crisis management rather than running their organisations effectively. Nor did frequent structural reorganisations (*see* below) that forced them to reapply for jobs do much to improve their morale. Rising pay for chief executives did little to compensate for their growing sense of insecurity: running an NHS trust had become a high-risk occupation, as they saw it.

More generally, the evidence of perverse effects – in particular the impact on front-line morale in the NHS – seems to have been yet another contributory factor to ministerial disillusionment with the command-and-control style of managing the NHS and the consequent search for a new model. Before turning to the various components of the new model in more detail, however, the next section discusses yet another factor. This was the continuing gap between policy ambitions and policy achievements, testifying to the sheer difficulty of changing the way in which the NHS works: the intractability of the organisational marble which Ministers were trying to shape.

The implementation gap

As money flooded into the NHS in the new millennium, Ministers had much to boast about. And boast they did. Already by 2002 the Secretary of State, in his foreword to the Department of Health's annual report, could point out that the extra resources were producing results.[45] In the five years since 1997, the NHS had taken on 31,000 more nurses and 9,000 more doctors; 21 new hospitals had been opened; high street walk-in centres and the NHS Direct helpline had been introduced. Outcomes, too, had improved: waiting times had been cut, so that nine out of 10 people now had their operations within three months. Over the next three years the litany was to expand with more success stories to report. By 2005 the targets for waiting times had been cut; the graph showing the number of patients waiting over six months for admission had fallen steeply; the decline in premature deaths from cancer and coronary heart disease had continued.[46] The NHS appeared to be on course to achieve the goals set by Ministers.

Official publications reinforced the statistical message by vignettes of changing practice within the NHS. The 2002 departmental report peppered its text with such examples. Eastbourne Hospitals NHS Trust had introduced a fast-track referral pathway for cancer scans which had cut waits from 14 to five days; Peterborough had cut waiting times for cataract operations from 12 months to four weeks by introducing a one-stop service, which allowed opticians to refer patients directly to the hospital for surgery so cutting out visits to GPs and outpatient clinics; Heatherwood and Wrexham Park Hospitals Trust had introduced a system which allowed all day-surgery patients to pre-book their appointments, with the result that the number of missed appointments had been cut and patient satisfaction had risen from 45 per cent to 81 per cent.

Statistics and vignettes combined to give a picture of a service bubbling with local initiatives – new ways of organising the provision of care – and with a rising tide of improvements in access and quality for patients.

It was an accurate picture, as far as it went. But there was another side to it. On the one hand, quite a few of the policy initiatives launched by Ministers – and hardly a month went by without Ministers announcing an initiative of some kind or another – disappointed or foundered on the rocks of implementation. Policy euthanasia often followed, though with less publicity than at the launch. On the other hand, as in the past, the NHS remained a service where it was possible to make two contradictory statements, both of which would be true. The missionaries of the Modernisation Agency may have won many converts, but the gospel of modernisation was not universally embraced. There were indeed examples of outstanding achievements in terms of both service delivery and organisational innovation, such as the cancer networks which brought together the various strands of care. But there were also examples of inadequacy in the services offered and poor standards. The average level of performance might well have risen, but it was far from clear that the gap between the best and worst performing service providers was closing. Generalising the best remained an elusive goal.

Consider the case, first, of a policy initiative that foundered. In 1997 *The New NHS* announced what was advertised as a trail-blazing initiative. This was the creation of Health Action Zones (HAZs). Their aim was to be to find 'new ways to tackle health problems and reshape local services' in areas of deprivation, with a special emphasis on tackling health inequalities. In the event 26 such Zones were set up. They were intended to have a seven-year lifespan. But by the beginning of 2003, they were in effect wound up. A highly sophisticated evaluation of the scheme, sponsored by the Department of Health, concluded that 'there is no escaping the fact that they did not do what they set out to achieve'.[47] The conclusion was qualified. At their best HAZs demonstrated the possibility of change; they also made a contribution to the development of local strategic partnerships. They were also the victims of unrealistic expectations: modestly financed, they were asked to take on tasks of great complexity. Nevertheless, in the eyes of policy-makers, they were clearly a failure: hence the euthanasia.

The next example is of a rather different kind. It illustrates the rocks in the road to implementation. In 1998 the Department of Health set up a National Patients' Access Team (precursor of the Modernisation Agency) to redesign hospital services. One of its first tasks was to pilot a national booked admissions programme, to design a system whereby patients could book their admission date. Again the Department of Health funded an evaluation of the pilots. This came to two conclusions.[48] First, while the pilots did demonstrate progress in increasing booking, much of this improvement was subsequently lost. Second, there were wide variations in what was achieved: 'The local context had more influence on what was achieved than the national context.' The findings underlined 'the power of physicians' as well as 'the inertia built into established ways of working', with much emphasis on the former. It was no doubt a conclusion that the leader of the research team took with him when he subsequently became director of the Department's Strategy Unit. In this case, the experience with the pilots did not lead to the abandonment of the programme – which went ahead full steam – but it did illustrate powerfully the scale of the effort (and resources) needed to bring about change in the NHS.

Our third example is of the unintended, sometimes perverse, effects of policy. In the drive for greater efficiency, and cutting management costs, the Labour Government continued and, if anything, accelerated its predecessor's policy of encouraging mergers between NHS trusts. Between 1997 and 2002 there were 99 such mergers. A sample study of the mergers[49] concluded that these 'had a negative effect on the delivery and development of services' and that the savings in management costs were much less than predicted. Ramming the message home, there was an inquiry by the Healthcare Commission into poor quality clinical services at a Yorkshire trust[50] that was the product of a merger between three different hospitals. This found that one of the factors contributing to the trust's failure to deal with 'significantly higher' mortality rates in one specialty was the lack of managerial capacity to bring together three different hospitals' cultures, while at the same time trying to deal with a dire financial situation. The mergers, clearly, had created at least as many problems as they had solved.

The persistence of variations in the rate of progress towards achieving higher standards was illustrated by a series of reports published by the Healthcare Commission in 2005. Consider, for example, the quality of care in A&E departments.[51] Professional guidelines recommend that patients with a hip fracture should receive an X-ray within 60 minutes of arrival. A few hospitals achieved this target for all their patients, many more did not: the median figure for the proportion of patients X-rayed within 60 minutes was less than 40 per cent. Again, 'there was extreme variation in performance between departments with no obvious explanation' in the percentage of children in pain receiving analgesia within 60 minutes of arrival in A&E (the professional standard): 100 per cent in the best departments, less than 20 per cent in quite a few and a median of 55 per cent. Or consider the case of day surgery.[52] The target set by *The National Plan* in 2000 was that 75 per cent of elective surgery admissions should be day surgery, and the Modernisation Agency actively promoted this goal. Yet four years later, the figure was still only 67.6 per cent, with once again (no surprise) great variations between trusts – touching 100 per cent at one end of the distribution, less than 10 per cent at the other end. In the case of one specific procedure the range was from 96 per cent to 2 per cent. The same story emerged when the Healthcare Commission inspected a sample of hospitals for cleanliness.[53] Of the 37 NHS acute hospitals inspected, 11 got a clean bill of health, with high standards of cleanliness across the board, but in four cases the report commented that 'the lack of cleanliness is widespread and standards are unsatisfactory'. Mental health and community hospitals got an even worse report, while independent sector hospitals did better.

Variations in the way resources were used echoed the variations in standards. Here a single example, taken from the report on day surgery, will illustrate the point. On average, just 16 hours of surgery was performed per week in the average dedicated day-surgery operating theatre. But while the most efficient units used their theatres for 23 hours a week, the least efficient used them for only eight hours. Across England, the report reckoned, there was a capacity to do 46 per cent more day-surgery cases in NHS hospitals, simply by achieving the level of efficiency recorded by the 25 per cent best performing units.

Despite the extra billions, despite the extra machinery of control, regulation and inspection, the NHS therefore appeared to have changed little in this one, crucial respect: variations in performance continued, as in the past, to be the norm in the NHS (as they are, perhaps, in all health care systems). The picture of continuing improvement, however accurate, had a flaw that diminished its overall impact: the persistence of pockets of poor, or at least lagging, practice. It was a particularly damaging flaw politically in that one example of poor practice – particularly when illustrated by an individual case amplified through the media, as in some of the cases already noted – was likely to weigh more heavily in the public's balance sheet than the statistics which showed solid, all-round progress. Like the projections of the future funding burden, like the growing disillusion-ment with a target-setting command-and-control strategy, this helps to explain a central puzzle. If the improvements in the NHS were as great as Ministers claimed them to be, why did they continue to cast around for new solutions and turn towards a mimic-market model?

Enter the regulators

The organisational logic of the mimic-market model, as we have seen, was that improvement would be driven not by ministerial fiat but by the twin forces of patient choice and competition between providers, with payment by results providing the necessary dynamic. Conversely, the political logic was that Ministers would no longer be held accountable for everything that happened in the NHS. The noise of dropped bedpans would no longer reverberate through the corridors of Whitehall. It was thus as much a strategy of blame diffusion as an attempt to introduce a new set of dynamics into the NHS. The emphasis switched from ministerial direction to regulation.[54]

One key element in the new model was the introduction of NHS Foundation Trusts, first unveiled by Alan Milburn at the beginning of 2002. These were modelled on co-operative societies and mutual organisations.[55] They were to be independent public-interest organisations and would 'replace central state ownership with local ownership'. A majority of their Boards of Governors would be elected by local people, while others would be elected by staff. They would enjoy autonomy in running their financial and other affairs. Their income would depend on their ability to attract patients. Initially only three-star trusts would be candidates for FT status, but eventually all NHS organisations would be eligible. Translating these notions into legislation proved highly contentious, provoking much opposition within the Parliamentary Labour Party, where many saw FTs as a threat to the integrity of the NHS. The Treasury, too, was suspicious – as it was about many of the changes introduced in the NHS – and insisted on limiting the freedom of FTs to borrow money in the market. However, in 2004 the first wave of FTs – 20 in all – was launched, the first of a succession of such waves.

The reality of governance in FTs challenged much of the political rhetoric.[56] Boards of Governors were elected by self-selected 'members', but recruiting such members from patients and the public at large proved hard in many cases: in eight out of the first 20, the total electorate was under 2000. There was much confusion about the relationship between the Boards of Governors and the Boards of Directors. The directors exercise the powers of the NHS Foundation Trust; the governors have the power to appoint or dismiss directors. But neither the Board of Directors not the chief executive is accountable to the governors: this model was explicitly rejected during the policy-making process (as was the New Zealand model of having health boards elected at the same time as local government elections and by the same voters). So is the role of governors supervisory or advisory? Are they there to voice the concerns of patients and public about the day-to-day operations of the trust or are they supposed to focus on strategic issues? If they are, in effect, no more than an advisory body – as suggested by the decision of many FTs to restyle Boards of Governors as Members' Councils – what is then left of accountability to the local community? And without accountability to the local community, does 'local ownership' mean anything in practice? In this, as in other respects, the FT model appears to reflect the influence of a group of trust chief executives whose demands for more autonomy helped to prompt this institutional innovation in the first place and who subsequently formed a highly active lobby pressing for ever more freedom to expand the scale and scope of FT activities: they clearly did not want a governance system which would sit heavily on their shoulders.

If there was confusion about the 'downward' accountability of FTs to their local community, there was absolute clarity about their 'upward' accountability. The Boards of Directors are accountable only, and exclusively, to an Independent Regulator: a non-departmental public body designed to be a 'circuit breaker' between centre and periphery in the words of one policy-maker. It is Monitor, as the Independent Regular is now known, who decides on applications for FT status. It is Monitor who reviews the performance of FTs, with particular emphasis on their financial viability. It is Monitor who can insist on a change of leadership at a trust, as happened early in the history of the FT experiment when a troubleshooter was dispatched to Bradford FT to sort out its troubled finances. The chain of accountability to the Secretary of State has been broken: Ulysses is tied to the mast, no longer able to listen to voices tempting him to intervene in local matters. And, perhaps significantly, neither the Secretary of State nor the Prime Minister became involved in Bradford's fiscal troubles. Further, in 2004 the Secretary of State told MPs that in future Ministers would no longer be in a position 'to comment on, or provide information about, the details of operational management' in FTs. To the extent that the FT model becomes generalised through the NHS, so the Secretary of State will no longer have to answer for the day-to-day operations of the service and, in turn, the service will be insulated from the kind of ministerial pressures prompted by individual cases in the past. In theory at least, the telephone line has been cut. The long and much discussed option of turning the NHS into a quasi-independent Commission (*see* Chapter 5) will, in effect, have become largely irrelevant.

The emergence of Monitor represented a change of plan in the course of the policy-making process. When Alan Milburn first sketched out his plans for FTs, the role of regulator was assigned to the newly created Healthcare Commission.[57] In the event the Healthcare Commission kept a regulatory role, but one limited to inspecting the quality of care delivered to patients and the effectiveness of management. The Healthcare Commission was the successor of the Commission for Health Improvement, the product of the 1997 crop of institutional innovations (*see* previous chapter). The CHI's remit had been to inspect the implementation, and effectiveness, of clinical governance by NHS trusts.[58] The ministerial assumption was that good clinical governance could be equated with good quality of care. It was a highly questionable assumption: process did not equate to outcome. And while the CHI was successful in developing a system of inspection and making it acceptable in the NHS – no mean achievement – its style of inspection attracted criticism: the CHI's review teams imposed an excessive burden on trusts, it was argued, and there was too much inconsistency between its reports. So when the machinery of regulation for quality in the NHS came under review, following the report of the public inquiry into children's heart surgery at Bristol, the CHI was replaced by a new Commission with a new and rather different remit.

The public inquiry conducted by Ian (later Sir) Kennedy was as ambitious in scope as it was lengthy, detailed and expensive: its budget topped £14,000,000. The report was more than 530 pages long and had 198 recommendations.[59] Most of the recommendations were in line with Government policy and were, with few if significant exceptions, accepted.[60] Among the many issues covered were professional relations with patients, the role of trust boards, training in leadership skills, clinical negligence, better information for decision-making and public involvement. But one major theme ran through the recommendations. This was that the Government needed to establish a system of regulation to protect the interests of the people who received the service and that such a system should be independent of Government. It was not enough to rely on professional regulation to assure the quality of care being delivered, though Kennedy proposed changes in that as well. Explicit standards should be set, against which the performance of NHS providers would then be monitored. The system of routine one-off inspections should be replaced by a system of validation designed to promote continued improvement in the quality of care with the ultimate sanction of withdrawing validation. Both the standard-setting and the validation should be the responsibility of independent bodies.

Most of the Kennedy recommendations were in line with the Government's own policies for promoting quality. To this end the Department of Health had already set up two new bodies. One was the National Clinical Assessment Authority, a body to which NHS employers could refer doctors whose performance was seen as problematic for review. The other was the National Patient Safety Agency, responsible for operating a national system of reporting and analysing adverse events and 'near misses'. On one point, however, the Department of Health was not prepared to follow the Kennedy line: it would not delegate responsibility for setting standards to an independent body. It was the Department which in 2004 produced a set of national standards.[61] They were presented by John Reid, who had succeeded Milburn as Secretary of State for Health, as part of a new focus: more emphasis on achieving standards across the service and less emphasis on achieving specific targets – the number of the latter being cut. The standards came in two categories: 'core standards' which required immediate and universal implementation and 'developmental standards' which were more aspirational in character. The standards were something of a ragbag based on a trawl of previous departmental policies and guidance. For example, one standard was that 'clinicians continuously update skills and techniques', while another one required health care organisations to have a system in place to ensure 'staff treat patients, their relatives and carers with dignity and respect'. They were criticised for demanding that clinicians should base their practice on evidence while seemingly having been designed without any evidence base.[62] Nevertheless, for the first time in the history of the NHS there was a set of explicit standards against which performance could be assessed. Applying them was now the task of the Healthcare Commission, which on 1 April 2004 had replaced the CHI. Its chairman was none other than Sir Ian Kennedy.

The Healthcare Commission was more independent of Government than its predecessor. Its members were chosen not by Ministers but by the NHS Appointments Commission. This had been set up in 2001 to vet candidates for trust boards and other NHS bodies in order to dispel the well-founded suspicion that political affiliations influenced the process. The Healthcare Commission also evolved into an ever more all-embracing regulatory body. It became the court of appeal for patient complaints. It swallowed up the National Care Standards Commission, which had been set up to regulate the independent health care sector: it seemed only logical, given the NHS's increasing use of private providers, that the same standards should apply across both sectors. The Commission for Social Care Inspection was set to follow. The Audit Commission's work on the efficiency, effectiveness and economy of health care was taken over.

In these respects the Commission appears to have been the beneficiary of a cross-government reaction – led by the Cabinet Office – against the explosion of regulation and a consequent drive to reduce regulatory overlaps and burdens. Rationalisation through amalgamation appeared to be the answer in this case, though the example of hospital mergers might have sounded a warning note. The new philosophy of regulation – that it should be proportionate to risk and light-handed – also helped to shape the Commission's strategy. The 'radically new approach to assessing and reporting on the performance of healthcare organisations'[63] began to be put into operation at the end of 2005. No longer was there to be a routine, triennial visit to trusts as in the days of the CHI. The new 'annual health check' was based on self-assessment by trusts, using the framework of the national standards as elaborated by the Commission.[64] Only 20 per cent of trusts were to be visited: a random sample of 10 per cent and a further 10 per cent where there was reason for concern. Sir Ian's vision for regulation was on the way to being achieved.

Successfully surviving this round of institutional reinvention was another regulator: the National Institute for Clinical Excellence (*see* previous chapter), where the most obvious change was the addition of 'Health' to its designation and the creation of an advisory Citizens' Council. By 2005 it had published 86 technology appraisals (of pharmaceuticals and specific health interventions) and 23 clinical guidelines (about the management of particular conditions) based on an analysis of clinical and cost effectiveness. NICE had two implicit political objectives, quite apart from its overarching goal of promoting evidence-based practice. The first, implicit goal was to screen Ministers from decisions about rationing resources – to provide a technical rationale for denying particular drugs or treatments to patients. In the event, Ministers responded to public outcry or pressure from the pharmaceutical industry – if only on very rare occasions – by asking NICE to reconsider a thumbs-down decision rather than to shelter behind it. Or, as in the case of Patricia Hewitt, who replaced John Reid as Secretary of State in 2005, to ignore NICE altogether: which is what she did when encouraging PCTs to fund an expensive drug for early-stage breast cancer, herceptin, if a clinical case could be made.[65] This followed the much publicised case of a patient, Barbara Clark, who had been prepared to sell her house to fund a course of herceptin. NICE was involved only after the event. Overall, the record suggests an asymmetry in the use of NICE as an independent arbiter: Ministers will always be tempted to take credit for generosity, even while seeking to avoid blame for parsimony.

The second and explicit goal was that NICE should end postcode rationing. If everyone followed NICE decisions and guidance, there would no longer be the variations in practice and the availability of drugs that had marked the NHS from the start. And indeed in January 2002 the Secretary of State directed PCTs to fund NICE technology appraisal guidance (though not clinical guidelines) within three months of an appraisal's publication. As it turned out, though, implementation proved spotty.[66] One reason was that following NICE guidance usually means spending more: overall, the cumulative cost of NICE's technology appraisals had risen to £800 million a year by 2005. Other reasons cited in an Audit Commission study of the take-up of NICE guidance[67] include apathy and resistance to change. The DoH core standards, now being used by the Healthcare Commission to appraise trusts, require that health care organisations ensure that they conform to NICE technology appraisals, while the developmental standards require them to conform not only to NICE guidance but also to National Service Frameworks and agreed national guidance on service delivery. It remains to be seen whether this will bring about the desired degree of national conformity.

How the money flows

Central to the development of the new model NHS, and the retreat from a command-and-control style of management, was the introduction of a system of payment by results. 'The history of the NHS is that it has had weak or perverse incentives and as a result has relied on top-down instruction', Milburn argued when first unveiling his plans in 2002. 'For example, hospitals that are doing well in getting waiting times down are often forced not to use their spare capacity to treat more patients because that breaks through the budget ceilings they have been set. Conversely, poor performers in the NHS are often bailed out with extra financial help.'[68] It was a diagnosis which echoed that made in Mrs Thatcher's 1989 White Paper.[69] 'The present system of funding offers only limited incentives for hospitals to satisfy the needs and preferences of patients or to take on additional work by improving productivity', this had argued. And the remedy offered was not so very different. In future rewards and sanctions would be automatic as money followed the patient: providers who were successful in attracting patients and efficient in using their resources would reap the benefits, while trusts who failed to attract custom or whose costs were too high would risk financial failure if they did not improve their performance. But whereas the Thatcher reforms had never achieved the desired goal – block contracts, insensitive to changes in activity, remained the norm – the Labour Government adopted a more radical approach: a 'complete change to NHS funding', as the Audit Commission described it.[70]

The introduction of the new system was a cautious, step-by-step process. But the intention is that by 2008/9 it will cover all NHS activities. Key to the system is a national tariff: prices are set nationally for individual procedures (Healthcare Resource Groups), and apply to all NHS providers as well as private providers treating NHS patients. The prices are based on an average of all hospital costs for that procedure; national funding will compensate for unavoidable regional variations in costs. In this, there is a significant change from the contracting system adopted by the Conservative Government and subsequently perpetuated, which involved often acrimonious negotiations between providers and purchasers both about the price and the quantity of services to be provided. No longer will local purchasers haggle over prices: a change designed to cut administrative costs and to focus attention exclusively on the quality and appropriateness of the services being provided.

There were worries about the methods and quality of the data used to calculate the tariff; the appointment of an independent regulator to determine prices seemed only a matter of time.[71] But while the change was revolutionary for the NHS, it was not so in the comparative context of other health care systems. The USA, Canada, Australia and the Netherlands are among the countries that have adopted payment by results: the ancestry of Healthcare Resource Groups can be traced back to the Diagnosis Related Groups first introduced in the USA. And while international evidence demonstrated the feasibility of such a system, it also illustrated the risks that it carried, as the Audit Commission pointed out.[72] There was the risk of gaming by providers. For example, they might select the most expensive diagnosis for a patient: what is known in the US as DRG creep. Or they might deliberately keep patients in hospital for more than 48 hours to attract the full (rather than short-stay) tariff. Above all, there was the risk that the system gave providers, operating in a competitive environment with spare capacity, an incentive to drum up custom: 'to increase both volume and complexity', as the Audit Commission put it. Even while promoting the efficiency of individual providers, payment by results might therefore create upward pressures on total NHS spending.

Much therefore depended on the purchasers if the NHS was to retain its reputation, won during the first 50 years of its existence, for being able to control spending more effectively than any other health care system. Here the role of primary care trusts, through whom 80 per cent of all NHS funding now flowed, was central. But were PCTs up to the task? The Audit Commission thought not: 'PCT commissioning is not currently fit for purpose', it concluded. Its doubts were shared by Ministers, among many others. In 2005 they announced proposals for 'reconfiguring' PCTs, through amalgamations, to make them more effective as purchasers (*see* section on organisation change, below). But it was not clear that this could solve the underlying problem: how to control the total volume of demand in an era of patient choice and spare capacity, when waiting-lists were no longer an effective way of rationing demand. However effective PCTs might be managerially, they ultimately had no direct way of controlling demand short of announcing that they would no longer fund certain activities: a step highly embarrassing for Ministers.

Hence the resurrection of what was in all but name (shunned by Ministers) fundholding: practice-based commissioning as it was rechristened. All GPs were to be given indicative budgets. The rationale was clear. 'GP practices are one of the main determinants of health care utilisation', the Government argued when launching its proposals in 2004.[73] But practices did not need 'to consider how they are using health care resources'. Under the new system, GPs have to balance their budgets over a three-year period. They therefore have a direct incentive to limit patient demands or to substitute less expensive interventions for high-cost hospital procedures – so supporting another Government goal, that of moving an increasing proportion of services into the community. Cost control is internalised, as it were, and once again rationing is disguised as clinical discretion. The politically unacceptable is replaced by the politically invisible.

From voice to choice

As from the start of 2006 patients have had the right to choose from at least four providers selected by their GP for planned hospital care, including an option to be treated in a private hospital. By 2008 they will have the right to choose from any health care provider that meets the Healthcare Commission's standards and charges the NHS price. Individual decisions by patients will (in theory at any rate) drive the configuration of health care services, determining which hospitals thrive and which hospitals go under. The logic of the new NHS model is, in short, that it is the market which will determine the menu of options available to patients: so, for example, it may reduce the options available in any geographical area if it leads to the closure of local hospitals or a cut in the range of the services they provide.[74] This raises the question of whether there are any balancing mechanisms which allow collective – as distinct from individual – preferences to be articulated. Will the market trump politics?

In a publicly funded service like the NHS, it is clearly the responsibility of Ministers to represent collective interests. In this respect, the command-and-control model conformed to their constitutional position and their accountability to Parliament. The new model still presumes that Ministers will be responsible for determining priorities, strategy and the direction of travel for the NHS. But it is not clear how far Ministers will push the doctrine of insulation from day-to-day decisions at the periphery – reflecting not only market forces but also evolving professional practices – when it is precisely those decisions which will help to determine what the NHS looks like. In the 1990s Conservative Ministers (as we saw in Chapter 6) intervened when market forces threatened dislocation in London's health services and imposed a planned reconfiguration, contrary to the rationale of the mimic market which they had introduced. In 2001, the Government set up an Independent Reconfiguration Panel to review contested service changes, while leaving the final decision to the Secretary of State. For the future, it remains to be seen how far Ministers will accept changes in the NHS, such as hospital closures, driven by the market: a hard test for the rhetoric of devolution of responsibility to the front line and the primacy of patient choice.

There are, of course, some mechanisms for articulating collective community interests. PCTs have two roles: to implement national priorities – where they remain accountable to the centre – and to plan services on behalf of their local communities. But their ability to carry out the latter role must be in doubt, even if their managerial capacity improves as a result of amalgamations. The combination of practice-based commissioning and patient choice means that they have only limited control over the configuration of local services: if GPs and patients prefer to use providers in other parts of the country, there is little they can do about it. There are other voices which can claim to speak on behalf of the local populations. In 2000 the Government announced that it would give local government the power to scrutinise local health services.[75] At the same time, however, it abolished Community Health Councils. In doing so, it argued that it was transferring power from an unelected body to elected local authorities, which would inherit the right to refer major planned changes to the Secretary of State. It remains to be seen how local authorities will use this power in an era when service 'reconfiguration' is likely to become ever more frequent, and whether this move will strengthen community voice.

However, one of the few goals of Government policy to have been consistently pursued since 1997, reiterated in almost every policy document published since, has been the encouragement of patient voice. And indeed before expanding capacity made it possible for the Government to make choice its major theme, the emphasis on patient voice was dominant. New Labour has been good for the survey industry. Regular surveys of patients, designed to elicit their experience and degree of satisfaction, have become part of the NHS landscape, both nationally and locally, covering all aspects of the service. These, in turn, have fed into the performance rating exercises of first the CHI and subsequently the Healthcare Commission. Further, every NHS trust now has its Patient Forum, over 500 of them. And major Government initiatives tend to be prefaced by extensive public consultations: one such involved getting together 1000 people in Birmingham's Convention Centre.[76] The extent to which such exercises actually shape Government policy – as distinct from giving it added legitimisation – remains an open question.

All this is impressive evidence of ministerial dedication to the notion of listening to the patient's voice. But if voice is so central to the Government's vision of a patient-centred NHS, why has it been found necessary to reinforce it by introducing choice? The invocation of choice as a guiding principle for the organisation of public services is far from unique to the NHS: it became one of the mantras of the latter-day Blair Government, flowing from the initial New Labour diagnosis (*see* previous chapter) that in a consumerist society the public expect to make their own decisions about what school or hospital to use. So it was very much a general theme being played out in the specific arena of the NHS. In the case of the NHS, the general thesis is reinforced by two arguments, one instrumental and the other political.

The instrumental argument has already been explored. It is, as we have seen, that the combination of patient choice and payment by results will provide the incentives required to make hospitals more efficient and more responsive to patient preferences. The political argument is that Government policy is accurately reflecting public preferences; more fundamentally, political theory would suggest that the ability to exercise choice is the mark of an autonomous citizen.[77] A variety of evidence bears on the political argument. There is the evidence that patients are becoming active consumers, using the web and other sources to inform themselves about treatment options: a trend supported by the Government's policies for providing more information about the services available. There is survey evidence showing that a majority of the public do indeed value choice: one survey reported that 66 per cent of the public considered choice of hospitals to be very or fairly important to them.[78] However, there are problems about interpreting such results. So, for example, it may be that patients attach more importance to choice of treatment, and access to it, than to choice of where to be treated or by whom. Another survey asked the public what factors they considered most important in choosing a hospital for treatment.[79] This found that 50 per cent of the sample considered waiting times to be most important; only cleanliness scored more highly at 52 per cent. In contrast, the reputation of the hospital and of consultants scored 34 per cent and 18 per cent respectively, while choice of consultant scored a mere 10 per cent. One conclusion might well be that to the extent that Ministers succeed in achieving their policy goals of eliminating waiting-lists and ensuring quality care – let alone cleanliness – in all hospitals, so the public will attach less importance to choice between providers. So while the introduction of choice in the NHS may well prove to be a necessary instrument in the drive to 'generalise the best', it may yield diminishing political returns the nearer the Government comes to achieving its ambitions. Even though the public may still value the *option* of choice as a weapon of last resort, its exercise will have been made largely redundant. And if the day ever comes when all health care providers offer high quality, quick access and good amenities, what will be the currency of competition between them?

The private sector to the rescue

Extending choice and encouraging competition depended, as already noted, on increasing capacity. And while channelling more money to the NHS was easy, training and recruiting extra doctors and nurses was not. New medical schools were set up, but it would take time before their graduates would be at the cutting edge of the NHS. So, starting in 2000 with *The National Plan*, Ministers began to look to the private sector. In October the same year a Concordat was concluded with independent providers specifying the terms of engagement.[80] The private sector's spare capacity was to be used for public purposes. New Labour's pragmatism had won over Old Labour's suspicions of private medicine.

There was nothing new about the NHS buying services from independent providers. Long before 2000 the NHS had been buying between 60,000 and 80,000 procedures annually, at a cost of some £100 million.[81] The new twist was that the occasional flirtation had been turned into an official co-habitation. The volume of contracting by NHS purchasers went up, contributing to the fall in waiting times. But continuing expansion was constrained in two respects. First, operations in the private sector were carried out by NHS consultants whose time was not infinitely expandable. Second, the private sector was exploiting the pressure on NHS managers to cut their waiting-lists by charging over the odds: the public sector was paying something like 40 per cent more than the average cost of performing the same procedures in the NHS.

The next step for Ministers therefore was to invite overseas providers, importing their own specialists rather than using NHS consultants, to enter the field. Starting in 2002, these were invited to bid for the setting up of Independent Treatment Centres: specialised clinics for carrying out elective surgery and diagnostic procedures. By the end of 2005, there were 32 such ITCs, run partly by independent operators and partly by NHS trusts, and a second wave was on the horizon. The number of operations performed by the newcomers was modest – an estimated 50,000 procedures out of the 5,500,000 elective operations that the NHS carries out each year – but they appear to have made a disproportionate impact: their competition seems to have persuaded NHS trust managers operating in the same localities to raise their game, while making it easier to persuade their consultants to reorganise services in order to cut waiting times (and charge lower fees for extra work carried out in the NHS trusts themselves).

Overall, the role of the independent sector remains modest: in 2005 it was estimated that it carried out 10 per cent of elective surgery at a cost of 1 per cent of the total NHS budget. However, its role is growing and independent operators are moving into new territory: for example, bidding to provide general practice services in under-doctored areas.[82] The process of expansion provoked complaints and criticism. For example, PCTs were pushed by the Department of Health into guaranteeing ICTs a specified level of activity as an inducement to enter the market. They therefore had to pay, much to their fury, for the guaranteed volume of activity even in those cases where the number of contracted procedures had not been carried out.[83] Critics also have argued that ITCs represent poor value for money if paid at the national tariff rate, inasmuch as they tend to take the simpler cases while the NHS is left to deal with the more complex ones, and that training is being damaged as routine surgery moves out of the NHS. Undeterred Ministers, however, pushed ahead with their policies, giving independents 'preferred provider' status in the bidding for new developments to the exclusion of NHS trusts. The assumption is that the spur to NHS efficiency prompted by competition from independents – and the challenge they offer to existing practices – will yield dividends that outweigh the costs of introducing more diversity and pluralism into the health care system.

In any case, the terms of trade between the NHS and the independent sector may well change. In 2005 one-fifth of the activity in acute independent hospitals was funded by the NHS (while the figure for independent sector mental health hospitals was already over 80 per cent). By 2008 this proportion is, on present trends, likely to double.[84] In short, the independent sector will become increasingly dependent on NHS funded patients even while the NHS itself is expanding its capacity. The NHS should therefore be able to strike tougher bargains: competition cuts both ways. In turn, to the extent that independent providers – and insurers – come under pressure to cut costs, so they are likely to apply pressure on consultants to reduce their fees. At present specialist fees in England are among the highest in the world:[85] for example, the average specialist fee for a coronary artery bypass graft in 2002 was $3,545 in the UK, $2,324 in Australia, $1,936 in the US and $1,068 in Canada (all at the purchasing power parity rate).

Consultants, and the independent sector generally, may come under increasing pressure for another reason as well. To the extent that the Government achieves its policy goals for the NHS, and waiting times cease being an all-important issue, so the incentive to take out private health care insurance will weaken. Why pay to be a patient in a private hospital – either through insurance or out of one's own pocket – if the NHS is prepared to pick up the bill for the same treatment in the same place? The boom in private insurance was clearly over and there were already complaints from some consultants about falling income from private practice. The number of individual policy holders fell from a peak of 1,457,000 in 1996 to a low of 1,175,000 in 2003, with a very slight rise the following year,[86] while the number covered by corporate schemes for employees remained steady. In total, some 7,500,000 people were still covered by some form of health care insurance. Future trends in these figures will provide a sensitive barometer of public perceptions of the Government's success or otherwise.

The most long-standing use of private resources for public purposes remained, however, the Private Finance Initiative: using private finance to build hospitals. Inherited from the Conservatives and embraced in 1997 – if only because the money invested did not swell the Chancellor of the Exchequer's borrowing requirements – a large PFI programme followed. But by 2005 there were signs of disillusionment.[87] Some PFI funded trusts were running into financial trouble; a flagship PFI project in London was abandoned. Most important of all, though, there was a growing awareness of policy dissonance: different streams of

Government policy were not running in the same direction. On the one hand, PFI projects usually assumed a 30-year life expectancy and committed the trust concerned to paying for the capital cost over the same period. On the other hand, Government policy was increasingly directed to promoting new initiatives such as ICTs and out-of-hospital care. In a fast-changing NHS, PFI funded hospitals threatened to lock the service into a pattern of delivery that was becoming obsolete. Yesterday's policy solution had – not for the first time – become tomorrow's policy problem.

The State and the profession

In the controversies about the transformation of the NHS in the new millennium, there was one significant absentee: the medical profession. Most of the opposition came from within the Labour Party, as in the case of Foundation Trusts. Not that all was harmony in the relations between the Government and the profession. The profession clashed with Government policy on issues that affected it directly, notably pay. But while Mrs Thatcher's introduction of the internal market had provoked an all-out confrontation between the Government and doctors (*see* Chapter 6), the reinvention of that model by New Labour produced scarcely more than an occasional whimper. What explains this puzzle? One reason might be that by brushing aside the profession's opposition, Mrs Thatcher had also convinced it of the futility of battling governments on matters of high politics. Another explanation might be that the profession had realised that the Conservative reforms had not produced the predicted disaster and had indeed brought benefits, like fundholding, to its members: the experience may therefore have acted as a kind of vaccination against the shock of new ideas. Again, the metamorphosis of the NHS under New Labour was a gradual, step-by-step process, as we have seen, providing little opportunity for a confrontation on the principles underlying the model that finally emerged. The fact that New Labour's 'tectonic' policy shift took place at a time when extra billions were flowing into the NHS no doubt also helped to ease, if not to dispel, any reservations the profession might have had.

Further, the Labour Government took pains to win the support of the medical profession for its policies. To the extent that those policies were directed at promoting new patterns of practice and service provision in the NHS, so the support of doctors (among others) was seen as essential. Ministers therefore made determined efforts to engage the medical profession in the process of change. As we have already seen, various medical dignitaries were involved in the preparation of *The National Plan* in 2000. Subsequently, too, Ministers looked to leaders of the profession to lead the process of change. For example, in 2002 Sir George Alberti – a former President of the Royal College of Physicians – was appointed to lead a programme of action designed to improve emergency services.[88] However, the relationship remained a see-saw one, with periods of co-operation followed by periods of friction. Two sets of issues, in particular, were calculated to sour the atmosphere. The first was the always contentious topic of pay. The other was the accountability of doctors, both individually and collectively.

Negotiating a new GP contract was, for once, a relatively undramatic affair. It started with the BMA in an aggressive mood, demanding a new contract. Negotiations were ostensibly conducted by the NHS Confederation, the NHS employers to whom the Department of Health had delegated responsibility for pay bargaining, but with close involvement by Ministers and officials. They ended with a complex deal which appeared to give something to both sides.[89] On the one hand, the BMA achieved one of its main objectives: to end the open-ended commitment of GPs to look after their patients and to limit the hours they worked and the services they provided. In future, for example, PCTs would be responsible for providing weekend services and home visits at night, if practices chose not to take responsibility. On the other hand, the Department of Health could claim that it had negotiated a contract that rewarded quality. The new contract linked pay to 76 indicators, ranging from the quality of the practice's written record to the proportion of patients whose blood pressure has been recorded. In a ballot 75.8 per cent of GPs voted in favour of the new contract, conditional on the pricing being acceptable. In the event the pricing was found to be acceptable. Indeed the deal turned out to be a great deal more expensive than the Department of Health had reckoned.[90] The incentives worked, all too well. The earnings of GPs soared: the cost of implementing the new contract rose from £5.8 billion in 2003/4 to £7.5 billion in 2005/6. More GPs than expected reached the quality standards, suggesting either that these were set too low or that the incentives offered were too generous. Peace with the BMA had been expensively bought but at least Ministers could argue that the new contract framework gave them scope to adapt it to their goals in future.

In contrast, negotiations with the consultants proved stormy. Here the Department of Health had two objectives. The first was to strengthen managerial control, by defining the responsibilities of consultants more precisely. The second was to limit the time spent by consultants on private practice, particularly by obliging newly appointed consultants to work full time for the NHS for seven years (Ministers had earlier considered buying out the right to private practice but rejected this option as too expensive). In the event, neither goal was achieved: 'The Department was shafted', as one policy-maker put it when reflecting on the conduct of negotiations by officials. Conversely, from the BMA perspective, 'It was like taking candy from a baby' in the words of one of its representatives.

The negotiations took place over two rounds. In the first round, the consultant leadership agreed to a contract that would have given the Government at least something in return for the extra money it was proposing to spend. Not for the first time, the leadership was overwhelmingly repudiated by the rank and file in England (though not Scotland and Wales). One consultant, in calling on his colleagues to reject the contract, called it 'a charter of enslavement'.[91] Milburn initially refused to renegotiate. However, the risks of all-out confrontation were judged to be too great, and eventually a revised contract was negotiated. The restrictions on new consultants were dropped. Above all, consultants were not to be subject to 'the excessive and inappropriate managerial control' that had been the 'major sticking point' in the original contract, to quote Dr Paul Miller, Chairman of the BMA's Consultants' Committee.[92] Under the new deal, there would be a more relaxed regime: 'the focus would be', he pointed out, on 'joint planning where consultants and managers work out what needs to be done'. A majority of consultants voted in favour of acceptance and the new contract was implemented in 2004.[93]

Like GPs, consultants did well financially out of the new contract. Their salaries rose by 15 per cent and, in some cases, considerably more. Like other employees of the NHS, they were the beneficiaries of a more open-handed attitude bred of the extra billions pouring into the service. And the new contracts reinforced the position of NHS doctors as among the best paid in Europe relative to the earnings of the rest of the population.[94] But in neither of the contract negotiations was money, as we have seen, the only currency of dispute. In the case of GPs, their aim was to win more freedom to arrange their working lives as they wished. In the case of consultants, their aim was to resist 'excessive and inappropriate managerial control'. In short, the argument was as much about accountability as about pay.

There was, in the first place, the accountability of individual consultants for the resources they used. Were they accountable to the managers? The dividing line between clinical judgements (which everyone agreed was an exclusively medical prerogative) and resource-use judgements (where managers might well claim a say) was often difficult to draw. With managers under ever-increasing pressure to achieve the targets set centrally, some of the pressure inevitably spilled over into the medical domain. Hence the complaints from consultants, noted above, that they had been forced to subordinate clinical priorities to the achievement of waiting-list targets: treating patients at the top of the list rather than patients with the greatest clinical need. There were other factors which helped to explain why doctors felt both over-worked and under-appreciated.[95] For example, a European Union work directive, limiting the number of hours that could be worked by doctors in training, meant that consultants had to carry extra responsibilities. But running through the complaints was one theme: loss of control following on from a more demanding system of accountability. Clinical discretion was being circumscribed by NICE guidance; medical autonomy was threatened by audit and annual reviews of practice under the evolving system of clinical governance monitored by the CHI.

Collectively, too, the medical profession was under pressure to strengthen the machinery of accountability (*see* previous chapter). The pressure increased following the Kennedy report's diagnosis of a failure in the profession's own system of self-regulation. The General Medical Council, pushed by the Government (at one stage Ministers had even thought about abolishing the GMC) and pulled by medical radicals like Sir Donald Irvine, reformed itself. The transformed GMC, which took office in July 2003, was much reduced in size with a much higher proportion of lay members: the latter rose from 25 per cent to 40 per cent of the total membership. It set about reforming its disciplinary procedures and introducing a system of revalidation: the notion that doctors would periodically be required to demonstrate their continued competence to remain on the medical register. Further, the Government set up a Council for Health Care Regulatory Excellence, whose remit was to review the performance of all professional self-regulatory bodies in the health care field: so, for example, it could (and did) review the disciplinary decisions of the GMC – as of the other bodies – and refer them to the High Court if it considered the regulator's decision to be unduly lenient.

Nor has the story of collective medical self-regulation yielding, step by step, to the State's demands for ever-tighter accountability to the public ended. In 2005 the issue was again put on the agenda. Just as the Bristol case had prompted the catalytic Kennedy Inquiry, so the case of the murderous GP, Dr Harold Shipman, had prompted another, equally ambitious inquiry. This was led by Dame Janet

Smith who, following a series of reports on various aspects of the case and after taking 2,500 witness statements that filled 270,000 pages of evidence, in 2004 eventually published her conclusions on the role of the GMC.[96] These were damning. Despite the many improvements in its procedures, she argued, the GMC had not changed its culture: the balance was still weighted towards protecting the profession rather than the public. The leopard, she remarked, had not changed its spots. Ranging well beyond the issues raised directly by the Shipman case – where she cleared the GMC of any direct blame – she made two radical recommendations, as well as proposing some fine tuning in the disciplinary system. The number of GMC members elected by the profession should be cut; the proposed system of revalidation was not demanding enough and required toughening up. And indeed the GMC's system of revalidation represented a watered-down version of what had initially been conceived, the result largely of pressure from the BMA: evidence once again that the medical profession often seeks to regain lost ground in the process of implementation.

The Shipman Inquiry's report led, in turn, to the appointment of a committee to inquire into the future of professional self-regulation. This was headed by the Chief Medical Officer, Sir Liam Donaldson. His report's 44 recommendations[97] imply a radical transformation of professional accountability. The GMC's composition and role would change. None of its members would be elected by the profession (so much for professional *self*-regulation) and it would lose its judicial role to an independent tribunal and its control of medical education. At the same time, the GMC and the Royal Colleges would become responsible for developing 'clear unambiguous and operationalised standards' to be incorporated into NHS contracts with doctors and the annual assessment process; specialist certification would be reviewed every five years against those standards. Implementation of these proposals will be contentious, but clearly the medical profession will have to accept further, perhaps unpalatable, changes.

Reorganising yet again

Although the focus of policy switched from anatomy to physiology in the new millennium, this did not stop the 'cycle of perpetual change', as the House of Commons Health Committee termed it,[98] in the organisational structure of the NHS and the Department of Health. There was perhaps one difference from the past. Structural change was the by-product of the transformation of the NHS rather than being seen as a driver of that transformation. With the balance of roles changing – as between the Department and the regulators, between centre and periphery – so it was inevitable that there would be organisational reform as well. As policy changed, so did the organisation.

In 2001 Alan Milburn announced far-reaching changes in the management structure of the NHS as part of his new commitment to shifting 'the centre of gravity to the NHS front line'.[99] The NHS, he acknowledged, was seen as 'top heavy' by PCTs and trusts; the lines of accountability were confused, with trusts reporting to the Department's regional offices and PCTs reporting to health authorities. Accordingly, the 95 health authorities were to be replaced by 28 strategic health authorities, responsible for the performance management of both trusts and PCTs. At the same time, the NHS Executive and its eight regional offices were to be abolished: there were still to be Regional Directors for Health and Social Care, but they would no longer be a link in the chain of accountability.

By 2003 these changes had been implemented. Two years later, however, came another round of reorganisation designed to reflect the fact that the NHS was moving 'from being a provider-driven service to a commissioning-driven service'.[100] PCTs were to be 'reconfigured', i.e. amalgamated. Their number was to be reduced from 302 to about a third of that figure – the precise outcome depending on local consultations and the views of the Independent Reconfiguration Panel. The new PCTs were to be, as near as possible, coterminous with the boundaries of local authority social services: an echo of one of the preoccupations that had shaped the 1974 reorganisation of the NHS (*see* Chapter 3). Strategic health authorities, too, were expected to follow the path of amalgamation, with the aim of shrinking their number to eight or so: what looked remarkably like the reinvention of the regional offices that had been abolished earlier.

In proposing the amalgamation of PCTs, Ministers were in effect endorsing the widespread view that these were – with few exceptions – not up to the tasks set for them in the new, patient-driven NHS. Not only were PCTs responsible for controlling the total budget, even while devolving the commissioning process to GP practices and their patients, but they were also the custodians of the local population's health, charged with improving the health of the community and reducing health inequalities (*see* next section). One solution, Ministers thought, would be for PCTs to divest themselves of the community services for which they were responsible – by contracting with independent providers – in order to concentrate on their commissioning role. But, in any case, larger PCTs would be managerially more effective. It was not an argument which convinced the House of Commons Health Committee: its report on the Government's proposals, quoted above, was highly critical. There was little or no evidence, the Committee pointed out, that size correlated with effectiveness in commissioning, while larger PCTs would be more remote from their populations. Many of the intended benefits could be achieved by a process of gradual evolution, without yet another 'hugely disruptive' restructuring. And the Committee was deeply sceptical of the Department of Health's claim that reconfiguration would cut administrative costs by £250 million.

The last point introduces another theme of Government policy, one first developed in 1997 and consistently reiterated subsequently. This was the theme of saving money by cutting bureaucracy, invoked in support of all organisational changes. This persistent emphasis on administrative parsimony was somewhat at odds with New Labour's equally consistent enthusiasm for creating new agencies, among them NICE and the Healthcare Commission. By 2003/4 there were 38 such 'arm's length bodies' (departmental agencies with varying degrees of independence) – some inherited, many newly created – employing 25,000 people at a cost of £1.8 billion a year. A cull followed that reduced their number to 20.[101] It was a combination of forced marriages for some and euthanasia for others: for example, the Healthcare Commission, among others, took on extra responsibilities while the recently created Commission for Patient and Public Involvement was axed. Not only would it ease this regulatory confusion and burdens, the Government claimed, but it would save £500 million a year. As with the other organisational changes, there was no attempt to quantify the costs – as distinct from the benefits – of the consequent redundancy payments and disruption.

In all this, the Department of Health led by example. In 1997, the Department had a core staff of 4,000. By 2004, this figure had been cut in half. In part, of course, this was a statistical illusion: some of the reduction was the result of transferring staff to arm's length agencies. In the main, however, the cuts accurately reflected the changing role of the Department: its abandonment of the command-and-control model, the retreat from the supervision of front-line operations and the reliance on regulators. But if the Department was clear that it had changed its role, it was less clear about how best to organise itself to perform that role. The 'cycle of perpetual change' characterised the Department itself as it continued to experiment with various organisational permutations. In 2004, it switched from 14 directorates to a streamlined structure of three business groups. In January 2006 the cards were shuffled again, with a series of new appointments to an enlarged Departmental Board.[102] Given the continued contraction in numbers and organisational instability, the Department's institutional memory began to decay: those who could not remember the past were at risk of repeating its mistakes. Ministers were even heard lamenting the loss of traditional civil servant expertise – like policy analysis – in a Department where graduates from NHS management had come to occupy many of the top positions, including that of chief executive. With management consultants once again called in, further changes seemed inevitable.

In all this, did the Government succeed in achieving its overall 1997 goal of cutting bureaucracy? As a proportion of the total NHS budget, management costs fell from 5 per cent in 1997/8 to 3.8 per cent in 2003/4. But this was because the total budget had gone up sharply not because spending on management had been cut: in fact, it rose from £1,728 million to £2,387 million over the same period,[103] excluding the administrative costs of the various regulators and arm's length bodies. So the Government could claim a qualified success in cutting the costs of bureaucracy in the Department and the NHS: a conclusion which, however, begged the more interesting question of whether it was a more effective machinery for devising and delivering policy as a result.

On this score, there was scope for scepticism. At the turn of 2005 the NHS found itself in a familiar situation. With the end of the fiscal year approaching, the NHS's auditors warned that it was overspending its budget. Overall the threatened over-spend – some £500 million, though estimates fluctuated month by month – was small change in the NHS's multi-billion budget. However, it was heavily concentrated in a minority of PCTs and trusts. As these struggled to balance their books, there was en epidemic of headlines about delayed operations and cuts in staff and services.[104] Such end-of-fiscal-year crises were far from new in the history of the NHS. What was new, and highly embarrassing for Ministers, was that the delays and cuts were taking place at a time when extra billions were flowing into the NHS. Ministers squarely put responsibility on the managers of the trusts and PCTs in trouble: 'turn-around teams' were sent out by the Department of Health to sort out their finances. Managers blamed the Government for introducing badly costed pay schemes and imposing over-rigid targets.[105] And in March 2006 Sir Nigel Crisp took early retirement from his combined post of Chief Executive and Permanent Secretary, a casualty of fiscal turbulence and the consequent recrimination. The spectacle was not calculated to induce confidence in the way the NHS was run.

Nor did the evidence of policy incoherence. Only consider the much-trumpeted

White Paper published in January 2006,[106] announcing 'a radical and sustained shift in the way services are delivered'. Much was not new, but expanded on the Government's long-standing commitment to shifting the balance of care from expensive hospital care to more accessible community services. Nothing was said, however, about the implications for trusts committed to expensive and long-term PFI schemes, whose financial viability might well be threatened if the promised 'radical and sustained shift' were to cut demand for their services. Further, the White Paper announced the introduction of 'incentives to GP practices to offer opening times and convenient appointments' in order to promote accessibility and choice. Yet such incentives were required chiefly because a few years earlier the Department of Health had negotiated a contract that allowed GPs to limit opening times to suit their convenience rather than that of patients.

In short, the impression was of a Department which appeared to be more anxious to satisfy the desire of Ministers to achieve politically salient targets and to launch new initiatives than to ensure that the various policy goals fitted together in a coherent pattern: hyperactivity claiming its own price. The pathology of the traditional Whitehall culture, as many Ministers saw it, was that it put more emphasis on analysis than on drive, so often frustrating their ambitions to change the world. The pathology of the new Whitehall can-do culture of delivery – a transformation that started under Mrs Thatcher and continued under Tony Blair – may turn out to be that it does not frustrate Ministers often enough. The risk is that when policies disappoint, this will be seen as failure of delivery rather than of design – so that the question of whether, in the first place, they were compatible with other goals and realistic in the means chosen is never asked.

Beyond the Department of Health

In one respect, continuity rather than change was the hallmark of Government policy in the post-2000 era. New Labour, like Old Labour, remained committed to reducing health inequalities and improving population health (*see* previous chapter). And this commitment was reiterated in a succession of policy documents and initiatives in the new millennium. Exploring this policy theme underlines, however, the limits of the Department of Health's role. Most of the levers for bringing about improvements lay outside the direct control of the Secretary of State for Health: they were in the hands either of other government departments or of local agencies which could be prompted but not compelled to act.

In 2001 the Secretary of State announced a target for reducing health inequalities: by 2010 the social class gap in health outcomes, as measured by infant mortality and life expectancy at birth, was to be cut by 10 per cent. From the start, it was recognised that a complex challenge required a co-ordinated programme of action across government.[107] A set of 12 national indicators was developed to monitor progress on each of the components of the programme.[108] A third fell clearly within the remit of the Department of Health: reducing smoking prevalence, increasing the uptake of influenza vaccinations, improving access to primary care, and reducing mortality from cancer and circulatory diseases in areas with poorer outcomes than the rest of the population. The others did not. These included: the proportion of children living in low-income households and the proportion of households living in 'non-decent housing', the rate of decline in road accident casualties in disadvantaged communities, the proportion of people in the lowest quintile of income distribution consuming five or more portions of fruit and vegetables per day, and the percentage of schoolchildren getting five GCSE qualifications at 16 and spending a minimum of two hours a week 'on high quality PE'.

The Department of Health, in turn, translated the national indicators within its remit into targets for PCTs and trusts. But could it (or they) be held answerable for the achievement of the national target of reducing inequalities by 10 per cent by 2010? Clearly not: too many others were involved. Experience of the Joined Approach to Social Policy initiative in the late 1970s, i.e. collaboration between different departments nationally and different agencies locally, had suggested that success could not be taken for granted.[109] So it proved again 25 years later, when the experiment was repeated under the label of 'joined-up government'. A study of the first years of the local implementation of the inequalities project found that it was 'hampered by deficiencies in performance management, insufficient integration between policy sectors, and contradictions between health inequalities and other policy streams'.[110] Faced with a plethora of priorities, local NHS managers put achieving hard targets such as reducing waiting times before softer targets such as reducing inequalities; similarly, other local agencies were primarily concerned with the policy imperatives of their sponsoring departments. Subsequently, pressure increased on both PCTs and local authorities to move the inequalities project up their list of priorities: so, for example, PCTs were required to carry out health equity audits. However, the ability of the Department of Health to steer local priorities remained limited. Only in matters falling exclusively under its remit could the Department act decisively. So, for example, the Department adapted its resource allocation methods to accelerate the process of bringing PCTs in deprived areas up to target. Even so, the 10 PCTs most below target were overwhelmingly in deprived areas, while the 10 PCTs most above target included a high proportion of better-off areas.[111] Overall, progress across the 12 national indicators was slow. But there was one important exception: there had been a significant improvement in child poverty between 1997 and 2005.[112] Here the key player was the Treasury and not the Department of Health, a reminder that it is easier to implement policies that involve money transfers than policies that involve changes in organisational behaviour or service delivery.

Much the same story can be told about policies for improving the population's health: here, too, there was a multiplicity of policy actors involved in devising and implementing a complex programme under conditions of uncertainty about what would work. In 2002 the Wanless report, as we have seen, had underlined the economic case for improving the population's health – and its use of health services – if demands on the NHS were to be restrained. In February 2004, he produced a further report[113] analysing the challenges involved and the policy tools available. Two aspects of this Wanless report are particularly relevant for our analysis of Government policy. First, there is the report's stress on ignorance and uncertainty. While there had been many interesting innovations in the field of health prevention and promotion – and the report gave many examples – their cost-effectiveness had not been evaluated for the most part. Absent such evidence, policy-makers could not know where best to put their money. The second is the report's review of the many different types of policy options with a bearing on the population's health. As in the case of health inequalities, these quite predictably ranged across the whole spectrum of Government activity: from tax policy to the regulation of advertising, from the installation of cycle lanes to the provision of free fruit in schools.

Six months later the Government produced its own White Paper,[114] mirroring much of the Wanless analysis. The White Paper appeared to be the product of a Whitehall trawl where all Departments were asked what they were doing to improve health or prevent disease; with only a little ingenuity, these were able to present many of their existing projects (such as encouraging flexible working hours or establishing the Cycle Training Reference Group) under the new rubric. And while the resulting picture of a Government buzzing with enthusiasm for initiatives to improve health may have been over-drawn, the exercise did underline yet again the fact that the Department of Health was only one player among many in achieving the Government's goal. In some areas of policy, the Department did have the key role. It was the Department which introduced legislation to stop smoking in public places. It was the Department which negotiated a contract with GPs that rewarded preventive medicine. It was the Department which introduced health trainers, accredited by the NHS, to advise and support people in deprived areas in the search for a healthier lifestyle. And so on. But enhancing people's ability to choose a healthier lifestyle (the White Paper's main theme) depended on two sets of factors outside the Department's control. To the extent that the ability to choose depends on income, so the Treasury's decisions about the distribution of income are crucial.[115] And to the extent that choice is shaped by what is on the shelves, so the Departments which determined licensing hours for the sale of alcohol or the salt content of food become crucial. In both cases the actors in the NHS policy arena are, for the most part, little more than spectators: they may well advise, but they do not decide. As the scope of Government policy-making expands, so does the set of actors involved: for example, new, powerful commercial interests come into play. So does a new set of political considerations: for example, worries about the level and incidence of taxation and arguments about the extent to which the State can or should interfere with the people's pleasures. In effect, the politics of the NHS end when the politics of population health begin.

References

1. See, for example, Julian Le Grand, *Motivation, Agency and Public Policy*, Oxford UP: Oxford 2003. Le Grand was subsequently to become Tony Blair's policy adviser. For a sceptical view of the new ideas, see Theodore Marmor, *Fads in Medical Care Management and Policy*, The Nuffield Trust: London 2004.
2. Sally Ruane, 'The Future of Healthcare in the UK: Think Tanks and their Policy Prescriptions', in Martin Powell, Linda Bauld and Karen Clarke (eds), *Analysis and Debate in Social Policy, 2005*, Social Policy Review No.17, The Policy Press: Bristol 2005, p. 159.
3. Pre-Budget Report Statement to the House of Commons delivered by the Rt. Hon. Gordon Brown MP, Chancellor of the Exchequer, HM Treasury: London December 2005.
4. The 2001 figures come from a poll conducted by MORI for *The Economist* between 10 May and 14 May 2001; the 2005 figures from a poll conducted by MORI for *The Evening Standard* between 7 April and 11 April 2005. See: www.mori.com.

5. *Ambitions for Britain*, The Labour Party: London 2001.
6. *Time for Common Sense*, The Conservative Party: London 2001.
7. *Britain Forward, Not Back*, The Labour Party: London 2005.
8. *Are You Thinking What We're Thinking?* The Conservative Party: London 2005.
9. Sam Coates, 'Cameron Breaks with Thatcherite Past in About-turn over Health Policy', *The Times*, 2 Jan. 2006, p. 7.
10. The indignant protester making the headlines was Sharron Storer. See James Landsdale, 'Blair Taken to Task by Cancer Woman', *The Times*, 17 May 2001, p. 13.
11. Anthony Seldon, *Blair*, Free Press: London 2005, pp. 630–1.
12. Secretary of State for Health, *The NHS Plan*, The Stationery Office: London 2000, Cm. 4818.
13. Interview with Alan Milburn cited in Brian Edwards and Margaret Fall, *The Executive Years of the NHS*, Radcliffe Publishing: Oxford 2005, p. 170.
14. 'A National Plan for a National Health Service: Five Teams to Focus on NHS Challenges', Press Release, Department of Health: London 23 March 2000.
15. Department of Health, *Health Reform in England: Update and Next Steps*, DoH: London December 2005.
16. Patricia Hewitt, Annual Health and Social Lecture, London School of Economics, 13 Dec. 2005, DoH: London 2005.
17. Secretary of State for Health, *Delivering the NHS Plan*, The Stationery Office: London 2002, Cm. 5503.
18. Department of Health, *Practice-based Commissioning*, DoH: London October 2004.
19. Secretary of State for Health, *The NHS Improvement Plan*, The Stationery Office: London 2004, Cm. 6268.
20. Simon Stevens, 'Reform Strategies for the English NHS', *Health Affairs*, vol. 23, no. 3, May/June 2004, pp. 17–43. This account by one of the architects of policy, as adviser successively to the Secretary of State for Health and the Prime Minister, provides an illuminating if somewhat over-tidy account of the successive stages in the reform programme.
21. Trevor Jackson, 'Coming Up Roses', *British Medical Journal*, vol. 324, 2 Feb. 2002, p. 306.
22. Chris Ham, 'From Targets to Standards: But Not Just Yet', *British Medical Journal*, vol. 330, 15 Jan. 2005, pp. 106–7.
23. Stevens, op. cit., p. 43.
24. Alan Milburn, 'Redefining the National Health Service', Speech to the New Health Network, 15 January 2002, DoH: London; 'Shifting the Balance of Power in the NHS', Speech at the Launch of the Modernisation Agency, 25 April 2001, DoH: London.
25. Derek Wanless, *Securing our Future Health: Taking a Long-term View*, Interim Report, HM Treasury: London 2001.
26. Derek Wanless, *Securing our Future Health: Taking a Long-term View*, Final Report, HM Treasury: London 2002.
27. Clive Smee, *Speaking Truth to Power*, Radcliffe Publishing: Oxford 2005. Smee's account of the Wanless Inquiry is drawn on in what follows.
28. Strategy Unit, *Health Strategy Review: Analytical Report*, 27 June 2002, www.cabinet office.gov.uk.
29. Smee, op. cit., pp. 62–5.
30. Office of National Statistics, *Public Service Productivity: Health*, ONS: London October 2004.
31. House of Commons Health Committee, *Department of Health Written Evidence to the Committee*, The Stationery Office: London 2005, HC 736-lll.
32. Sir Nigel Crisp, *Chief Executive's Report to the NHS*, DoH: London December 2005.
33. Department of Health, *Healthcare Output and Productivity: Accounting for Quality Changes*,

DoH: London December 2005. See also Phillip Lee, *Public Service Productivity: Health*, Office for National Statistics: London February 2006. This gave the results of using different methodologies – and incorporating quality measures – for calculating NHS productivity. Depending on the assumptions made, NHS productivity either fell by 1.5 per cent or rose by 1.6 per cent a year between 1999 and 2004 (with other methods producing figures in between these extremes).

34. The illustrative example used is the 2003 exercise: Commission for Health Improvement, *NHS Performance Ratings for 2002/2003*, Commission for Health Improvement: London 2003.

35. Department of Health, *Departmental Report, 2005*, The Stationery Office: London 2005, Cm. 6524, p. 65.

36. Neil Carter, Rudolf Klein and Patricia Day, *How Organisations Measure Success*, Routledge: London 1992.

37. For a balance sheet of the strengths and weaknesses of the star rating and target-setting strategy, see Gwyn Bevan and Christopher Hood, 'Have Targets Improved Performance in the English NHS?', *British Medical Journal*, vol. 332, 18 Feb. 2006, pp. 419–22.

38. House of Commons Public Administration Select Committee, *On Target? Government By Measurement*, The Stationery Office: London 2003, HC 62-1.

39. Royal Statistical Society Working Party on Performance Monitoring in the Public Services, *Performance Indicators: Good, Bad and Ugly*, Royal Statistical Society: London 2004.

40. Audit Commission, *Achieving the NHS Plan*, Audit Commission: London 2003.

41. Alan Milburn, 'Shifting the Balance of Power in the NHS', Speech at the Launch of the Modernisation Agency, DoH: London 25 April 2001.

42. Comptroller and Auditor-General, *Inappropriate Adjustments to NHS Waiting-lists*, The Stationery Office: London 2001, HC 452.

43. Audit Commission, *Waiting-list Accuracy*, Audit Commission: London 2003.

44. The phrase is that of Ken Jarrold, a former member of the NHS Executive and chief executive of a strategic health authority. Cited in Jeremy Davies, 'NHS Held Back by Lack of Strategy, Veteran Warns', *Health Service Journal*, 24 November 2005, www.hsj.co.uk. My comments also draw on my experience over several years when lecturing to chief executives attending Lancaster University's annual leadership course: a dispirited, low morale group if ever there was one.

45. Department of Health, *Departmental Report, Expenditure Plans 2002–03 to 2003–04*, The Stationery Office: London 2002, Cm. 5403.

46. Department of Health, *Departmental Report, 2005*, The Stationery Office: London 2005, Cm. 6524.

47. Lin Bauld, Ken Judge, Marian Barnes, Michaela Benzeval, Mhairi Mackenzie and Helen Sullivan, 'Promoting Social Change: The Experience of Health Action Zones in England', *Journal of Social Policy*, vol. 34, no. 3, 2005, pp. 427–45. For a fuller account, see Marian Barnes, Linda Bauld, Michaela Benzeval, Ken Judge, Mhairi Mackenzie and Helen Sullivan, *Health Action Zones*, Routledge: London 2005.

48. Chris Ham, Ruth Kipping and Hugh McLeod, 'Redesigning Work Processes in Health Care: Lessons from the National Health Service', *The Milbank Quarterly*, vol. 81, no. 3, 2003, pp. 415–39.

49. Naomi Fulop, Gerasimos Protopsaltis, Andrew Hutchings *et al.*, 'Process and Impact of Mergers of NHS Trusts: Multicentre Case Study and Management Cost Analysis', *British Medical Journal*, vol. 325, 3 Aug. 2002, pp. 246–9.

50. Healthcare Commission, *Investigation into Mid Yorkshire Hospitals NHS Trust*, Healthcare Commission: London 2004.

51. Healthcare Commission, *Acute Hospital Portfolio Review: Accident and Emergency*, Healthcare Commission: London August 2005.

52. Healthcare Commission, *Acute Hospital Portfolio Review: Day Surgery*, Healthcare Commission: London July 2005.
53. Healthcare Commission, *A Snapshot of Hospital Cleanliness in England*, Healthcare Commission: London December 2005.
54. For a general review of the growth of regulation, see Christopher Hood, Colin Scott, Oliver James, George Jones and Tony Travers, *Regulation Inside Government*, Oxford UP: Oxford 1999; for a review of regulation in health care, see Kieran Walshe, *Regulating Healthcare*, Open University Press: Maidenhead 2003.
55. Department of Health, *A Guide to NHS Foundation Trusts*, DoH: London December 2002.
56. Patricia Day and Rudolf Klein, *Governance of Foundation Trusts: Dilemmas of Diversity*, The Nuffield Trust: London 2005.
57. Alan Milburn, Speech on NHS Foundation Trust, 22 May 2002, DoH: London 2002.
58. Patricia Day and Rudolf Klein, *The NHS Improvers: A Study of the Commission for Health Improvement*, King's Fund: London 2004.
59. Ian Kennedy, *Learning from Bristol: The Report of the Public Inquiry into Children's Heart Surgery at the Bristol Royal Infirmary 1984–1995*, The Stationery Office: London, Cm. 5207.
60. Secretary of State for Health, *Learning from Bristol: The Department of Health's Response to the Report of the Public Inquiry into Children's Heart Surgery at the Bristol Royal Infirmary*, The Stationery Office: London 2002, Cm. 5363.
61. Department of Health, *National Standards, Local Action*, DoH: London 2004.
62. Charles D Shaw, 'Standards for Better Health: Fit for Purpose?', *British Medical Journal*, vol. 329, 27 November 2004, pp. 1250–1.
63. Healthcare Commission, *Our Progress: One Year On*, Healthcare Commission: London December 2005.
64. Healthcare Commission, *Assessment for Improvement: Understanding the Standards*, Healthcare Commission: London 2004.
65. Mary-Louise Harding, 'Hewitt, Herceptin and the £100m Bill PCTs Can't Afford to Pay', *Health Service Journal*, 8 Dec. 2005, www.hsj.co.uk.
66. Trevor A Sheldon, Nick Cullum, Diane Dawson *et al.*, 'What's the Evidence that NICE Guidance has been Implemented?', *British Medical Journal*, vol. 329, 30 Oct. 2004, pp. 999–1003.
67. Audit Commission, *Managing the Financial Implications of NICE Guidance*, Audit Commission: London September 2005.
68. Secretary of State for Health, 2002, op. cit., p. 19.
69. Secretary of State for Health, *Working for Patients*, HMSO: London 1989, Cm. 555, p. 33.
70. Audit Commission, *Introducing Payment by Results*, Audit Commission: London 2004.
71. Simon Stevens, 'On Regulation', *Health Service Journal*, 17 February 2005, p. 19.
72. Audit Commission, *Early Lessons from Payment by Results*, Audit Commission: London 2005.
73. Department of Health, *Practice-based Commissioning*, DoH: London October 2004.
74. Chris Ham, 'Does the District General Hospital Have a Future?', *British Medical Journal*, vol. 331, 3 Dec. 2005, pp. 1331–3.
75. Secretary of State for Health, 2000, op. cit., p. 94.
76. Daniel Martin, 'Public Flexes its Muscles on Health Care Outside Hospital', *Health Service Journal*, 10 Nov. 2005, pp. 12–13.
77. Albert Weale, *Political Theory and Social Policy*, Macmillan: London 1983.
78. Cited in Public Administration Select Committee, *Choice, Voice and Public Services*, The Stationery Office: London 2005, HC 49, p. 18.
79. MORI, Patient Choice: Final Topline Results, 1 February 2005, www.mori.com.
80. Department of Health, *For the Benefit of Patients*, DoH: London October 2000.

81. Nicholas Timmins, 'Use of Private Health Care in the NHS', *British Medical Journal*, vol. 331, 12 Nov. 2005, pp. 1141–2; Nicholas Timmins, 'Challenges of Private Provision in the NHS', *British Medical Journal*, vol. 331, 19 Nov. 2005, pp. 1193–5. What follows draws on these articles.

82. John Carvel, 'US Health Giant to Run GP Practices as Hewitt Looks for Competition', *The Guardian*, 13 Jan. 2006.

83. Tom Smith, 'The Early Experience of NHS Commissioning of Independent Provision', *Health Policy Review*, vol. 1, no. 1, Autumn 2005, pp. 36–51.

84. Laing & Buisson, *Market Analysis of the Independent Healthcare Sector in England*, A report prepared for the Healthcare Commission, Laing & Buisson: London May 2005.

85. NERA Economic Consulting, 'Cross-country Comparison of Specialist Fees, 2002', NERA: London December 2003.

86. Laing & Buisson, 'Individual PMI Demand Holds Firm in 2004', Press Release, Laing & Buisson: London 21 July 2005.

87. Rifat A Atun and Martin McKee, 'Is the Private Finance Initiative Dead?', *British Medical Journal*, vol. 331, 8 Oct. 2005, pp. 792–3. See also 'Buildings – PFI Special Report', *Health Service Journal*, 26 Jan. 2006, www.hsj.co.uk.

88. 'Sir George Alberti Appointed National Clinical Director for Emergency Access', Department of Health Press Release, 10 Sept. 2002.

89. British Medical Association, *Your Contract, Your Future*, BMA: London April 2002.

90. House of Commons Health Committee, 2005, op. cit., Table 1.2.3.

91. Jonathan D Beard, 'What About Consultants in Front-line Specialties?', *British Medical Journal*, vol. 325, 7 Sept. 2002, p. 546.

92. Zosia Kmietowicz, 'Consultants Vote in Favour of a Revised Contract', *British Medical Journal*, vol. 327, 25 Oct. 2003, p. 945.

93. For a critical review of both the new GP and the new consultant contracts, see Alan Maynard and Karen Bloor, 'Do Those Who Pay the Piper Call the Tune?', *Health Policy Matters*, Issue 8, Oct. 2003. Their answer to the question of the title is 'no'.

94. Organisation for Economic Co-operation and Development, *Health at a Glance*, OECD: Paris 2005, Chart 2.9, p. 43. The level of remuneration is calculated as a ratio to GDP per capita.

95. Richard Smith, 'Why are Doctors so Unhappy?', *British Medical Journal*, vol. 322, 5 May 2001, pp. 1073–4. See also Chris Ham and KGMM Alberti, 'The Medical Profession, the Public and the Government', *British Medical Journal*, vol. 324, 6 April 2002, pp. 838–41.

96. Dame Janet Smith, *Safeguarding Patients, Lessons from the Past – Proposals for the Future*, Fifth Report of the Shipman Inquiry, The Stationery Office: London 2004, Cm. 6394.

97. Sir Liam Donaldson, *Good Doctors, Safer Patients: A report by the Chief Medical Officer*. Department of Health: London July 2006.

98. House of Commons Health Committee, *Changes to Primary Care Trusts*, The Stationery Office: London 2006, HC 646.

99. Alan Milburn, 25 April 2001, op. cit.

100. Sir Nigel Crisp, *Commissioning a Patient-led NHS*, Circular to all NHS Chief Executives, DoH: London 28 July 2005.

101. Department of Health, *Reconfiguring the Department of Health's Arm's Length Bodies*, DoH: London July 2004.

102. Department of Health, *Transition Arrangements in the NHS and the Department of Health*, Special Bulletin, DoH: London 26 January 2006.

103. House of Commons Health Committee, 2005, op. cit., Table 3.7.1.

104. For example, Robert Carvel, 'Operations Go-slow Forced by NHS Crisis', a front-page story in *The Guardian*, 3 Dec. 2005.

105. Daniel Martin, 'Managers Lay the Blame at Door of Government', *Health Service Journal*, 19 Jan. 2006, www.hsj.co.uk.

106. Secretary of State for Health, *Our Health, Our Care, Our Say: A New Direction for Community Services*, The Stationery Office: London 2006, Cm. 6737.
107. HM Treasury/Department of Health, *Tackling Health Inequalities: Summary of the 2002 Cross-Cutting Review*, DoH: London 2002.
108. Department of Health, *Tackling Health Inequalities: A Programme for Action*, DoH: London 2003.
109. Rudolf Klein and William Plowden, 'JASP meets JUG: Lessons of the 1975 Joint Approach to Social Policy for Joined-up Government', in Vernon Bogdanor (ed.), *Joined-up Government*, Oxford UP: Oxford 2005, pp. 107–13.
110. Mark Exworthy, Lee Berney and Martin Powell, 'How Great Expectations in Westminster May Be Dashed Locally: The Local Implementation of National Policy on Health Inequalities', *Policy and Politics*, vol. 30, no. 1, 2002, pp. 79–96.
111. Healthcare Commission, *State of Healthcare, 2005*, Healthcare Commission: London 2005, pp. 69–70.
112. Department of Health, *Tackling Health Inequalities: Status Report on the Programme for Action*, DoH: London 2005.
113. Sir Derek Wanless, *Securing Good Health for the Whole Population: Final Report*, HM Treasury: London 2004.
114. Secretary of State for Health, *Choosing Health: Making Healthy Choices Easier*, The Stationery Office: London 2004, Cm. 6374.
115. JN Morris and C Deeming, 'Minimum Incomes for Healthy Living', *Policy and Politics*, vol. 32, no. 4, 2004, pp. 441–54.

Chapter 9

From church to garage

The world into which the NHS was born no longer exists. The half century that separated Clement Attlee and Tony Blair as Labour Prime Ministers witnessed, to sum up the argument of previous chapters, a transformation in the social, economic and political environment of the NHS. The industries nationalised in the Attlee years have been sold off. Britain's class and industrial structure has changed dramatically; the new economy is based not on digging coal or building cars or ships but on services and information technology. Real incomes per head have more than doubled: the era of post-war austerity has given way to a flamboyant consumerism. The credit card culture has replaced the piggy-bank culture. Although Britain has not become a more egalitarian society, as many hoped in the flush of post-war optimism, its people have become much better housed, better educated and better able to make their own lifestyle decisions. With greater resources, and infinitely greater access to information, the sphere of personal autonomy has expanded for most (though by no means all) of the population: the ability to make choices has, to an extent which would have astonished in 1945 or 1950, been democratised. In turn, there has been a transformation in the assumptive world of policy-makers. The commitment to collectivism and faith in central planning that marked the Attlee epoch – and shaped the NHS – have both gone. A new public philosophy – certainly more sceptical about the role of the State and perhaps more individualistic – has emerged.

Not only has the environment of the NHS altered dramatically, so has the role of the NHS itself, for reasons that have little or nothing to do with decisions of Ministers about its funding, organisation or structure. The pattern of demand for health care and the technology of medicine have both changed.[1] On the one hand, coronary heart disease and cancer have become the new epidemics, largely displacing infectious diseases, while chronic degenerative conditions like arthritis and dementia have become ever more significant in an ageing population. On the other hand, new drugs and innovations in surgery and diagnostic equipment have not only revolutionised medical practice but have also created possibilities of treatment where there were none before. Long hospital stays belong to the past while drop-in repairs are the new reality: 80 per cent of operations are done as day cases. The point is obvious enough. But it has been stressed because it underlines the fact that much Government policy-making is a response to challenges or opportunities created by the process of continuously evolving practice at the coalface of the NHS. So the creation of the National Institute of Clinical Excellence can be seen as a response to the fiscal challenge of an ever-expanding medical armoury, while the introduction of Independent Treatment Centres can be seen as exploiting the opportunities created by day surgery. Like other health care systems, the NHS has its own momentum and rhythm:

Ministers waving their conductor's baton can exhort the brass to blare out more loudly or tell the strings to make the *allegro* more *furioso*, but they don't write the score when it comes to medical practice.

Nor does the importance of changes endogenous to the NHS end there. More than half the graduates from medical school are women and, whether as a result or not, attitudes within the medical profession are changing. The rising generation of doctors see medicine as a career rather than a vocation, are more inclined than their elders to regard medicine as a job like any other and believe that work should be organised to balance career and family life.[2] They also accept corporate responsibility for their colleagues and are ready to share responsibility for patient care with other health professionals.[3] At the same time the balance between different health professionals is shifting, in recognition that the delivery of health care is a team effort. In the emergent health care system, it has been argued, 'nursing is the key profession'.[4] While nurses have been significant absentees on the scene of high politics, they are key players in the micro-politics of day-to-day life in hospitals and community care. If Government-sponsored changes in professional regulation over the past 20 or so years have encountered less opposition than might have been expected from the early history of the NHS, it is at least in part because the professions themselves have changed.

To emphasise the transformation in the NHS's environment, and within it, is also to suggest that what needs explaining is less the series of radical changes introduced first by Mrs Thatcher and then by Tony Blair than the fact that its defining features have survived unscathed in the process. It remains a tax-financed, universal service where health care is available free to all at the point of delivery. The waves of change have swirled around the NHS but have not swept it away. An institution that often seemed to be a national problem – its history punctuated by crises and prophecies of impending collapse, as we have seen – has survived as a national treasure. Public support remains rock solid: political parties compete to proclaim their faith in the service and their role as guardians of its future.

For Old Labour believers in Creationism this is not, of course, a puzzle. The NHS's survival, and its unique place in the hearts of the British people, are seen as testimony to the wisdom of the founding fathers. Institutions not only reflect the values of the time that gave birth to them but also shape the values of the future. In symbolising the commitment to social solidarity of the post-war era, the NHS has helped to perpetuate that commitment. If the NHS often failed to deliver the goods – if long since it ceased to be the envy of the world – it was simply because it had been under-funded over the decades:[5] an argument which, however, begs the question of why the founding fathers had devised a funding system which institutionalised parsimony for most of the NHS's existence. For New Labour (and other) believers in evolution, this is at best a partial truth. For them the survival of the NHS is contingent on adaptation to a changing external and internal environment: the battle for public support is a continuing one. The believers in intelligent design see the NHS as a church; the believers in evolution see it as a garage.[6] The different elements, and characteristics, of the two models of the NHS are summed up in Table 1.

Table 1 The competing models

Model I: health care as church	Model II: health care as garage
Paternalism	Consumerism
Planning	Responsiveness
Need	Demand
Priorities	Choice
Trust	Contract
Universalistic	Pluralistic
Stability	Adaptability

The model of health care as a secular church represents the tradition maintained and carefully tended over the decades by the disciples of Aneurin Bevan:
indeed it was one of those disciples, Barbara Castle, who explicitly invoked the
religious metaphor as we saw in Chapter 4. Creating the NHS was seen as an
act of social communion, celebrating the fact that all citizens were equal in the
sight of a doctor.[7] But it was also a model based on the assumption that it
would be the doctor who would determine who should get what. The vision
informing the design of the NHS, to recapitulate the argument of Chapter 1,
was as much one of technocratic rationality as one of social justice. Indeed
technocratic rationality was equated with social justice. It was the experts who
would determine needs, frame priorities accordingly and implement their
policies universalistically throughout the NHS. The model was based on trust:
the professionals working in the NHS would, it was assumed, put the interests
of patients before their own and quality would be assured by the dedication of
doctors, nurses and others.

The alternative model of health care as a garage has never been articulated as
clearly or explicitly. It is implicit, however, in the invocation of a patient-driven
NHS and the design of a mimic market for health care. In this model decisions are
driven not by experts but by consumer preferences: the body is taken in for repair
by its owner, who retains control over what happens to it. The ability to choose
between garages becomes crucial, as does access to information about how the
garages perform. Given the multiple preferences of consumers, diversity of
provision is to be encouraged. Choice and competition will, in turn, lead to
greater responsiveness (as well as efficiency). Professional providers cannot be
trusted to be selfless altruists, so appropriate incentives and quality tests are
required.[8] Consumer sovereignty, however, is also seen as carrying consumer
responsibilities: the garage model implies a responsibility for looking after our
bodies, in the same way as we look after our cars – hence an emphasis on self-care
and the importance of leading healthier lives. There is as yet no equivalent of the
MOT – the compulsory annual test carried out on cars above a certain age to test
their safety on the road – but the new GP contract provides for regular check-ups
for the elderly.

Like all models, these over-simplify a complex reality. The evolution of model I
into model II has not only been gradual but also partial. The NHS's centre of
gravity has indeed shifted from paternalism to consumerism, from need to
demand, from planning to choice. Equally, the decision-making system of the
NHS has shifted over the decades from relying primarily on collegial control by

professionals to one based on bureaucratic, hierarchic control, which in turn has yielded to a more market-orientated approach.[9] But in no case has the shift been complete. National priorities continue to be proclaimed; hierarchic control has not ceased. Paternalism has migrated from the health service to health promotion: there may be more choice about where to go for treatment but there is less choice about where to smoke. Above all, policies are still shaped by the values that gave birth to the NHS as an instrument of social justice. The policies of the Blair Government can therefore best be described as an attempt to combine the best features of the church with the most attractive characteristics of a garage: to design, as it were, a drive-in church.

The next section examines the state of the NHS as the drive-in church model was in the process of being introduced, but before it was in operation: an interim balance sheet. The following section asks to what extent New Labour policies reflected the special circumstances of the NHS – and British politics – as distinct from trends common to all health care systems in rich countries. The concluding section looks at the implications of the Blair legacy for the future: the tensions that have to be resolved and the challenges that have to be met.

The record so far

By 2006 Ministers could indulge in occasional triumphalism. 'NHS waiting will be history', the Secretary of State for Health proclaimed.[10] Government policies had delivered 'the fastest ever access to NHS treatment'. Waiting-lists had fallen below 800,000 for the first time since records began. New, more demanding targets had been introduced: by the end of 2008 no one should have to wait for more than 18 weeks from the time of seeing their GP and treatment. To the extent that waiting-lists and times were an appropriate or accurate measure of the NHS's performance – as distinct from having high political visibility – the Government could therefore claim success for its policies: the extra billion had produced the promised outcome. But, of course, assessing the NHS's performance is a complex, multi-dimensional matter,[11] with trade-offs between the different goals of policy: success in achieving one goal may be bought at the expense of another. Not surprisingly, therefore, widening the scope of analysis produces a more qualified verdict.

Consider the report of the Healthcare Commission on the state of the NHS in 2005.[12] The report found much to celebrate. Access to services had improved. So had outcomes of treatment for people with coronary heart disease and cancer. But it also pointed out that 'the extent of improvement is less clear in areas . . . that are not subject to national targets or regular public scrutiny'. National standards were not being met in services that were not considered high priority such as mental health and maternity. In the case of maternity services, the Healthcare Commission's investigations had 'uncovered significant problems' such as poor standards of cleanliness and overcrowding. Despite the emphasis of Government policy on providing seamless care, 'for patients services can still seem fragmented and designed more to suit the needs of those delivering them rather than those using them'. Other reports reinforced the message that while there had indeed been significant improvements, performance was often patchy. For example, the House of Commons Public Accounts Committee found much to criticise in the implementation of the Government's cancer plan: almost a third of the cancer networks visited by the National Audit Office, it reported, 'did not have comprehensive plans for providing cancer services in their locality'.[13] Partnership working, like seamless care, was difficult to deliver. Further, the Public Accounts Committee concluded that patients were still diagnosed with cancer at a later stage in the UK than in other European countries, particularly so in deprived areas. The story of huge variations in performance – albeit around a rising norm – was much the same as it had been five years earlier (and as it had been throughout the NHS's existence).

Add such evidence of a continuing gap between achievements and policy aspirations to the financial troubles of many trusts and PCTs (*see* previous chapter), and there seemed relatively little to show for the extra billions poured into the NHS, the many extra staff recruited (and paid more generously than ever before) and the countless initiatives taken. But, paradoxically, there was reassurance for Ministers in this outcome. It supported the diagnosis that had led to the embrace of a mimic market in the first place: the dynamics of the NHS would have to be changed if the extra billions were to produce a commensurate improvement in performance. While targets and pressure from the centre might succeed in bringing results, as the record on waiting-lists showed, they also had perverse effects, as the relative neglect of services not covered by them demonstrated. So enter competition and choice as the drivers of change, as we have seen. As of 2005, the new system was still largely on the drawing board, with only some of the elements in place; no wonder then that progress was halting and that the process of implementation remained an often frustrating exercise in rolling boulders uphill. The lesson for Ministers seemed clear: ever onward towards the promised land of the mimic market. Once on the high wire, there was no turning back.[14]

There remains another element in the balance sheet. What were the Government's political dividends for its investment in the NHS? History suggested that there was a direct relationship between the financial and political costs of the NHS. Parsimonious NHS budget translated into political unpopularity: money saved meant votes at risk. That certainly was the experience of Mrs Thatcher's Government in the 1980s. Would the Blair Government, conversely, get political credit for its generosity? There was every reason to expect so: there had been strong public support for spending more on the NHS even if this meant higher taxes,[15] as in the event it did. But the evidence is ambiguous. As in the past, the public and patients spoke with different voices about the NHS. The public at large was critical: in a 2004 survey, for example, 59 per cent of those interviewed agreed with the statement that fundamental changes were needed to make the service better – up from 52 per cent in 1988.[16] But patients consistently reported a high degree of satisfaction with the services they received, whether from GPs or in hospital. There were quite a few peas under the mattress: for example, survey questions about the extent to which staff involved patients in decisions and provided information elicited more critical responses.[17] Overall, though, the divergence between public and patient views remained.

It is therefore difficult to interpret survey evidence showing continuing public pessimism about the NHS's prospects, despite rising expenditure and falling waiting-lists. In a survey conducted in September 2005, 37 per cent of those interviewed thought that the NHS would get worse over the next few years, as against 26 per cent who thought that it would get better.[18] Seemingly Government policies were not translating into public confidence or support. However, a chart of the responses to the same question over the years shows a puzzling pattern, with rapid swings from month to month. In May 2002 the optimists outnumbered the pessimists by 14 per cent, yet by June 2003 the pessimists outnumbered the optimists by 10 per cent. In May 2005, when Patricia Hewitt took office, there was a positive balance of 9 per cent; four months later, this had turned into the negative balance of 11 per cent noted at the beginning of this paragraph.

Only one conclusion would seem to follow: which is that public attitudes, as revealed in surveys, are shaped not by the performance of the NHS – which does not vary from month to month – but how that performance is presented in the flickering, volatile searchlight of the media. When the media highlight scandal or failure, confidence in the NHS (and Government policy) slumps. Bad news displaces good news.[19] Public perceptions lag behind achievements while, in turn, those achievements lag behind the expectations cranked up by ministerial rhetoric. Once again, therefore, the lesson for Ministers seemed clear, reinforcing the case for devolving responsibility from the centre. The more they succeed in insulating themselves from the day-to-day operations of the NHS, the less vulnerable they will be politically.

Policy-making in an international context

Explaining the evolution of health care policy in England in terms of the special characteristics of the NHS and the national political system, as this account has done, carries a danger. It is that the account will fall into the trap of ethnocentric over-explanation. What if all health care systems in rich countries are moving in the same direction? Would this not suggest that policy is being driven by the dynamics of health care – the effects of the ever-expanding technology of medicine, compounded by demography as populations everywhere age – rather than country-specific institutional or political factors? To address these questions, this chapter therefore looks briefly at the international experience.

There are indeed common themes, just as there are common pressures, across most if not all the rich countries of the West. With ever-increasing levels of spending on health care, the preoccupation with making the system more efficient and effective is universal. The twin concepts of choice and competition, 'the master myth of modern societies',[20] appear to be guiding policy-makers in Europe and the United States, pushing them in the same direction. Reform of health care systems has become an international phenomenon. For example, Germany, the Netherlands and Sweden are among the countries to have adapted their systems to widen choice and competition since the 1990s.[21] Other themes, too, have crossed frontiers. There has been a trend towards devolution, as in the case of Italy and Spain. There has been increasing emphasis almost everywhere on putting primary care in the driver's seat.[22] Many of the same policy instruments, too, have been introduced: for instance, systems of payments to hospitals adapted from the American DRG (diagnostically related groups) model have spread through Europe. So what, if anything, is different about Britain?

In answering this question, the most important point to note is that the convergence of countries towards a common, market-like model is more apparent than real.[23] The vocabulary of policy discussion may be much the same, but the meaning of the words depends on national context.[24] For example, the Dutch and the Germans (like most other West European nations) have long enjoyed free choice of doctors and hospitals under their social insurance models of health care. The new element introduced in those countries was choice of insurer. The expectation was that insurance funds competing for subscribers would have an incentive to keep their subscription rates down and to exert pressure on health care providers to cut costs, as well as tailoring the packages on offer to the preferences of consumers. The case of Sweden is rather different. Its publicly funded, universal system is first cousin to Britain's NHS, albeit based on local government. In Sweden, in contrast to the Netherlands and Germany, choice of doctor was conspicuous by its absence until the 1990s when patients were given the right to choose their primary care physician and some county councils gave patients the option of seeking care from public or private providers outside their area if their local hospital could not offer treatment within three months, with money following the patient. Nor has change been a one-way street.[25] In France, where traditionally there has been almost unlimited choice of both primary care physicians and specialists, policy has switched to introducing financial incentives designed to encourage patients to sign up with a specific GP and to limit their choice of specialists.

So the notion that Britain is simply being swept along by an irresistible, universal wave of change does not stand up to scrutiny. Shared concerns do not necessarily mean shared solutions; the march of medical technology and the geriatrification of society do not compel the adoption of a particular model of health care. Even within Britain, following devolution, health care policy-making in Scotland and Wales has followed a divergent path from that pursued in England despite the shared framework of the NHS.[26] Local politics and local culture clearly matter, a point further explored below. But so do the ideas in good currency – the assumptive world of Ministers and civil servants – that feed into policy-making. And in this respect there is indeed good reason to think that the policies pursued by successive British Governments reflect international trends. No account of the evolution of NHS policy in Britain can ignore the globalisation of ideas that has taken place over the past decades, a phenomenon which has little or nothing to do with the specific circumstances of health care systems. The consequent transformation of the world of ideas is at least as important as the transformation in the social, economic and political context of the NHS in explaining the direction of change if not the precise form of that change.

Some of the characteristics of the new, international language of policy discourse have already been explored (*see* Chapter 5). It is heavily accented by economic theory. Its vocabulary is that of incentives, choice and competition. It is the language of international institutions like the World Bank and the Organisation for Economic Co-operation and Development (OECD), whose analyses and recommendations span the whole range of Government activity – from economic management to health care. It is also a language with a strong American accent. To the extent that many of its leading exponents are American economists (or European economists trained in the United States), so it is an instrument for exporting American-style analysis and prescription: the role of Alain Enthoven, who introduced the notion of an internal market to British audiences, is a case in point (*see* Chapter 6). But, as the example of Alain Enthoven also shows, intellectual influence does not necessarily translate into policy output: the internal market that actually evolved under Mrs Thatcher was very different from that which he had envisaged and bore the imprint of a wide range of institutional and political factors. Again, therefore, it must be stressed that none of the international trends identified – whether demography, medical technology or intellectual change – *determine* policy. The new language of discourse certainly enlarged the repertory of options and instruments for policy-makers, probably affected the way in which they interpret the world around them and perhaps also imparted a bias towards economistic, market-style solutions, but it did not dictate their decisions: free will still reigned, as the variations in national policies underline.

How to explain those variations? The role of ideology, and competition between parties of the Left and Right, was much invoked to explain differences in the original design of health care systems. However, change (or its absence) in mature systems calls for a somewhat different explanatory strategy. Here an ever-expanding academic industry provides a number of competing tools of under-standing.[27] Dominating much analysis is the notion of path dependency:[28] the notion that the structure of institutions – in the widest sense to include the norms of policy-making – and interests created at one point in time will constrain future policy choices. History matters. The difficulty is that this theory is better at explaining policy inertia than at helping us to understand policy change. Enter the notion of 'windows of opportunity'.[29] These open when Governments with a new policy agenda, forged perhaps under economic pressure, come into office. Mrs Thatcher's reform of the NHS provides a neat example; Tony Blair's commanding parliamentary majority provides another, less neat case since he could have used the size of that majority to maintain the status quo. When the windows open, the entrepreneurs of new ideas can seize the opportunity. Other institutional factors may still frustrate them. In countries such as France or Germany where the legislative system has many veto points or where there is a tradition of policy-making through consensus – so allowing interest groups like the medical profession to block or modify initiatives – change may be more difficult, and certainly slower, to achieve.[30] Conversely, countries with a Westminster-style constitution, where Governments can use their majorities to ram legislation through the legislature, offer fewer obstacles: Britain and New Zealand are cases in point, both offering examples of a rapid cycle of change.

But there is an all-important difference between explaining why change does or does not take place and explaining the actual nature of the policies that are or are not adopted. Here the model of policy as a learning process (the approach adopted in this book) is helpful.[31] This sees policy-making as puzzle-solving: a quasi-experimental strategy, with policy-makers learning from both success and failure. Inherited institutions define the landscape within which those policy experiments take place: perceived problems and possible solutions will be different in a tax-funded, centralised system like the NHS from those in a social insurance based, pluralistic system like Germany's, in a system which is con-sidered to be under-funded from one which is seen as over-spending. But while institutions may constrain policy choices, they leave space for autonomous decision-making by policy-makers: were it not so, there would be no scope for political debate about the course of action to be taken and policy would be on automatic pilot. What policy-makers learn, and the implications they draw, depends on who they are: the lenses through which they see the world. Thus the lessons which Frank Dobson, the first Secretary of State for Health in the Blair administration, drew from his experience of running the NHS were very different from those of his successor, Alan Milburn, as Old Labour lenses were replaced by New Labour ones.

The learning process also has an international dimension.[32] An explosion in the availability of comparative information about health care systems has meant that 'learning about other countries is rather like breathing – only the brain-dead are likely to avoid the experience'.[33] But until the 1980s the experience of other countries tended to reinforce complacency about the NHS: no other country appeared to have a health care system which delivered universal, comprehensive health care as parsimoniously as the NHS. While other countries appeared to be on an unstoppable escalator of rising spending, the NHS was a model of successful cost containment. When civil servants were sent to look at alternative systems of funding health care in Europe, as they were from time to time, they brought back the reassuring message that the disadvantages of social insurance outweighed the claimed advantages. So what was there to be learnt, apart from the fact that the British system was the best? From the 1980s onward, however, the Department of Health became 'much more willing to learn from others', in the words of its former Chief Economic Adviser.[34] By the turn of the millennium, international comparisons were used not for self-congratulation but for self-criticism, as we have seen. In making the case for higher spending on the NHS, the Wanless Inquiry asked the question 'How does the UK match up to other countries?'. The answer was that, in important respects, the standards of the NHS – as measured by outcomes – were below those achieved in many European countries.[35] International comparisons had helped to turn the NHS's fabled virtue – parsimony – into a vice: 'A new mechanism for the upward ratcheting of health expenditure had been born.'[36]

Not only did the experience of other countries provide benchmarks against which the performance of the NHS would be measured, it also fed into the process of developing new policy instruments. When the Department of Health set about devising its payment by results scheme, it looked to the lessons to be drawn from those countries which were already operating such a system. Similarly, when it was designing its Performance Assessment Framework, it looked at the methods developed in the United States to compare the performance of health plans. And there were many other such examples. Further, international experience widened the menu of policy options. For example, from Sweden came the notion of NHS trusts imposing financial penalties on local government social services if the latter were responsible for late discharges from hospital. Such direct transplants were very much the exception, however. More usually, and perhaps more importantly, knowledge of other health care systems served to underline the singularity of the NHS and to extend the range of ministerial thinking about alternative futures. So when Milburn announced his conversion to devolution, and the launch of Foundation Trusts, he invoked the example of other European countries, pointing out that the NHS was unique in the degree of centralisation and the uniformity of its ownership of providers: plurality of provision was the norm.[37]

Interpreting the experience of other countries was not, of course, a straightforward matter. For example, there was much interest in the performance of Kaiser Permanente, a United States health maintenance organisation, following the publication of an analysis in 2002 which showed that it had hospital admission and utilisation rates well below those of the NHS and thus appeared to provide better value for money.[38] In turn, this prompted a rush of policy-makers to California to dig in the statistics and investigate how this had been achieved. The Director of the Department of Health's Strategy Unit concluded that the NHS could indeed learn much from Kaiser's integrated approach ' . . . and the leadership provided by doctors in developing and supporting this model of care'.[39] But it was less than self-evident precisely *how* the Kaiser model could be translated into the very different context of the NHS or indeed what lessons should be drawn from it. Was the lesson that primary and secondary care should be integrated – and, if so, did this mean that primary care trusts should take over hospitals or that hospitals should expand into primary care?[40] Or did the key to Kaiser's success lie in its organisational structure, and the sense of ownership this gave doctors?[41]

International experience thus rarely spoke without ambiguity, all the more so since few of the reforms and models had been rigorously evaluated in their countries of origin. It was used selectively by Ministers and other policy-makers. It influenced the design of policy instruments, not policy goals. It provided not so much lessons, i.e. clear messages about what ought to be done, as prompts to the policy imagination. Its influence was mostly indirect and perhaps all the more powerful as a result: it helped to shape the lessons which Ministers drew from their own experience of running the NHS by challenging the assumption that everything that was unique about the NHS was also necessarily desirable.

The Blair legacy: shooting the rapids

The outlines of the design for the new model NHS are sharp and clear. No longer will the NHS be unique among European health care systems in the degree of its centralisation. Instead, Ministers will be insulated from responsibility for the day-to-day operations of the service by a battery of regulators. No longer will the collective funding of health care require the collective ownership of provision. Instead, there is to be a plurality of diverse providers, with choice and competition providing the dynamic of what remains a universal system providing comprehensive care. Technocratic paternalism has given way to consumerism in a mimic market. It is the kind of more loosely articulated health care service that might have evolved if the plans of the war-time coalition (*see* Chapter 1) had been put into effect, with the notable exception that there is still no role for local government despite much ministerial invocation of localism. A halting process of policy improvisation and discovery has seemingly produced a new model with a compelling logic of its own: a transformation of the NHS mirroring the transformation of society noted at the beginning of this chapter.

The coherence, solidity and durability of the model remain to be demonstrated, however. The foundations of the new building reach deep into the history of the NHS, a history which has shaped the culture of the service and the attitudes of those working in it. If the new model is to work, both will have to change. Indeed one of the explicit aims of policy is to bring about precisely such a cultural revolution. In turn, the success of policy depends on the extent to which the NHS adapts to the new language of consumerism and competition. But what if policy change and cultural change do not run according to the same timetable, and a gap opens between the expectations of change on which the success of policy is premised and the speed at which it is actually achieved? If policy can modify culture, does not the converse also follow? Further, there are strains and tensions within the reinvented NHS, some common to all health care systems, some inherited from the past and some created by inconsistencies in the new model: strains and tensions which are explored in the rest of this chapter. The test of the new model is therefore still to come as Ministers ride the rapids of implementation – steering towards the promised land of a service that will once again be the envy of the world, even while coping with swirling currents that threaten to drive them onto the rocks.

Central to the new model is devolution, as already noted. Ministers, insulated from the day-to-day operations of the NHS, are to limit themselves to a strategic role. That, at any rate, is the theory. Will it also be the practice? There is cause for scepticism. A pattern of swings from centralisation to devolution, and back again, has characterised the NHS throughout its history as previous chapters have shown. And Ministers will have to resist the strong gravitational pull to the centre if they are to translate the rhetoric of devolution into reality. There is the pull of parliamentary scrutiny: Ministers will still be accountable for the NHS's performance, even if they do not answer questions about day-to-day operations. There is the political pressure to respond to public anxieties about the reconfiguration of services: pressure which is likely to grow if the effect of competition in the new mimic market threatens the survival of local hospitals. Here the experience of the Conservative Government under John Major carries a warning (*see* Chapter 7): when competition threatened to undermine the viability of some central London hospitals, Ministers did not allow the logic of the market to play itself out but instead imposed a planned reconfiguration. Markets need to be managed.

History will not necessarily repeat itself. The New Labour version of the mimic market is different from the Conservative model in significant respects. The introduction of regulators and an inspectorate has meant that there is less reason for direct Ministerial intervention. But this carries a different danger.[42] This is that the new system of regulation and inspection will be superimposed on the existing machinery of central control rather than replacing it. And here there is a real dilemma. If the Department of Health is to fulfil its strategic role, in setting the direction of the NHS and determining priorities, it must inevitably set targets and standards. It may reduce the number of targets, as indeed it already has. It may leave the monitoring of progress towards achieving standards to the regulators and inspectors. But whose responsibility is it – if not the Department's – to intervene if national priorities are not implemented locally? While the system of regulation and providers may allow the Department to withdraw from direct supervision of providers, and intervention in their affairs, it will not absolve it from responsibility for seeing that local purchasers implement national policies effectively. Given uncertainty about the capacity of primary care trusts to carry out that role, it may be that a twin-track system will evolve: relaxed oversight of providers but continued central control over purchasers. This leaves another issue unresolved, however. Policy rhetoric emphasises the virtues of local decision-making. But what kind of deviations, and on what scale, from national norms are acceptable? How much discretion should be enjoyed locally, and in what respects? And what kind of legitimacy have PCTs, anyway, to act as the guardians of public sector commissioning[43] on behalf of their populations? If there is a democratic deficit in the NHS, it is surely at the local rather than national level.[44] The greater the degree of devolution, the more urgent will these questions become.

The balance between centre and periphery has provided one recurring theme in the history of the NHS; the relationship between the Government of the day and the medical profession provides another. That relationship remains critical for the success of the new model. The medical profession has lost much of its political clout, no longer exercises veto power over matters of high policy and has lost its ability to prevent issues even getting onto the agenda. In all these respects, there has been gradual but cumulatively important shifts of power within the health care policy arena, as a multiplicity of other actors have come on stage. The era of 'oligarchic élitism',[45] the union between technocratic paternalism and the medical profession, is over. But a rather different picture emerges when it comes to policy implementation, as distinct from policy formulation. To the extent that the new model is designed to change the way services are organised and care is delivered, so the Government needs the co-operation of those working in the NHS – starting with doctors: in this respect, nothing has changed. Yet, at the same time, implementing the new model may mean challenging the medical profession.

If the new model means strengthening the machinery of professional accountability, and challenging the doctrine of professional self-regulation, so it will create resentment among doctors. If new ways of working mean changing the distribution of tasks within the NHS, so once again there will be resentment among doctors: thus a Government proposal to give nurses and pharmacists extensive powers to prescribe drugs immediately prompted strong protests from the BMA.[46] In future, as in the past, there will therefore have to be a careful balancing act: policies which risk antagonising the medical profession will have to be balanced by strategies for reconciling it to the new model. The task will be all the more difficult since one of those strategies – generous pay settlements – has proved so expensive that it is unlikely to be repeatable. Moreover, there is an asymmetry in the relationship between Ministers and the medical profession, which puts politicians at a disadvantage. The public trusts doctors but not politicians to tell the truth.[47]

The role of the medical profession is crucial in another respect as well. Rationing in some form or other will continue to be a fact of life in the new NHS, as it is in the better equipped, better staffed and better funded health care systems which provide the model.[48] Some highly visible forms of rationing, like waiting-lists, may fade away. Other forms of rationing, like limiting access to expensive new drugs, may become increasingly significant. With the creation of the National Institute of Clinical Excellence, Ministers now have a technocratic screen behind which they can shelter. However, NICE guidance requires interpretation: doctors still enjoy a wide degree of discretion, if within guidelines, in determining who gets treated and how. How will that discretion be used? Will doctors internalise resource constraints in their clinical practice, as they have in the past? Or will the expanding budget of the NHS encourage them to expand also their definitions of appropriate treatment? These questions are all the more important because of another feature of the new model NHS. The payment by results system means, as noted in the previous chapter, that providers have an incentive not only to be more efficient but also to maximise activity. The ability of the NHS to operate within its budget – which long made it the envy of countries struggling to control rising costs – may thus be put under strain.

Compared to most other countries, the NHS also ranks high on equity:[49] i.e. access to health care according to medical need, irrespective of social class, income or other extraneous factors. The picture is not clear-cut. The evidence suggests that while access to the system is indeed equitable, in that use of primary care reflects need, there is a middle-class bias once patients are in the system.[50] When it comes to cardiac, diagnostic and surgical care, the middle classes do better than lower socio-economic groups: so for example, the latter have hip replacement rates 20 per cent lower than the former, despite having roughly 30 per cent higher need. So the expectations of the founding fathers have been only partially realised. Will those hopes be further betrayed by the introduction of choice into the NHS? Here the argument is that the middle classes, because they have better access to information and transport, as well as the social confidence required to exploit the system to their advantage, will use the opportunities offered by choice to increase their advantage. Against this, it has been argued that such an outcome is not inevitable: if choice were to be supported by the introduction of patient care advisers, and help with transport costs, there might indeed be an increase in equity.[51] In any case, it remains to be seen how choice will be exercised in practice: if a patient is rushed to hospital with a stroke or a heart attack, there is little scope for choice.

The policy implementation process will throw up other issues as well. Some policy streams are, as previously noted, inconsistent with each other. For example, the introduction of competition appears to be at odds with the emphasis on integrating different strands of health care.[52] Reconciling the different policy streams will thus be a major challenge to policy-makers. But, above all, there is the challenge of funding the NHS. The Government's commitment to a historically unprecedented rate of growth in the NHS's budget ends in 2008. Thereafter the NHS will once again, as in the past, have to compete with other claims on national resources.[53] The extra billions invested since 2000 were presented, and justified, as a catching-up exercise designed to bring Britain's health care system up to the level of comparable European countries. Once Britain has achieved that level – moving target though it may be – a more modest growth rate might appear to be appropriate. But just how modest should it be? And who would carry the pain of deceleration? If waiting lists diminish to the point of near invisibility, will public willingness to pay higher taxes to support the NHS leach away? Or will the dynamic of the new model – the expectations it creates among both users of the service and those working in it – stoke pressure for continuing high rates of spending growth? Will the introduction of choice, and the increasing assertiveness of informed con-sumers, lead to patients themselves defining what they need? And what would be the financial implications if a need-led NHS were to evolve into a demand-driven service? Can it survive in its present form while repudiating the notion of professional paternalism? And if the new model were to prove an escalator for rising fiscal demands, would the political consensus survive or would there be a revival of the debate about what the scope of a publicly funded health care service should be and how the NHS should be funded?

The questions pile up; the answers belong to the future. The new model for the NHS is intended to solve the problems of the 1948 design; the transformation of

Index